Biochemical Toxicology - Heavy Metals and Nanomaterials

Edited by Muharrem Ince, Olcay Kaplan Ince and Gabrijel Ondrasek

Published in London, United Kingdom

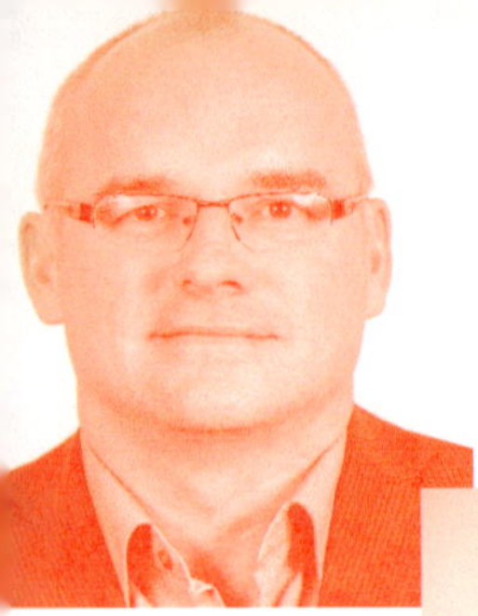
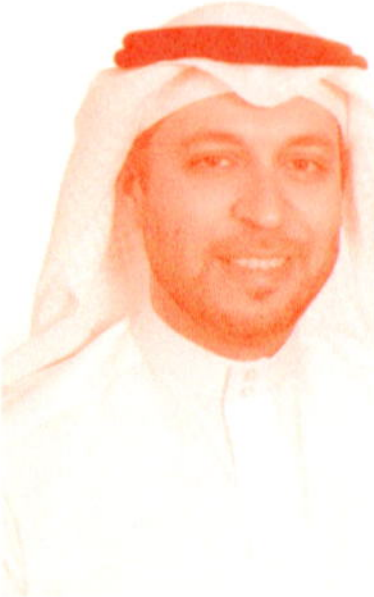
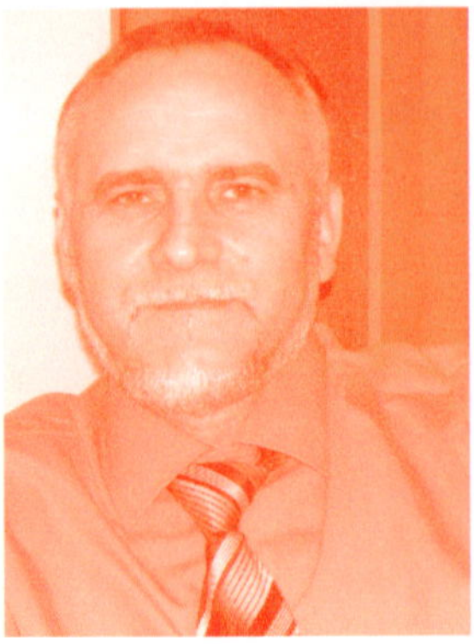
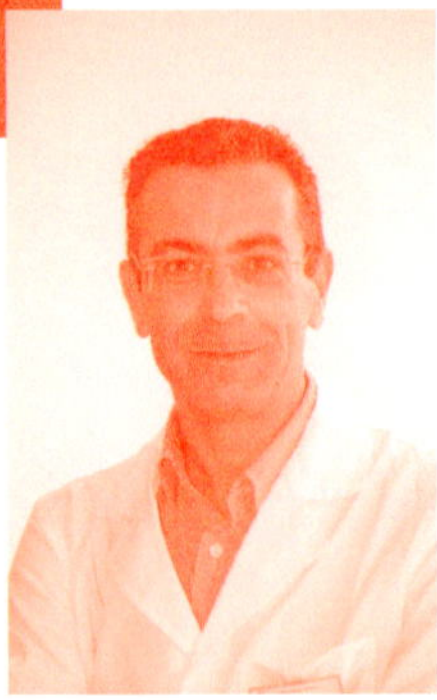
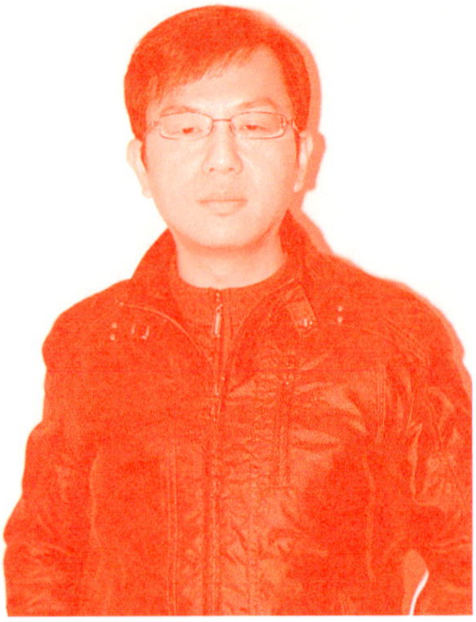
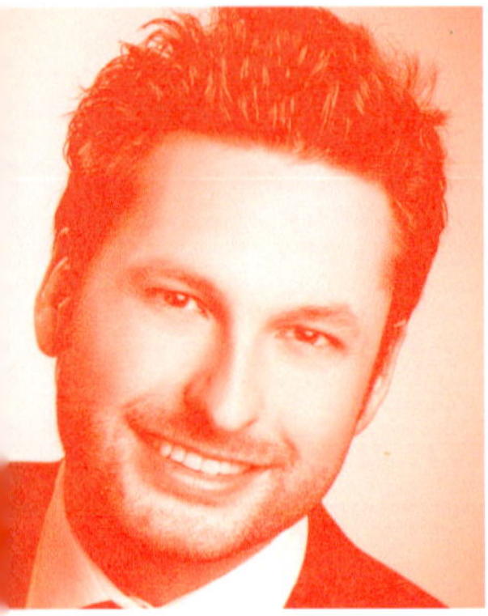
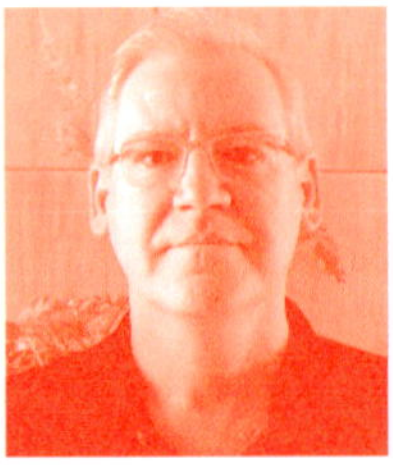

IntechOpen

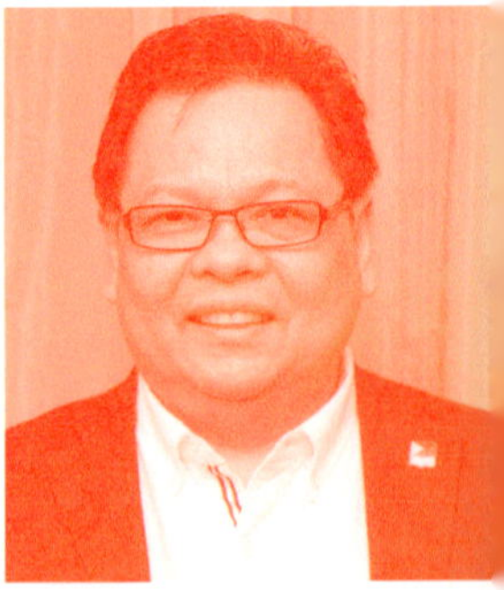
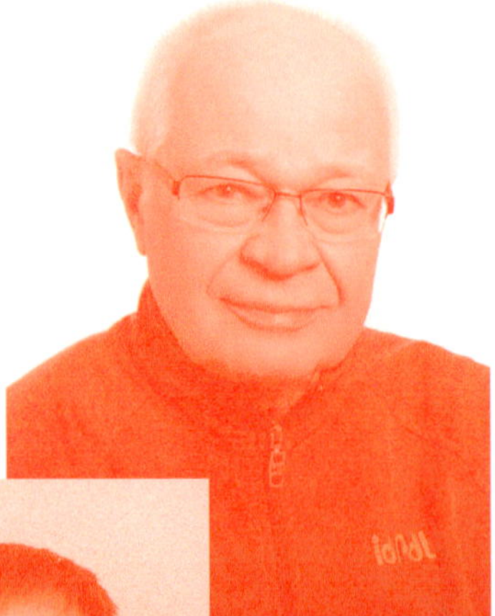
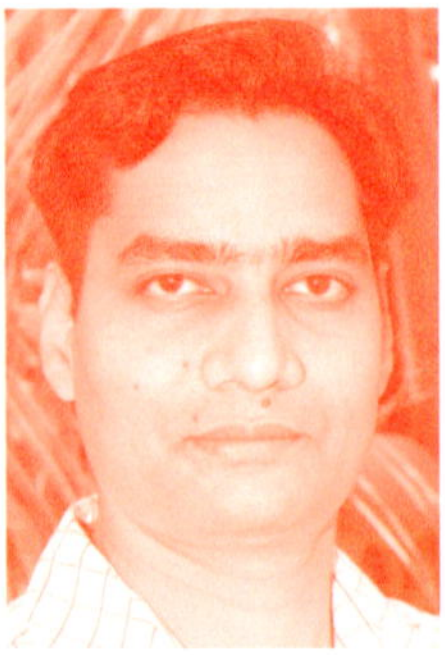
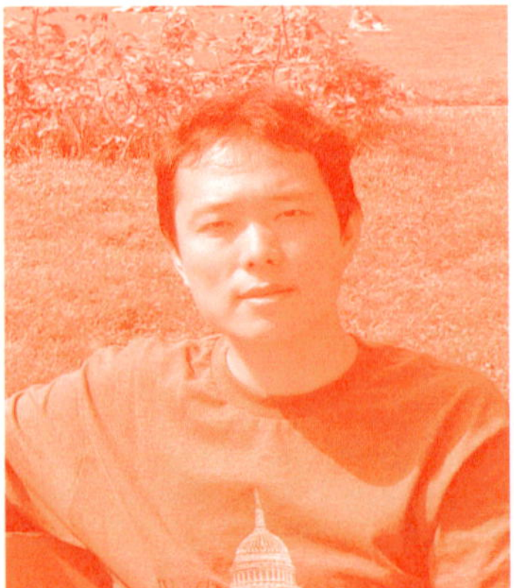
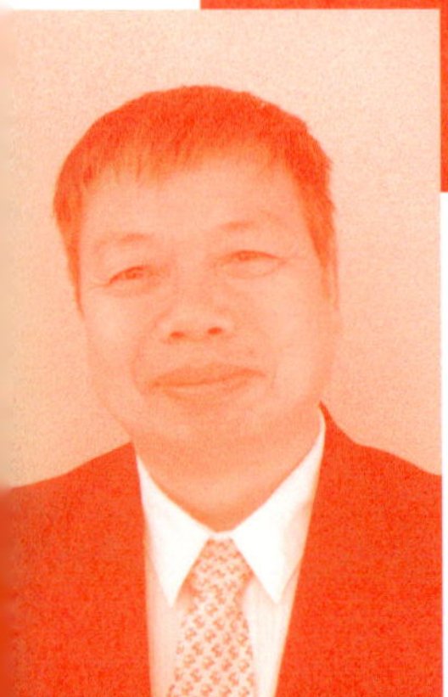
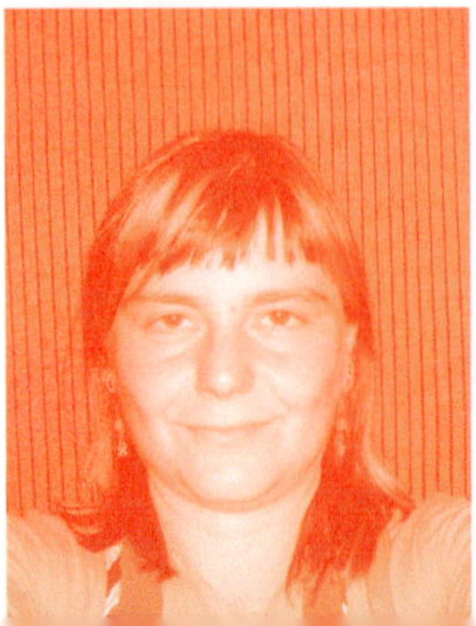

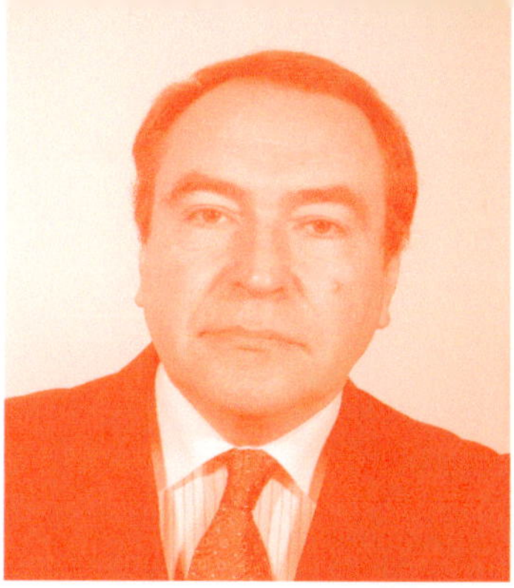
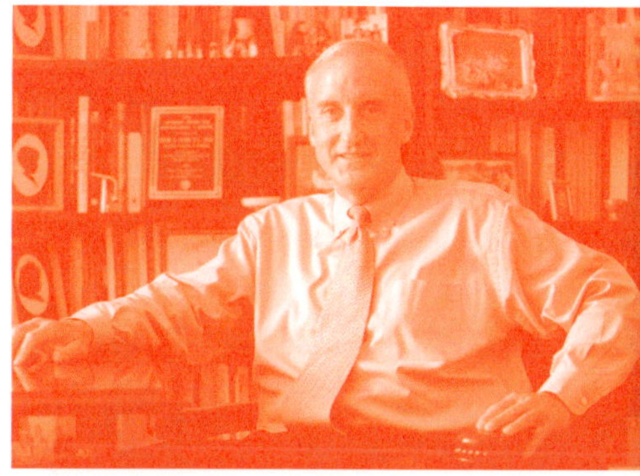
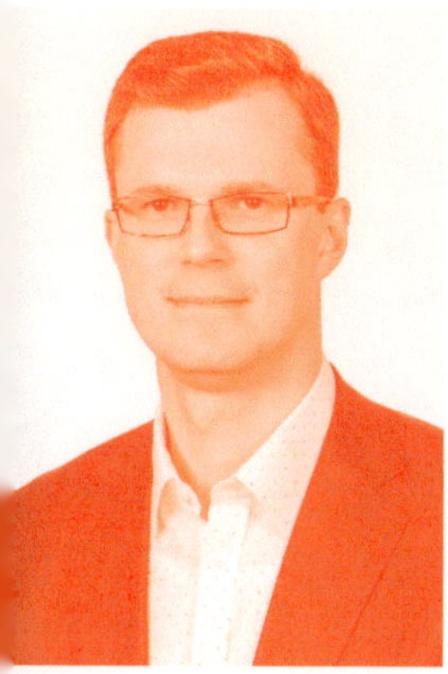
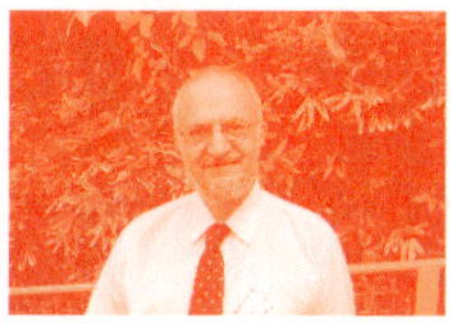
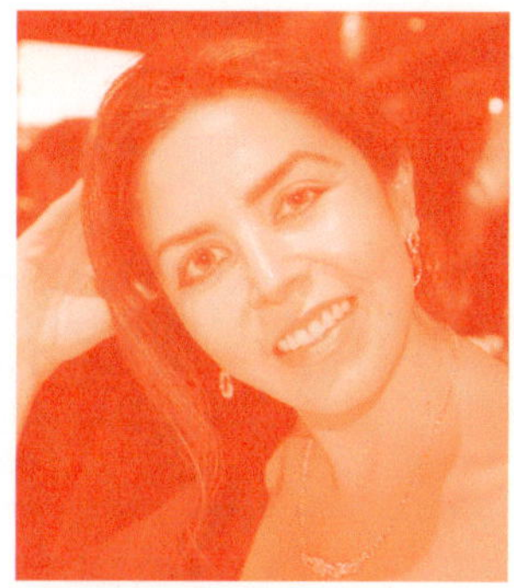

Supporting open minds since 2005

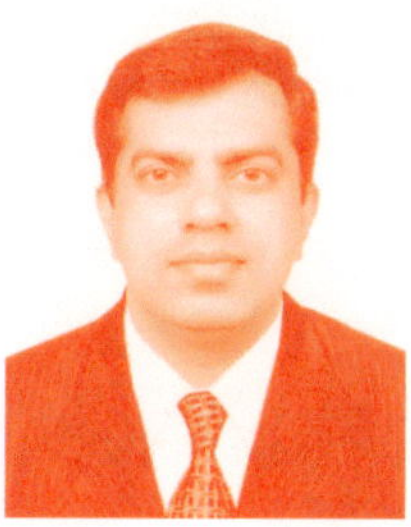
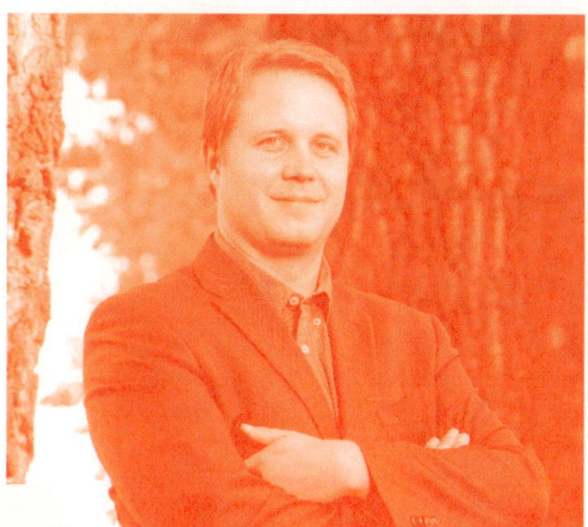
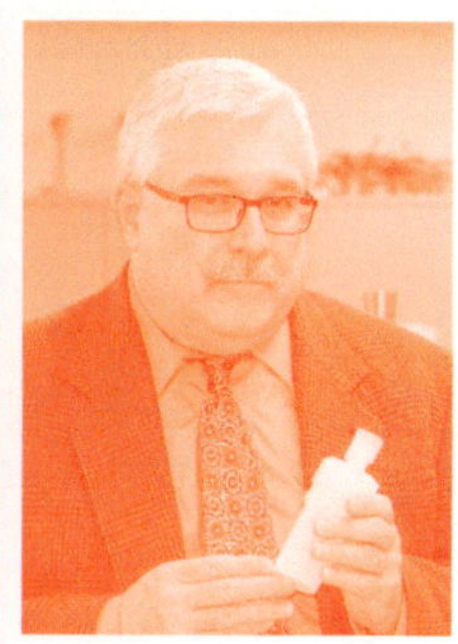
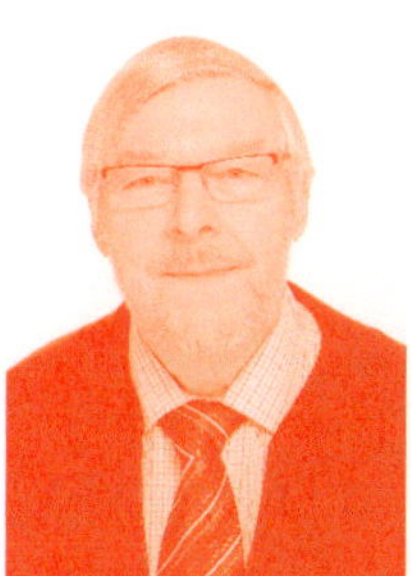
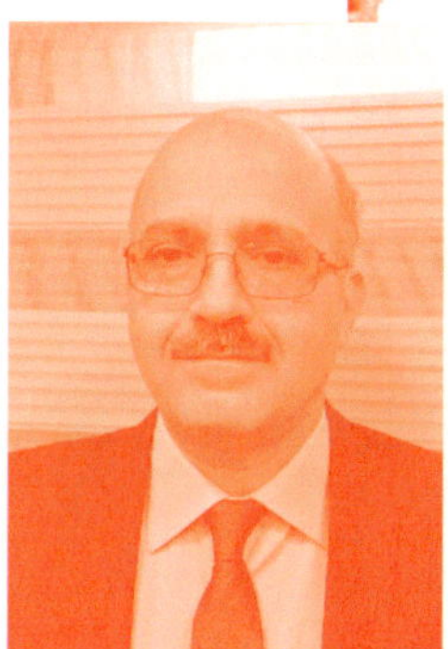
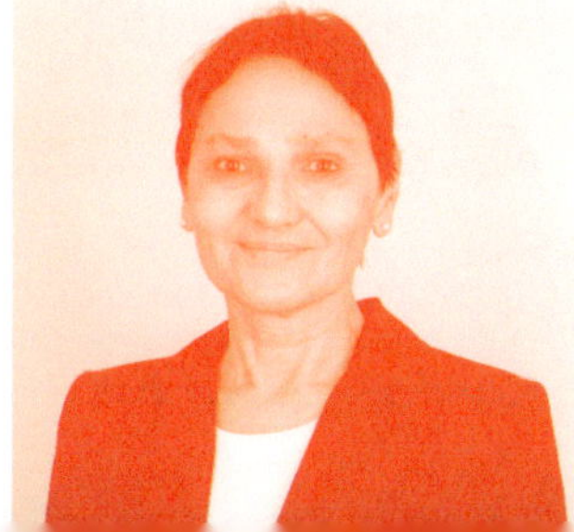
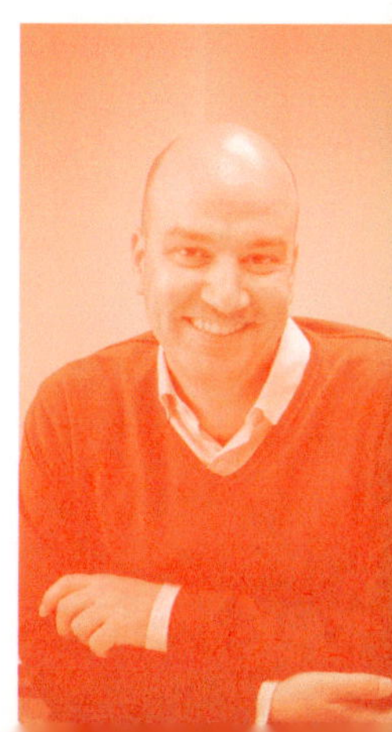

Biochemical Toxicology - Heavy Metals and Nanomaterials
http://dx.doi.org/10.5772/intechopen.85340
Edited by Muharrem Ince, Olcay Kaplan Ince and Gabrijel Ondrasek

Contributors
Bruno Bastos Gonçalves, Thiago Lopes Rocha, Percilia Cardoso Giaquinto, Jorge Laço Portinho, Douglas dos Santos Silva, Carlos de Melo e Silva Neto, Amanda Alves de Lima, Adriano Antonio Brito Darosci, Wanessa Fernandes Carvalho, Kassio Ferreira Mendes, Ana Paula Justiniano Régo, Vanessa Takeshita, Valdemar Tornisielo, Toan Vu Duc, Chi Do Thi Lan, Mai Ngo Tra, Nuriye Tuna Subaşı, Ayoub Baali, Ahmed Yahyaoui, Carlos Alberto Méndez-Cuesta, Cuauhtémoc Pérez-González, Miguel Martell-Mendoza, Roberto José Serrano-Vega, Hiram Isaac Beltrán, Jitendra Kumar, Chander Datt, Surya Kant Verma, Kavita Rani, Yuvaraj Muthuraman, Kizhaeral Sevanthiyppan Subramanian, Muharrem Ince, Olcay Kaplan Ince, Vinod Kumar, Akanksha Gupta, Sanjay Kumar, Magdalena Jedrzejczak-Silicka, Martyna Trukawka, Katarzyna Piotrowska, Ewa Mijowska, Dhruv Kumar, Sibi Raj, Venkatesan Yuvaraj, Venugopal Arunkumar, Muthaiyan Pandiyan

First published in London, United Kingdom, 2020 by IntechOpen
IntechOpen is the global imprint of INTECHOPEN LIMITED, registered in England and Wales, registration number: 11086078, 7th floor, 10 Lower Thames Street, London, EC3R 6AF, United Kingdom
Printed in Croatia

British Library Cataloguing-in-Publication Data
A catalogue record for this book is available from the British Library

Additional hard and PDF copies can be obtained from orders@intechopen.com

Biochemical Toxicology - Heavy Metals and Nanomaterials
Edited by Muharrem Ince, Olcay Kaplan Ince and Gabrijel Ondrasek
p. cm.
Print ISBN 978-1-78984-696-6
Online ISBN 978-1-78984-697-3
eBook (PDF) ISBN 978-1-83880-921-8

For EU product safety concerns:
IN TECH d.o.o., Prolaz Marije Krucifikse Kozulić 3, 51000 Rijeka, Croatia, info@intechopen.com or visit our website at intechopen.com.

Meet the editors

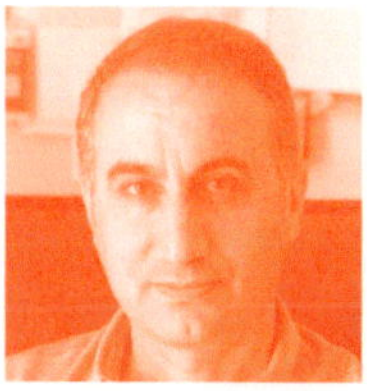

Dr. Muharrem Ince received his Ph.D. degree in analytical chemistry at Firat University, Turkey in 2008. From 2009 to 2012, he worked as a research analytical chemist at Mus Alparslan University, Turkey. He has been working at Munzur University since 2012. From 2013-2016, he served as a Head of Department of Chemical Engineering at Munzur University, Turkey. He is an Editorial Board member of several international journals as well as an author and co-author of more than 30 papers published in respectable international journals. Currently, he serves as an Associate professor at Munzur University, Turkey. His expertise lies in: Analytical Method Development, Spectroscopic and Chromatographic Techniques, Environmental Sciences, Food Analysis and Toxicology, Green and Sustainable Chemistry, Nanoscience and Nanotechnology.

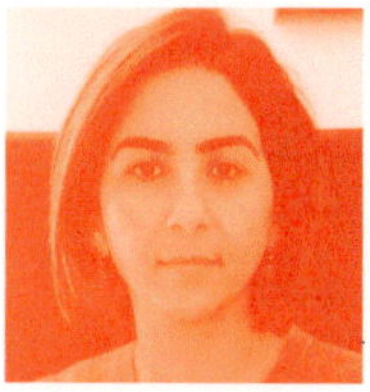

Dr. Olcay Kaplan Ince received her BS from Hacettepe University and PhD in Analytical Chemistry from Firat University in Turkey in 2008. Since 2009 she has been a research analytical chemist at Munzur University in the Food Engineering Department. She was head of the Department of Food Engineering at Munzur University from 2014 to 2015. Since 2019 she has served as editor-in-chief of the *International Journal of Pure and Applied Sciences*. Dr. Ince is the author of more than thirty-five papers published in respectable journals. Her research areas include trace and toxic element analysis, analytical chemistry, instrumental analysis, problem solving in analytical chemistry, food science and chromatography, nanoscience, and citotoxicology.

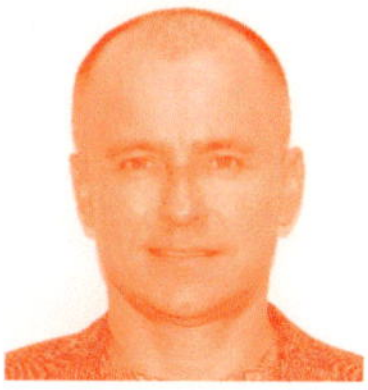

Gabrijel Ondrasek, PhD, is employed at the University of Zagreb, Faculty of Agriculture, Croatia, as a full professor and head of the Department of Soil Amelioration. His academic and scientific opus is orientated towards sustainable management of natural resources (water, soils) in the agro-environment, notably exposed to disturbed water balance on the soil–plant route, excessive salinity, metal contamination, and their environmental implications.

Contents

Preface

Over five sections, *Biochemical Toxicology - Heavy Metals and Nanomaterials* provides an overview of biochemical contamination, nanomaterials and toxic metals, and measurement techniques. It takes a broad view of organic and inorganic pollution and its effect on the ecosystem, and integrates a wide variety of approaches.

The first section of this book addresses heavy metal pollution, toxicity, and health effects. The second section addresses organic pollutants. The third section addresses the relationship of heavy metals – nanomaterials. The fourth section addresses nanoscience and nanoengineering. The fifth section addresses environmental management and risk assessment. Chapters cover such topics as industrial pollution, aquatic pollution, pollution evaluation, health risk assessment, and environmental impact. The aim of this book is to explain and clarify important studies and compare and develop new and groundbreaking measurement techniques. This book addresses the needs of graduate and postgraduate students, as well as chemists, other professionals, and readers interested in heavy metals, organic pollutants, soil, water and air pollution, and nanomaterials.

This book is edited by Dr. Muharrem Ince, Professor Olcay Kaplan Ince from Munzur University Rare Earth Elements Research and Application Center, Turkey, and Professor Gabrijel Ondrasek, Department of Soil Amelioration at the University of Zagreb, Faculty of Agriculture (UZFA), Croatia.

Muharrem Ince and Olcay Kaplan Ince
Munzur University,
Turkey

Gabrijel Ondrasek
University of Zagreb,
Croatia

Section 1

Heavy Metal Pollution, Toxicity and Health Effects

Chapter 1

Heavy Metal Removal Techniques Using Response Surface Methodology: Water/Wastewater Treatment

Muharrem Ince and Olcay Kaplan Ince

Abstract

Advanced water/wastewater treatment techniques including ion exchange separation, filtration separation, and adsorption are essential in the removal of non-biodegradable toxic wastes from water. In the current study, removal of heavy metal ions from water/wastewater and the use of response surface methodology (RSM) for experimental optimization were examined thoroughly. The objective of this work was to summarize the removal of heavy metal ions from water/wastewater using various chemical techniques and to emphasize the superiority of RSM in these studies.

Keywords: response surface methodology, water, chemical techniques, toxic wastes, optimization

1. Introduction

Due to the vital role of water for humanity, it is necessary to improve and maintain its quality. Environmental and global changes especially industrial wastes and domestic and agricultural activities are the main water pollution source. Worldwide, several water resources even underground water resources are contaminated, and they are not a suitable quality for drinking. Because of the rising living standards, growing world population, unconscious water consumption, and urbanization lead to increasing water supply costs. In most cases, as it contains different and large number of pollutants, wastewater lead to ecosystem hazards for being released around without being processed. So a few decades later, the world could face a major problem with freshwater supply [1]. In the past, very little financial resources have been allocated for wastewater because water supply received more priority than wastewater treatment (WWT). But, because of the increasing rapid population growth and trends in urbanization, WWT plays an important role in human life. Recently, because of the impact of sewage contamination of groundwater, rivers, and lakes, the growing awareness of wastewater treatment is now receiving greater attention from researchers and environmentalists. Research study results revealed that WWT, which is managed appropriately, has a large share in the growing economy when water resources treatment and supply are done in an appropriate manner [2, 3]. Safe, reliable, and sustainable treated WWT strategies have a vital role because of several challenges including adoption of low-cost WWT technologies. To prevent the spread of diseases, WWT systems are crucial, and they should have high levels of hygienic standards for reuse in agricultural and other areas. Lack of WWT can lead to environmental pollution, and it may cause a hazardous effect for the health of humans. To improve global health and to prevent spread of disease, reliable collection and treatment of wastewater are very important. Wastewater treatment and their reuse need innovative and appropriate technologies. Recently, WWT technologies including electrochemical technologies have regained their importance worldwide. In some cases, the electrochemical mechanism for metal recovery is very simple. These technologies have reached comparably with other technologies in terms of cost and efficiency [4]. Economic issues besides environmental and social aspects must be considered when choosing the most appropriate WWT method [5, 6]. All scientists and environmentalists desire widespread recognition of the need to implement more sustainable WWT techniques. Wastewater treatment technologies follow two main approaches: first is the development of a single indicator integrating different criteria and second is the development of a set of multidisciplinary indicators [7, 8]. When large volumes of treated wastewater contain low concentrations of chemical constituent discharge-receiving water body, it may still lead to water quality problem. Discharges from industrial activities have been identified as one of the major sources of aquatic pollution in industrialized countries. After 1990, to remove toxic pollutants in wastewater, scientists focused on persistent organic pollutants including PCBs, PAHs, and especially heavy metals due to destructive effects [9, 10]. People's anxieties also increase because of pollutions caused by heavy metals. Pollutions caused by heavy metals spread into the aqueous systems from many industries such as metal plating and smelters, eluents from plastics, mining, and textile industries [11]. Toxic heavy metals including mercury and chromium are discharged to the environment, and unfortunately they cannot biodegrade in nature [12, 13]. Heavy metals can be traveled through the food chain via bioaccumulation, the increase of heavy metals in human body causes some major diseases like brain, pancreas, and heart diseases, and they can lead to wide spread capillary damage and gastrointestinal irritation besides possibly necrotic changes in some tissue [14]. Even at low concentrations, heavy metals can cause serious toxic and harmful effects on the organism and the environment. The World Health Organization (WHO) limited heavy metal concentrations. Such as in drinking water, maximum acceptable limit of copper concentration is offered as 1.5 mg L^{-1}, when the limit concentrations of metals containing hazardous waste are different [15, 16]. Ion exchange, extraction, membrane filtration, and chemical precipitation especially adsorption techniques have been applied to remove heavy metals; on the other hand, generally adsorption technique is one of the most chosen method because of its simplicity, nontoxicity, cost-effectiveness, and local availability to remove toxic heavy metals from aqueous medium [12, 17–19]. In addition, heavy metal removal from different samples by natural adsorbents using adsorption is in the most appropriate technique, and the use of natural adsorbents has been the preferred choice for many researchers [20, 21]. In large number of studies, activated carbon, carbon nanotubes, clays, nanosized metal oxides, zeolites, and various biosorbents were used. However, statistical and optimization research using RSM with CCD or Box-Behnken design about heavy metal removal under various physicochemical parameters is restricted and very rare. Although numerous studies are in literature about heavy metal removal sorption using different materials, there are very little studies with the application of WWT using methodological approach. Classical and conventional methods cannot depict all factor combinations, which affect the experiment. At the same time, these methods take a lot of time to experiment for the determination of the optimum levels. Limitations can be eliminated using a statistical experimental design, which is optimizing all the effecting parameters collectively. In order for modeling of process parameters, RSM that contains a small number of experiments is widely used in various processes especially in adsorption [22]. Experimental design technique is a suitable tool for developing, improving, and optimizing process and multifactor experiments. It researches the common relationship between various factors for the most favorable conditions of the process, which helps to determine the interactions among optimized parameters [22, 23]. The primary target of RSM is to detect the optimum operational conditions for the system or to detect a region that compensates the operating specifications. The aim of this study was to present heavy metal removal from wastewater using RSM as a statistical technique. After discussion of wastewater treatment techniques as detail, several heavy metal removal methods from industrial wastewater will be presented.

2. The aim of wastewater treatment

There are two aims of wastewater treatment: firstly to purify wastewater without harming the public health and/or causing other nuisance and secondly to gain energy, nutrients, water, and other valuable resources from wastewater during purification steps.

3. Wastewater composition

Contaminated waters contain (**Figure 1**) various pollutants such as nutrients, various chemical compounds, and numerous pathogenic microorganisms besides toxic compounds. Inorganic solids, organic solids, and pathogenic microorganisms along with metals constitute a significant part of wastewater. While inorganic solids include salt, sediment, soil, and especially metals, organic solids contain food wastes, paper, and another household waste material. During WWT step, the removal of primarily organic particles especially suspended solids is vital prior to discharge to the environment. The proteins, lipids and carbohydrates are biodegradable components of wastewater. Biodegradable components contain carbon, and they can be converted to carbon dioxide. If these biodegradable organics are not removed from the wastewater, oxygen demand will exert

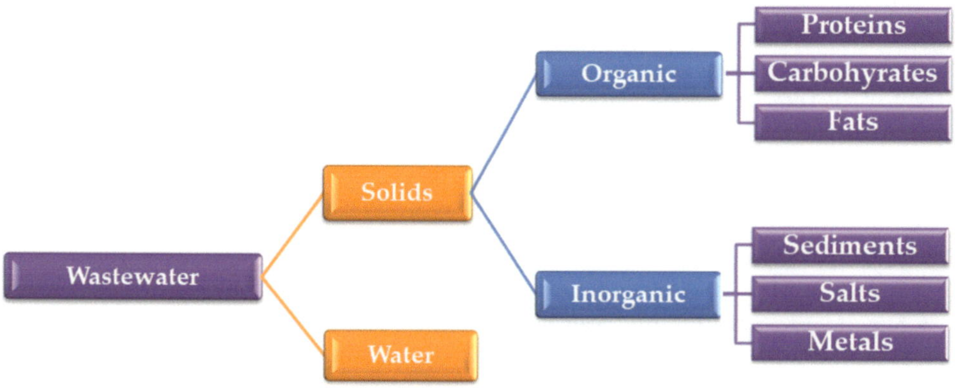

Figure 1.
Typical wastewater composition.

in the receiving watercourse. Biochemical oxygen demand (BOD) or chemical oxygen demand (COD) is typical measures of organic matter. BOD is the most widely used parameter to quantify organic pollution of water. BOD is the measurement of the dissolved oxygen that is used by microbes in the chemical oxidation of organic matter.

4. Water pollutants

It is important to understand the nature of water pollutants because wastewaters contain a large number of pollutants; however, toxicity is observed when the acceptable limits are exceeded. Wastewater contents depend on industrial, agricultural, and municipal wastewater. There are various water pollutants in nature, and they can be categorized as microbiological, radioactive, particulate, organic, and inorganic chemical contaminants. Harmful microbes such as viruses, fungi, bacteria, algae, plankton, and other microorganisms are basic components of bio-pollution in the water. These microorganisms may be responsible for various diseases. Organic toxic pollutants include many insecticides such as dichlorodiphenyltrichloroethane, herbicides, and other pollutants were manufactured for use in various industries. However, heavy metals are the most common inorganic water pollutants. Microbiological, radioactive, particulate, organic, and inorganic chemical water contaminants remain either in suspended, colloidal, or in solvated form.

5. Wastewater treatment methods

Because of the increasing population and rapid pollution of water resources, WWT and reuse are an important issue. The efficient use of existing water resources and treatment of polluted water resources with affordable and cheap technologies have been the focus of scientists. WWTs are needed for three reasons; these are water source reduction, WWT, and recycling. Recently, during purification step, while primary treatment includes preliminary physical and chemical purification processes, secondary treatment depends on biochemical decomposition of organic solids to inorganic or stable organic solids. Finally, after the third step called tertiary treatment processes, wastewater is converted into good-quality water, and it can be used for drinking or medicinal supplies. At the end of this step, almost all of the pollutants (up to 99%) can be removed from water. To producing good-quality and safe water, all these three processes should be combined together. Otherwise, it will not be possible to obtain safe water from the wastewater. Many advanced methods and techniques have been used for the recycle of safe water from wastewater, but economic and effective water treatment is still a serious problem. Treatment of wastewater and recycling technologies have been classified (**Figure 2**), and it is carried out in three stages. They are:

- Primary treatment methods
- Secondary treatment methods
- Tertiary treatment methods

These methods are briefly described below.

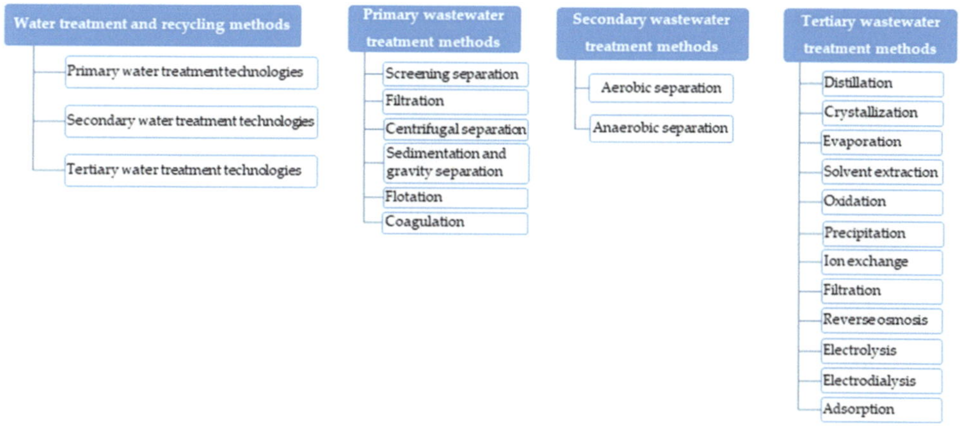

Figure 2.
Wastewater treatment and recycling methods.

5.1 Primary treatment methods

In order to remove organic matter and suspended solids from wastewater by means of physical operations, for example, sedimentation and gravity separation, they are done in primary treatment stage. Preliminary treatment, which is described as preparation for secondary treatment, is in fact intended to produce a liquid waste suitable for biological treatment.

5.1.1 Screening separation method

Screening separation method is used to remove solid wastes from wastewater. It is the process where suspended and floating materials including wood, paper, kitchen refuse, pieces of cloth, cork, hair, fibers, and fecal solids are removed from wastewater. In a WWT, screening is generally used as the first operation step. For this purpose, various size screens are used, and their size is selected as per the requirement. Finer particles such as sand and small pebbles can be eliminated by using screening separation method.

5.1.2 Filtration method

About 0.1–0.5 mm pore size is used in filtration separation method, water is passed through a medium having fine pores, and the filtration process is completed. Various membranes and filters, for example, cartridges, can frequently be used to remove suspended solids, greases, oils, and bacteria from the wastewater. The main purpose of filtration separation method is to separate the small solids and remove oil (they can be reduced up to 99%). Filtered water is used for many purposes such as ion exchange, adsorption, or membrane separation processes. In pharmaceutical and biotechnological industries, to the production of pure water, filtration separation method has become the main focus as promising separation tool for WWT. The used membrane has a key role due to selectivity, low fouling, and performance stability for long-term operation in the filtration separation method. Because of these advantages, this method and its performance are becoming more and more important. In addition, it is one of the important enrichment techniques for trace heavy metal ions along with simplicity and rapidity of the procedure. For all these reasons, many scientists have focused on this subject to develop and use alternative and effective membranes [24, 25].

5.1.3 Centrifugal separation method

This method is provided for separating components of a fluid or solid particles, but it is used especially for suspend solid from wastewater. Various types of centrifugal machines have been used to remove suspended noncolloidal solids in the centrifugal separation method. To separate solids from wastewater, centrifugal devices with various sizes are used. Density of suspended solids is the most important parameter when separating solid materials by centrifugation. In addition, oils and greases can be reduced and separated during application of centrifugal separation method.

5.1.4 Sedimentation and gravity separation method

Sedimentation and gravity separation method are based on the removal of suspended solids, grits, and silts from aqueous media. Suspended solid materials settle down to the bottom of the tank under the influence of gravity; this event may vary depending on solid size and density. Some chemicals can sometimes be added to accelerate sedimentation process. Although this method can reduce suspended solids only up to 60%, purification of wastes is a very useful separation application. Water treatment in this technique can be used in many areas such as water for membrane filtration processes and ion exchange method. It is generally applied out prior to conventional treatment.

5.1.5 Coagulation method

Coagulation processes are a particularly effective cleaning method for containing oil-in-water emulsions such as sea, lakes, and rivers besides most industrial wastes contain especially oil or petroleum. After sedimentation and gravity separation method, if there are non-settleable solids in wastewater, this is called processing coagulation with the addition of certain chemicals to precipitate these non-settleable solids and non-precipitating deposits. There are some natural coagulants such as aluminum salts, iron materials, alum, starch, and activated silica and also some polymers that can be used as coagulants. In this process, the most important controlling factors are contact time, temperature, and pH. In addition, during biological treatment processes, to remove microbes and any organics in the water, some certain coagulants can be added. Coagulation processes play an important role in recycling and removing pollutants from wastewater.

5.1.6 Flotation method

In order to remove suspended solid including oils, greases, biological solids, and other solids from wastewater, flotation separation method is used. In these processes, suspended solids are removed by adhering them with either air or gas. Various chemicals like alum and activated silica are used to successfully apply the flotation process to wastewater because they help flotation separation method. For paper and refinery industries, flotation separation method is an effective method for WWT because suspended solids that oil and grease is can easily be removed (up to 75–99%) by these processes. Recently, to separate mixed plastic is too difficult using gravity separation; therefore, for WWT and recycling purposes, plastic flotation method has been used as effectively [26].

5.2 Secondary treatment methods

Secondary treatment techniques have been used to remove soluble and insoluble pollutants from wastewater as biological. The main objective of this process is to convert the organic and inorganic solids into fluorinated residues that are finely divided and dissolved in the wastewater and to remove of soluble and colloidal organics and suspended solids besides reducing BOD and COD through biological process. When water has a high microbe concentration like bacterial and fungal strains, secondary treatment techniques should be selected for treatment because organic matter is converted into other products via these microbes; besides, they detoxify toxic inorganic matter. After this process is applied to wastewater, toxic organic and inorganic substances can be removed [27].

5.2.1 Aerobic separation method

In biological treatment processes, organic matter can be biodegradable by aerobic and facultative bacteria. Aerobic processes depend on temperature, the oxygen amount and availability of oxygen, and the biological activities of the bacteria. If bacterial growth is accelerated by adding some chemicals to the medium, the organic pollutant oxidation rate as biological will also be increased. Aerobic treatment techniques are the most effective method for removing suspended, volatile, and dissolved organics, nitrates, and phosphates besides BOD and COD. Because of the production of a huge amount of biosolids, aerobic treatment techniques have a big disadvantage; however, the biodegradable organic amount can be reduced substantially (up to 90%) using this method.

5.2.2 Anaerobic separation method

Anaerobic decomposition, called putrefaction, occurs when free dissolved oxygen is not present in wastewater, and this process is called as anaerobic treatment technique. In this treatment technique, organic matters convert into other organics including sulfur and carbon by anaerobic and facultative bacteria. There are two metabolic phases named acidogenic phase and methanogenic phase in the anaerobic separation technique. Some gases such as methane, hydrogen sulfide, ammonia, and nitrogen can be released. To reduce the biological load of wastewater, this method is very vital [1].

5.3 Tertiary treatment methods

For the production of safe water that people can consume, tertiary water treatment techniques are very important, and they should be applied to wastewater. In this last step, wastewater is subjected to final treatment using some vital techniques, and they are briefly summarized below.

5.3.1 Distillation method

The distillation method is based on the principle that the water is evaporated to the boiling point and the steam is distilled by cooling. After this process, purified water can be obtained free from impurities up to 99% in addition to wastewater is also freed from the volatile pollution. The obtained water by the distillation method is usable in levels of laboratory applications and medicinal preparations. In addition, to prepare potable water from the sea, distillation separation method is an effective tool.

5.3.2 Crystallization method

The crystallization method, which is based on the increasing principle of the concentrations of pollutants up to the crystallization point, is an effective method for obtaining quality water. Crystallization technique is useful to remove high concentrations of total dissolved solids including soluble organics and inorganics from wastewater, and it can be created either by mixing some solvents or by evaporation. This process is generally used for wastewater released to the environment from paper and dying industries. In addition, crystallization can be used for pH control because of other constituents including sulfite bicarbonate [1].

5.3.3 Evaporation method

When compared to other techniques, evaporation separation method is a natural process and suitable method but only for small wastewater volumes due to its high-energy consumption. However, this technique has some problems such as pollution, calcification, and foaming that have occurred in the presence of suspended solids and carbonates in the wastewater. Thus, to increase the evaporation rate and to reduce energy consumption, vacuum evaporation step can be used. Under natural conditions, water surface molecules escape from the surface, and they generally collected pure water. Recently, to recycle water process, mechanical evaporators and sometimes vacuum evaporation have also been used. Using evaporation separation technique is effective for the removal of pollutants including organic and inorganic compounds, but some volatile organic compounds may recirculate into the water during the evaporation phase. Evaporation treatment technique is applicated to various industry wastewaters like pharmaceutical, petroleum, and fertilizer industries. The obtained water from evaporation treatment technique has been used for different purposes including cooling in towers and boilers [28].

5.3.4 Solvent extraction method

Solvent extraction separation method is an important tool to dissolve pollutants from wastewater using various organic solvents like phosphoric acid. Acetone, methanol, hexane, ethanol, and acetonitrile are the most commonly used organic solvents. In this technique, some organic solvents are added to the wastewater to facilitate contaminant removal. The technique is very effective to remove oils, greases, and various organics. However, the process is often used for extraction and separation of heavy metals like lead, cobalt, and chromium using extraction and separation techniques from various industrial wastewater and effluents [29].

5.3.5 Oxidation and advanced oxidation method

To remove various toxic and hazardous chemicals especially endocrine-disrupting chemicals from wastewater, chemical oxidation techniques are preferred, and it is a promising technology for the treatment of wastewaters containing pharmaceuticals products. Organic compounds that are oxidized by oxidation of readily degradable species such as alcohols and carboxylic acids are the main components of this process [30]. Ozone, hydrogen peroxide, and Fenton's reagent are commonly used as chemical oxidation reagent. The chemical oxidation rate depends on some variables such as the presence of catalyst, temperature, and pH. Also, pollutants and nature of oxidants identify the rate of chemical oxidation. Various organic pollutants including hydrocarbons, dyes, and phenols can be removed from wastewater using chemical oxidation treatment technique. Recently, there has been a continuously increasing worldwide concern for the development of alternative wastewater reuse and recycling methods. Single oxidation separation method can sometimes be inadequate for the total decomposition of organic contaminants in wastewater. This requires advanced oxidation processes, which involve the use of more than one oxidation process at the same time [31]. Summarize, advanced oxidation process has big advantage because in this process all organic contaminants can be commonly oxidized to carbon dioxide form.

5.3.6 Precipitation method

The precipitation method based on the principle that the solubility of the contaminants is reduced and the precipitates which are converted into the solid form are easily separated from the water surface is an effective method for removing metal ions and various organic contaminants from wastewater. Chemical precipitation is a physicochemical process and a very flexible approach to various pollutant removals and can be applied at several stages during wastewater treatment. In industrial applications, precipitation has been the most common technology for metals [32]. In this process, to reduce solubility of the dissolved pollutants, it can be carried out either by lowering the temperature of the water or by adding some chemicals like sodium bicarbonates and ferric chloride, but chemical addition is not preferred because it increases the cost. Common applications of precipitation separation method are wastewater treatment from chromium and nickel plating industries and water recycling besides water softening and removal phosphate from water.

5.3.7 Ion exchange method

Ion exchange technique provides advantages due to it being technologically simple and enables efficient removal of even traces of impurities from solutions, high treatment capacity, high-removal efficiency, and fast kinetics when compared other usual methods. It can be applicable to various industrial wastewaters to remove hazardous materials. Ion exchange treatment technique depends on toxic or undesirable ions, which are replaced with others ions. There are two types of ion exchangers, which can be classified as cation and anion exchangers. Ion exchangers are natural or synthetic resins with active sites on their surface. Synthetic resins are widely preferred because of their effectiveness in removing heavy metals from wastewater [33]. In order to remove hazardous ions from wastewater, some resins including zeolites, sodium silicates, and acrylic and metha-acrylic resins are used as the most common. Reversible process and low-energy requirements are the most important advantages of this method. Using this method, organic and inorganic pollutants can be reduced about by 95%, but pretreatment may be needed if the wastewater contains oil or grease.

5.3.8 Filtration method

Recently, from the industrial sources, a large amount of oily wastewaters has been generated. The most serious pollutants are oil-in-water emulsions because of treatment cost and ineffective of using treatment methods [34]. Using microfiltration, a suspended solid pollutant that is a particle size from 0.04 to 1 mm can be removed. Microfiltration separation technique has been widely used to remove macromolecules, emulsion droplets, suspended particles, and microorganisms from various industrial fields including food, pharmaceutical, biotechnological, and petrochemical. In the last decade, membrane separations have been developed using various organic/inorganic membranes like ceramic membranes. It is becoming a promising technology for industrial processes and is utilized currently for oil field-produced WWT. When compared to traditional treatment methods, they have some advantages including high oil removal efficiency, low-energy cost, and compact design. Perhaps the most important advantage is that it does not require any chemicals. Some materials such as cellulose, fiberglass, and cotton can be used as filters in filtration method. Recently, several researchers focused on the new inorganic membrane development, for example, natural mineral-based ceramic membranes, carbon membrane, and zeolite membrane [35].

5.3.9 Reverse osmosis method

As membrane technology has been developed, membrane filtration mechanism became a feasible option for wastewaters. Reverse osmosis treatment technique that is called as hyperfiltration is the wastewater purification system that relies on the membranes' development technology. Using membrane filtration mechanism has shown results of very high efficiency in the filtration of wastewater. According to various studies from literature, when it is used, removal percentage has been achieved as at least 99.9% for COD, total organic carbon, suspended solids, coliforms, and pathogens. To achieve the required filtration, various membranes including cellulose, polyether, and polyamide are used in this process. In this process, the most important parameter is free energy, and other considerable parameters can be identified as pressure, pH, and operation time. To remove the soluble pollutants which contain macro- and microlevel nonpolar, ionic and toxic materials from the wastewater reverse osmosis is a very suitable separation technique. Reverse osmosis treatment technique is the most economic process because the water obtained from this process is of ultrapure water. It can be used in pharmacy and medicines because it can remove various microbes, bacteria, and viruses at high percentages (up to 99.99%) when compared other techniques [36].

5.3.10 Electrolysis method

Electrolysis method based on the redox reaction principle can be expressed as the separation and deposition of the dissolving materials on an electrode surface. During electrolysis separation method, metal ions are deposited on the electrode and separated from the wastewater. In the last decade, electrochemical oxidation methods have been an increasing interest because they can be applicable to WWT. In this process, various electrodes and anodes such as iron electrode, boron-doped diamond electrode, PbO_2 electrode, and graphite electrode [37, 38] have been used to remove different pollutants from wastewater.

5.3.11 Electrodialysis method

To remove various ions and other pollutants which have serious impact on the environment from wastewater, several methods have been used. Electrodialysis technique may be one of the most effective methods among these techniques because of recent progress in membrane technology. Electrodialysis, which is a membrane separation technology, depends on an electric potential difference, which is used to drive ion migration toward oppositely charged electrodes. In this process, under the influence of electric current, water-soluble ions pass through the membranes that are made of ion exchange material [39]. Certain factors, for example, nature of pollutants, applied current amount, temperature, and pH, must be kept in mind to remove dissolved solids. This method has been used to produce potable water from brackish water and for water source reduction [40].

5.3.12 Adsorption method

Adsorption separation method is an attractive process because it can be easily applied to WWT, which includes efficiency and flexibility. When it is compared with other treatment methods, it appears superior than others. Some factors that affect adsorption efficiency including the type of adsorbents, pollutant concentration, adsorbent particle size, pH, contact time, and temperature are very important for this process. A pretreatment may be needed to successfully apply the adsorption technique to wastewater because of the presence of suspended particles and oils. To remove pollutants especially heavy metals from wastewater, various adsorbents such as activated carbons from different materials [41, 42], Astragalus [19], carbon nanotubes [43], and a large number of biosorbents [44] have been used by different studies in the literature. However, novel and effective adsorbents with local availability besides economic suitability are still needed. Adsorption technique has two main problems: the first is the regeneration of columns and column life used as an adsorbent and the second is the management of the exhausted adsorbent.

6. Heavy metal removal from industrial wastewater using response surface methodological approach

Nowadays, because of rapid technological development especially in developing countries, environmental pollution is a serious problem for the ecosystem because wastewaters contaminated with toxic heavy metals are discharged directly or indirectly into the environment. Unlike most organic contaminants, heavy metals including As, Hg, and Cr are hazardous due to its nonbiodegradable nature [33, 45]. Thus, to protect the people and the environment, these hazardous ions should be removed from wastewater [46]. For example, while industrial wastewaters which contain Cr ions range from 0.5 to 270 mg L^{-1}, inland surface water tolerance limits 0.1 mg L^{-1}, and potable water Cr level should not exceed 0.05 mg L^{-1} according to various health organization such as the WHO and EPA [47, 48]. To remove heavy metal ions from wastewater, many conventional techniques such as membrane filtration, reverse osmosis, ion exchange, chemical precipitation, electrodialysis, electrochemical treatment, and adsorption have been employed. While most of these methods suffer from operational costs for the treatment process and high capital, the adsorption method is better than the other methods due to its flexibility in design, simplicity of operation, and facile handling, and it is considered more efficient and economical [45, 49]. Since the dynamic characteristics of the adsorption process are complex, it is essential to have optimum working conditions in order to achieve optimum pollution removal efficiency. Process optimization is crucial to determine design parameters value, which is achieving the optimal obtained response level. The RSM is one of the most used methods because of its developing, improving, and optimizing of the processes especially in the presence of complex interactions. It is also used to determine the ideal points of independent variables that are effective under optimum conditions and to evaluate the interactions of these variables [50]. Its greatest advantage is the decreased experimental trial number required to interpret multiple parameters. Therefore, RSM optimization process contains three main steps: (a) appropriate experimental design selection, (b) model coefficient estimation using analysis of variance (ANOVA), and (c) model validation based on prediction and experimental runs of the process response validation of the final model [51]. This experimental design method for an adsorption process is more practical than other approaches because it allows for the opportunity to monitor and interpret interactions between variables and to describe the overall effect of the parameters on the process. The RSM has been successfully used; in addition, its greatest applications have been in industrial research [52].

There are numerous studies, and different results were obtained using various adsorbents reported such as by Anupama et al. [53]. They used a CCD with RSM for removing Cr(VI) from aqueous medium [53]. They investigated the effect of some parameters including pH and temperature on adsorption, and the optimum pH, time, and adsorbent dose were found to be 2.32, 25.76 min, and 1.79 g L^{-1}. Also various adsorption kinetic models and isotherms were compared to find fit model. Jain et al. [54] studied Cr(VI) removal from aqueous solution using Box-Behnken model with combined RSM approach by chemically treated *Helianthus annuus* flowers. They investigated three effective factors for Cr(VI) removal. It was reported that the optimum pH, adsorbent dose, and initial concentration of Cr(VI) were found to be 2.0, 5.0 g L^{-1}, and 40 mg L^{-1}, respectively [54]. In an another study [55], Box-Behnken design has been applied to evaluate operating variables interaction for Cr (VI), Ni (II), and Zn (II) ions adsorption on *Bacillus brevis*. They carried out a total of 17 experiments and used a quadratic model. Based on this model, it was reported that the regression equation coefficients were calculated, and the data fitted to a second-order polynomial equation for these metal ions removal with immobilized on *B. brevis*. According to another study, to evaluate and optimize Cr ions, adsorption on activated carbon experimental conditions using RSM as an efficient approach for predictive model building was performed by Sahu et al. [56]. A full factorial CCD was employed, and based on ANOVA, a high coefficient (R^2 = 0.928) was obtained. In addition, satisfactory prediction of second-order regression model was derived. According to optimized process parameters, Cr(VI) removal percentage was obtained higher than 89% [56]. Kaplan Ince et al. [57] studied a batch experimental system for removal Pb(II) using clay, and optimized experimental approach was applied to some alcoholic beverages including beer and wine samples. Various effective parameters were investigated using a Box-Behnken experimental design methodology and RSM. They reported that the optimal conditions used for Pb(II) removal were pH of 5, contact time of 31 minutes, 75 mg for adsorbent dosage, and 100 rpm for agitation speed. Based on these results, maximum Pb(II) ion removal was calculated as 120 mg g^{-1} from aqueous medium using an ETAAS [57]. Balan et al. (2009) examined the efficiency of Cd(II) removal from aqueous solutions using sphagnum moss peat as biosorbent. They carried out a CCD for experimental design to evaluate an analysis of results and to optimize process parameters including the pH of solution, biosorbent dosage, and Cd(II) initial concentration. The optimum values of experimental parameters were obtained as 4.72 for pH, 14.7 g L^{-1} for biosorbent amount, and 13.64 mg Cd L^{-1} for initial concentration of Cd(II) [58]. In another study, removal of Cr(VI) from simulated wastewater using RSM was examined by Bhatti et al. [59]. They investigated the performance of a laboratory scale electrocoagulation system for the removal of Cr(VI) using Al-Al electrodes. They obtained an interaction between voltage × time and amperage × time coefficient of determination as 0.8873 and 0.9270, respectively. For the optimization of process variables including pH, voltage, and treatment time, the RSM was used. Prediction model results were validated through laboratory scale batch experiments [59]. In another similar study, to remove arsenic from contaminated water by arsenite, an electrocoagulation method with stainless steel electrode was used. A response surface methodology approach was performed to optimize significant process variables such as treatment time and solution pH. They obtained pH as 5.2, treatment time ¼ 20 min for 10, and 55–100 mg L^{-1} of initial arsenic concentration. It was stated that the waste elimination with electrocoagulation is a sustainable treatment technology with quick start-up, shorter treatment time, and minimum sludge generation [60]. An alginate-coated chitosan nanoparticle was carried out for heavy metal removal from industrial effluents by Esmaeili and Khoshnevisan [61]. To optimize the process of biomass for heavy metal removal from synthetic and industrial effluents containing nickel, an RSM approach was performed. Under optimum experimental conditions, which they obtained as a dose of 0.3 g biomass, pH of 3, 70 mg L^{-1} of initial concentration nickel, and 30 min contact time, maximum removal efficiency of biomass was found as 94.48% [61]. The Cd removal from wastewater and simulated aqueous solution was examined by Iqbal et al. [62] using a polyurethane material as adsorbent. The effect of operating parameters including adsorbent dosage, pH of solution, and metal ion concentration was modeled by RSM combined with CCD. Experimental runs and independent variables optimum values for Cd adsorption were obtained as 305 mg L^{-1} Cd ion initial concentration, pH 4.9, contact time 932 min, and adsorbent dose 1.3 g for polyurethane material. Based on the experimental results, to predict the response with good accuracy and reliability, it was mentioned that the RSM proved to be the best statistical model [62]. Ince and Kaplan Ince [63] examined the removal of Cr from industrial wastewater using RSM combined with CCD besides investigated as an efficient approach for examining predictive model building and optimization. To predictive regression models and optimize experimental variables, statistical design was modeled. The experimental parameters such as pH and agitation speed were selected for optimization. They obtained ideal Cr ion removal conditions as pH of 5.0, contact time 23.0 minutes, adsorbent dosage of 69.4 mg, and agitation speed of 135 rpm. The Cr removal efficiency was found at 23.16 mg g^{-1}. Also, significant independent parameters and their interactions were verified by means of the ANOVA. The proposed adsorption process was applied to various industrial wastewaters. It was stated that a CCD method was identified to yield a maximum Cr ion removal of 99% [63].

7. Conclusions

The choice of method to be used in the treatment of water/wastewater depends on the wastewater type and its composition besides the economic aspect. For example, high-grade contaminated water containing solid waste and poor color must be subjected to tertiary water treatment after primary and secondary water treatment processes. If the water does not contain any solids and is contaminated by other contaminants including inorganic, organic, and biological pollutants, the application of the tertiary treatment technique is sufficient. While surface waters are often polluted by organic, inorganic, and biologic pollutants, secondary and tertiary methods of treatment are needed in the treatment of these waters, and only tertiary methods of treatment should be used since groundwater is exposed to hazardous metal ions and anion pollution. The present study summarized removing heavy metal ions in various industrial wastewaters exposed to heavy metal pollution and was focused on optimizing the removal method and determining optimum experimental conditions.

Conflict of interest

The authors declare that they have no conflicts of interest in the research.

Author details

Muharrem Ince[1,2*] and Olcay Kaplan Ince[2,3]

1 Department of Chemistry and Chemical Processes, Tunceli Vocation School, Munzur University, Tunceli, Turkey

2 Munzur University Rare Earth Elements Application and Research Center, Tunceli, Turkey

3 Faculty of Fine Arts, Department of Gastronomy and Culinary Arts, Munzur University, Tunceli, Turkey

*Address all correspondence to: muharremince@munzur.edu.tr

References

[1] Gupta VK, Ali I, Saleh TA, Nayak A, Agarwal S. Chemical treatment technologies for waste-water recycling-an overview. RSC Advances. 2012;**2**:6380-6388

[2] El-Fadel M, Zeinati M, Jamali D. Water resources in Lebanon: Characterization, water balance, and constraints. International Journal of Water Resources Development. 2002;**16**(4):619-642

[3] Tahboub MA. Evaluation of Wastewater Treatment Alternatives for Hebron City. [Thesis]. Palestine: Birzeit University; 2000

[4] Chen G. Electrochemical technologies in wastewater treatment. Separation and Purification Technology. 2004;**38**:11-41

[5] Popovic T, Kraslawski A, Avramenko Y. Applicability of sustainability indicators to wastewater treatment processes. Computer Aided Chemical Engineering. 2013;**32**:931-936

[6] Møller KA, Fryd O, de Neergaard A, Magid J. Economic, environmental and socio-cultural sustainability of three constructed wetlands in Thailand. Environment and Urbanization. 2012;**24**(1):305-323

[7] Lozano-Oyola M, Blancas FJ, González M, Caballero R. Sustainable tourism indicators as planning tools in cultural destinations. Ecological Indicators. 2012;**18**:659-675

[8] Molinos-Senante M, Gómez T, Garrido-Baserba M, Caballero R, Sala-Garrido R. Assessing the sustainability of small wastewater treatment systems: A composite indicator approach. Science of the Total Environment. 2014;**497-498**:607-617

[9] Rizzo L, Manaia C, Merlin C, Schwartz T, Dagot C, Ploy MC, et al. Urban wastewater treatment plants as hotspots for antibiotic resistant bacteria and genes spread into the environment: A review. Science of the Total Environment. 2013;**447**:345-360

[10] Prasse C, Stalter D, Schulte-Oehlmann U, Oehlmann J, Ternes TA. Spoilt for choice: A critical review on the chemical and biological assessment of current wastewater treatment technologies. Water Research. 2015;**87**:237-270

[11] Fakhri A. Investigation of mercury (II) adsorption from aqueous solution onto copper oxide nanoparticles: Optimization using response surface methodology. Process Safety and Environment Protection. 2015;**93**:1-8

[12] Ince M, Kaplan Ince O, Asam E, Önal A. Using food waste biomass as effective adsorbents in water and wastewater treatment for Cu (II) removal. Atomic Spectroscopy. 2017;**38**:142-148

[13] Kaplan Ince O, Ince M, Yonten V, Goksu A. A food waste utilization study for removing lead (II) from drinks. Food Chemistry. 2017;**214**:637-643

[14] Chowdhury S, Saha PD. Biosorption kinetics, thermodynamics and isosteric heat of sorption of Cu(II) onto Tamarindus indica seed powder. Colloids and Surfaces. B, Biointerfaces. 2011;**88**:697-705

[15] World Health Organization (WHO), editor. Guidelines for Drinking Water Quality. 3rd ed. Vol. 1. Geneva, Switzerland; 2004. p. 334

[16] Kishor GR, Krishna D. Response surface modeling and optimization of Cu (II) removal from waste water using custard apple peel powder. international Journal of Elixir Chemical Engineering. 2013;**60**:16129-16134

[17] Ince M. Comparison of low-cost and eco-friendly adsorbent for adsorption of Ni (II). Atomic Spectroscopy. 2014;**35**:223-233

[18] Kaplan Ince O, Ince M, Karaaslan NM, Yonten V. Optimization of cadmium removal from water by hydroxyapatite using experimental design methodology. Analytical Letters. 2016;**49**:2513-2524

[19] Ince M, Kaplan Ince O. Box–Behnken design approach for optimizing removal of copper from wastewater using a novel and green adsorbent. Atomic Spectroscopy. 2017;**38**(6):200-207

[20] Rajic N, Stojakovic D, Jovanovic M, Logar NZ, Mazaj M, Kaucic V. Removal of nickel(II) ions from aqueous solutions using the natural clinoptilolite and preparation of nano-NiO on the exhausted clinoptilolite. Applied Surface Science. 2010;**257**:1524-1532

[21] Wang S, Peng Y. Natural zeolites as effective adsorbents in water and wastewater treatment. Chemical Engineering Journal. 2010;**156**:11-24. DOI: 10.1016/j.cej.2009.10.029

[22] Bingöl D. Removal of cadmium (II) from aqueous solutions using a central composite design. Fresenius Environmental Bulletin. 2011;**20**:2704-2709

[23] Alam MZ, Muyibi SA, Toramae J. Statistical optimization of adsorption processes for removal of 2,4-dichlorophenol by activated carbon derived from oil palm empty fruit bunches. Journal of Environmental Sciences. 2007;**19**:674-677. DOI: 10.1016/S1001-0742(07)60113-2

[24] Divrikli U, Arslan Kartal A, Soylak M, Elci L. Preconcentration of Pb(II), Cr(III), Cu(II), Ni(II) and Cd(II) ions in environmental samples by membrane filtration prior to their flame atomic absorption spectrometric determinations. Journal of Hazardous Materials. 2007;**145**:459-464

[25] Susanto H, Ulbricht M. Characteristics, performance and stability of polyethersulfone ultrafiltration membranes prepared by phase separation method using different macromolecular additives. Journal of Membrane Science. 2009;**327**:125-135

[26] Pongstabodee S, Kunachitpimol N, Damronglerd S. Combination of three-stage sink–float method and selective flotation technique for separation of mixed post-consumer plastic waste. Waste Management. 2008;**28**:475-483

[27] Pendashteh AR, Fakhru'l-Razi A, Chuah TG, Radiah ABD, Madaeni SS, Zurina ZA. Biological treatment of produced water in a sequencing batch reactor by a consortium of isolated halophilic microorganisms. Journal of Environmental Toxicology. 2010;**31**:1229-1239

[28] Gutiérrez G, Lobo A, Benito JM, Coca J, Pazos C. Treatment of a waste oil-in-water emulsion from a copper-rolling process by ultrafiltration and vacuum evaporation. Journal of Hazardous Materials. 2011;**185**:1569-1574

[29] Kumar V, Sahu SK, Pandey BD. Prospects for solvent extraction processes in the Indian context for the recovery of base metals. A review. Hydrometallurgy. 2010;**103**:45-53

[30] Esplugas S, Bila DM, Krause LGT, Dezotti M. Ozonation and advanced oxidation technologies to remove endocrine disrupting chemicals (EDCs) and pharmaceuticals and personal care products (PPCPs) in water effluents. Journal of Hazardous Materials. 2007;**149**:631-642

[31] Oller I, Malato S, Sánchez-Pérez JA. Combination of advanced oxidation

processes and biological treatments for wastewater decontamination-a review. Science of the Total Environment. 2011;**409**:4141-4166

[32] Brown PA, Gill SA, Allen SJ. Metal removal from wastewater using peat. Water Research. 2000;**34**(16):3907-3916

[33] Fu F, Wang Q. Removal of heavy metal ions from wastewaters: A review. Journal of Environmental Management. 2011;**92**:407-418

[34] Abadi SRH, Sebzari MR, Hemati M, Rekabdar F, Mohammadi T. Ceramic membrane performance in microfiltration of oily wastewater. Desalination. 2011;**265**:222-228

[35] Fang J, Qin G, Wei W, Zhao X, Jiang L. Elaboration of new ceramic membrane from spherical fly ash for microfiltration of rigid particle suspension and oil-in-water emulsion. Desalination. 2013;**311**:113-126

[36] Gupta VK, Jain R, Varshney S. Removal of Reactofix golden yellow 3 RFN from aqueous solution using wheat husk-an agricultural waste. Journal of Hazardous Materials. 2007;**142**:443-448

[37] Körbahti BK. Response surface optimization of electrochemical treatment of textile dye wastewater. Journal of Hazardous Materials. 2007;**145**:277-286

[38] Daneshvar N, Khataee AR, Amani Ghadim AR, Rasoulifard MH. Decolorization of C.I. acid yellow 23 solution by electrocoagulation process: Investigation of operational parameters and evaluation of specific electrical energy consumption (SEEC). Journal of Hazardous Materials. 2007;**148**: 566-572

[39] Abou-Shady A, Peng C, Juan Almeria O, Xu H. Effect of pH on separation of Pb (II) and NO_3 – from aqueous solutions using electrodialysis. Desalination. 2012;**285**:46-53

[40] Ottosen LM, Pedersen AJ, Hansen HK, Ribeiro AB. Screening the possibility for removing cadmium and other heavy metals from wastewater sludge and bio-ashes by an electrodialytic method. Electrochimica Acta. 2007;**52**:3420-3426

[41] Garba ZN, Afidah AR. Process optimization of K2C2O4-activated carbon from Prosopis africana seed hulls using response surface methodology. Journal of Analytical and Applied Pyrolysis. 2014;**107**:306-312

[42] Salman JM. Optimization of preparation conditions for activated carbon from palm oil fronds using response surface methodology on removal of pesticides from aqueous solution. Arabian Journal of Chemistry. 2014;**7**:101-108

[43] Sheibani M, Ghaedi M, Marahel F, Ansari A. Congo red removal using oxidized multiwalled carbon nanotubes: Kinetic and isotherm study. Desalination and Water Treatment. 2014;**53**:844-852

[44] Gutha Y, Munagapati VS, Naushad N, Abburi K. Removal of Ni(II) from aqueous solution by *Lycopersicum esculentum* (tomato) leaf powder as a low-cost biosorbent. Desalination and Water Treatment. 2015;**54**:200-208

[45] Ahmadi A, Heidarzadeh S, Mokhtari AR, Darezereshki E, Harouni HA. Optimization of heavy metal removal from aqueous solutions by maghemite (γ-Fe_2O_3) nanoparticles using response surface methodology. Journal of Geochemical Exploration. 2014;**147**:151-158

[46] Alslaibi TM, Abustan I, Ahmad MA, Foul AA. Application of response surface methodology (RSM) for

optimization of Cu^{2+}, Cd^{2+}, Ni^{2+}, Pb^{2+}, Fe^{2+}, and Zn^{2+} removal from aqueous solution using microwaved olive stone activated carbon. Journal of Chemical Technology and Biotechnology. 2013;**88**:2141-2151. DOI: 10.1002/jctb.4073

[47] World Health Organization, editor. Guidelines for Drinking-Water Quality. 3rd ed. Geneva, Switzerland: World Health Organization; 2006. p. 54

[48] Environmental Protection Agency (EPA). Environmental Pollution Control Alternatives. EPA/625/5-90/025, EPA/625/4-89/023. Cincinnati, US; 1990

[49] Han C, Pu H, Li H, Deng L, Huang S, He S, et al. The optimization of As(V) removal over mesoporous alumina by using response surface methodology and adsorption mechanism. Journal of Hazardous Materials. 2013;**254**:301-309

[50] Wantala K, Khongkasem E, Khlongkarnpanich N, Sthiannopkao S, Kim K-W. Optimization of As (V) adsorption on Fe-RH-MCM-41-immobilized GAC using box–Behnken design: Effects of pH, loadings, and initial concentrations. Applied Geochemistry. 2012;**27**:1027-1034

[51] Myers RH, Montgomery DC, Anderson-Cook CM. Response Surface Methodology: Process and Product Optimization Using Designed Experiments. Hoboken, New Jersey: John Wiley & Sons; 2009

[52] Amini M, Younesi H, Bahramifar N. Biosorption of nickel(II) from aqueous solution by Aspergillus Niger: Response surface methodology and isotherm study. Chemosphere. 2009;**75**:1483-1491

[53] Anupama K, Dutta S, Bhattacharjee C, Datta S. Adsorptive removal of chromium (VI) from aqueous solution over powdered activated carbon: Optimisation through response surface methodology. Chemical Engineering Journal. 2011;**173**:135-143

[54] Jain M, Garg VK, Kadirvelu K. Investigation of Cr(VI) adsorption onto chemically treated Helianthus annuus: Optimization using response surface methodology. Bioresource Technology. 2011;**102**:600-605

[55] Kumar R, Singh R, Kumar N, Bishnoi K, Bishnoi NR. Response surface methodology approach for optimization of biosorption process for removal of Cr (VI), Ni (II) and Zn (II) ions by immobilized bacterial biomass sp. *Bacillus brevis*. Chemical Engineering Journal. 2009;**146**:401-407

[56] Sahu JN, Acharya JK, Meikap BC. Response surface modeling and optimization of chromium(VI) removal from aqueous solution using tamarind wood activated carbon in batch process. Journal of Hazardous Materials. 2009;**172**:818-825

[57] Kaplan Ince O, Ince M, Onal A. Response surface Modeling for Pb(II) removal from alcoholic beverages using natural clay: Process optimization with box–Behnken experimental design and determination by Electrothermal AAS. Atomic Spectroscopy. 2018;**39**:242-250

[58] Balan C, Cojocaru C, Bulai P, Bilba D, Macoveanu M. Optimization of process variables for cadmium removal from synthetic wastewaters by sphagnum moss peat. Environmental Engineering and Management Journal. 2009;**2**:225-231

[59] Bhatti MS, Reddy AS, Thukral AK. Electrocoagulation removal of Cr(VI) from simulated wastewater using response surface methodology.

Journal of Hazardous Materials. 2009;**172**:839-846

[60] Gilhotra V, Das L, Sharma A, Kang TS, Singh P, Dhuria RS, et al. Electrocoagulation technology for high strength arsenic wastewater: Process optimization and mechanistic study. Journal of Cleaner Production. 2018;**198**:693-703

[61] Esmaeili A, Khoshnevisan N. Optimization of process parameters for removal of heavy metals by biomass of Cu and Co-doped alginate-coated chitosan nanoparticles. Bioresource Technology. 2016;**218**:650-658

[62] Iqbal M, Iqbal N, Bhatti IA, Ahmad N, Zahid M. Response surface methodology application in optimization of cadmium adsorption by shoe waste: A good option of waste mitigation by waste. Ecological Engineering. 2016;**88**:265-275

[63] Ince M, Kaplan Ince O. Application of response surface methodological approach to optimize removal of Cr ions from industrial wastewater. Atomic Spectroscopy. 2019;**40**(3):91-97

Section 2

Organic Pollutants

Chapter 2

Ecotoxicology of Glyphosate-Based Herbicides on Aquatic Environment

Bruno Bastos Gonçalves, Percilia Cardoso Giaquinto, Douglas dos Santos Silva, Carlos de Melo e Silva Neto, Amanda Alves de Lima, Adriano Antonio Brito Darosci, Jorge Laço Portinho, Wanessa Fernandes Carvalho and Thiago Lopes Rocha

Abstract

Glyphosate-based herbicides (GBHs) are chemicals developed to control unwanted plants such as weeds or algae. These chemicals act on EPSPS enzyme that blocks the production of tyrosine, phenylalanine, and tryptophan amino acids causing plant death. This biochemical pathway exists only in plant organisms. Despite the target use, GBHs have been related to toxic effects on nonplant organisms, such as invertebrates, fishes, amphibians, reptiles, birds, and mammals, including humans. This chapter is focused on ecotoxicological effects of GBHs on aquatic environment, showing a perspective of studies since this kind of product was developed until nowadays, an analysis of how many studies for each taxonomic group. Furthermore, we analyzed specifically the toxic effect of GBHs on each taxon, and finally, we discuss future perspectives and suggestions for a better regulation and application for this chemical.

Keywords: ecotoxicology, water quality, weed control, Roundup®, Monsanto

1. Introduction

Herbicides are chemical compounds used mostly to control weed (i.e., uncultivated) plants in agriculture and forestry and also for algae control [1, 2]. Herbicide formulations are designed to affect mainly plants, affecting specific plant biochemical pathways. However, it is common that this kind of pesticides affects nontarget organisms such animals, including aquatic organisms [3, 4].

The most used herbicide worldwide is glyphosate-based herbicide (GBH), such as Roundup® from Monsanto, and its usage has been increased [5] mainly due to the development of transgenic glyphosate-resistant crops [6]. Glyphosate (N-(phosphonomethyl) glycine (CAS no. 1071-83-6)) is a weak organic acid with a molecular weight of 169.09 M and has a half-life of 7–142 days in water and 76–240 in soil [6, 7]. Glyphosate has high solubility in water (10,000–15,700 mg L^{-1} at 25°C), and it readily dissolves and disperses in an aquatic environment.

IntechOpen

Glyphosate affects a specific plant biochemical pathway, inhibiting the action of the enzyme 3-enolpyruvylshikimic acid 5-phosphate synthase (EPSPS) that is necessary for biosynthesis of amino acids such as phenylalanine, tyrosine, and tryptophan [8] (**Figure 1**). Animals do not have this biochemical pathway, and hypothetically, they would be safe from glyphosate. However, the use of glyphosate requires that some other compounds as surfactants are added to the commercial formulation to increase adhesion to the leaf surface and absorbance by plants, trespassing the waxy cuticle [6]. There are a variety of surfactants, but the most common used on glyphosate-based formulations has been polyethoxylated amine (POEA). This surfactant is known to be more toxic to animals then glyphosate itself [6, 9].

As mentioned above, glyphosate *per se* has low toxicity when compared to its commercial formulation containing surfactants. However, those formulations are toxic to a large number of organisms due mainly to products added to the formulae. Many studies have reported tissue damages, DNA damages, enzyme inhibition such as acetylcholinesterase (AChE) and aromatase, endocrine disruption, development disruption causing malformations, and carcinogenesis caused by GBH in animals as fish, amphibians, and mammals, including humans [6, 10–17].

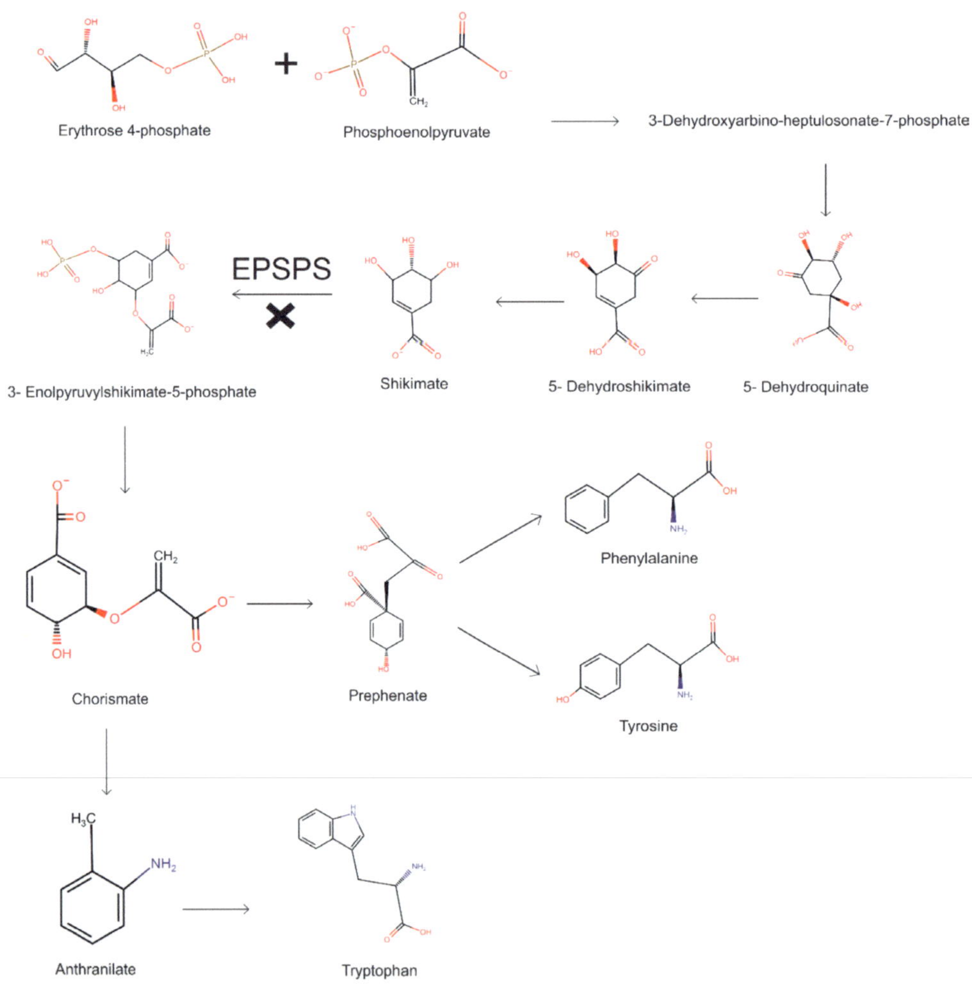

Figure 1.
Glyphosate action on the biochemical pathway of plants inhibiting 3-enolpyruvylshikimic acid 5-phosphate synthase (EPSPS) enzyme and production of essential amino acids as phenylalanine, tyrosine, and tryptophan, causing plant death.

In terrestrial animals, glyphosate reaches these organisms through direct application and contaminated food consumption. However, application of GBH in an aquatic environment is not so common when compared to terrestrial environments. Despite this, GBH can reach the aquatic environment through many ways. It can be applied directly on water bodies for algae control, although the opposite effect can be found, with proliferation of some species of algae due to the increase of phosphorus levels [18]. GBH can also reach the aquatic environment through leaching, run-off, and contaminated food source [6].

As mentioned, glyphosate has high solubility in an aquatic environment. Some studies say that 50% of glyphosate in natural waters dissipates by water flow and decomposition in a few days to 2 weeks [19–21]. Despite that, glyphosate binds to soil particles and solid surfaces [22], which makes its dissipation difficult. The by-products of glyphosate decomposition are sarcosine and aminomethylphosphonic acid (AMPA). The first one is known to be nontoxic [23] and the second one less or equally toxic for aquatic organisms than glyphosate [24, 25]. This substance has also a great solubility and dissipates in water in 7–14 days. POEA in natural environments degrades by microbial decomposition in 14 weeks and its half-life is estimated in 21–42 days [24].

Considering that glyphosate *per se* and the commercial formulations are widely used around the world, being the most popular herbicide, this chapter summarizes the available data from the literature on the ecotoxicity of glyphosate and its formulation compounds, as well as its degraded products, to aquatic organisms (aquatic plants, invertebrates, fish, reptiles, amphibians, and birds) and analyzes the worldwide politics about glyphosate use and environment safety.

2. Studies about glyphosate-based herbicides on the aquatic environment

One of the first studies that evaluated the effects of glyphosate and GBH in aquatic environments was performed by Folmar et al. [26]. According to Thomson's ISI WoS (Institute for Scientific Information, Web of Science) database, using keywords as "glyphosate," and "aquatic environment," since 1979 to the present day, 233 papers have been published that evaluated the toxicological effects of glyphosate in aquatic environments (**Figure 2**). These papers addressed the toxic effects of glyphosate on various types of organisms. The invertebrate group was the most studied, with 52 published articles (21.3%), followed by fish with 51 (20.9%), amphibians 40 (16.4%), plant 31 (12.7%), and aquatic environment 30 (12.3%).

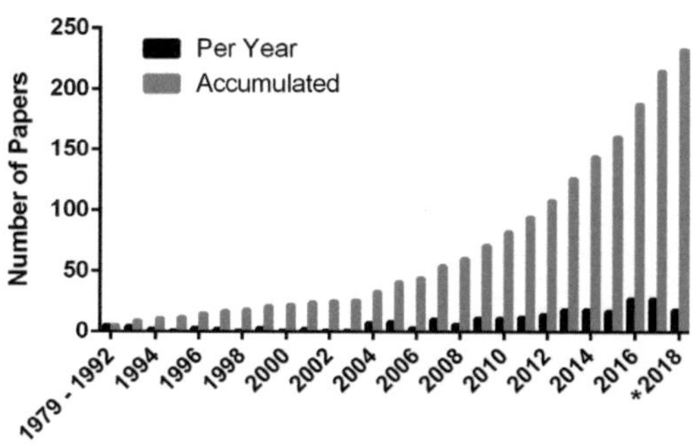

Figure 2.
Number of papers published per year. Black bars represent the number of papers published in each year. Grey bars represent the number of papers accumulated per year. (*) Papers published until August 2018.

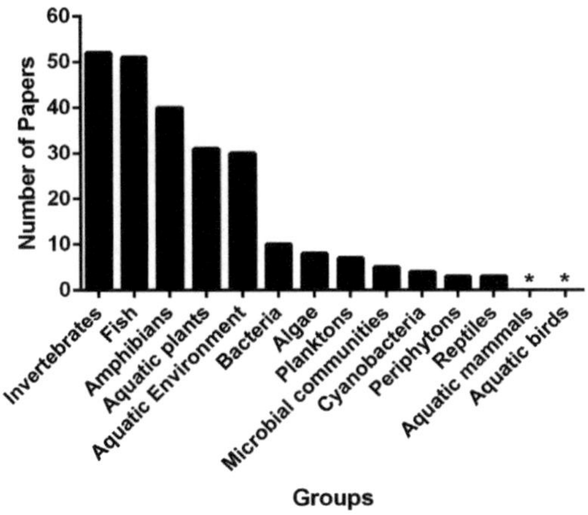

Figure 3.
Number of papers per organism group. Black bars represent the number of papers on toxicological effects of glyphosate published for each aquatic organism groups. Asterisk indicates lack of studies evaluating the toxicological effects of glyphosate in aquatic mammals and birds.

The other groups were present in 40 published articles (16.4%) (**Figure 3**). For the investigated period and database, there were no papers which have evaluated the toxicological effects of glyphosate in aquatic mammals and birds. This scarcity of studies demonstrates the lack of knowledge on the risk of exposure of these groups in aquatic environments contaminated by glyphosate.

2.1 Aquatic plants

Glyphosate in the aquatic environment causes the death of the macrophyte community, which serves as a microhabitat for zooplanktonic, phytoplanktonic, and periphytic communities, and this leads to top-down control of planktonic organisms, affecting refuge and feeding to fish [27], triggering a chain effect. Studies have evaluated the effects of glyphosate on aquatic lentils (*Lemna gibba*) [28] (**Table 1**), showing that larval mortality of tadpoles was caused by predation without their micro-habitats in the absence of macrophytes, due to contamination of water body by glyphosate.

Dörr [18] studied the effect of glyphosate on the growth and production of secondary metabolites by toxigenic strains of the cyanobacteria *Microcystis aeruginosa* and *Cylindrospermopsis raciborskii*. The author assessed the influence of different concentrations of glyphosate on the growth and production of these cyanobacteria and observed that toxin production and growth increased at 15 mg L^{-1}. When exposed to 20 mg L^{-1}, their growths and toxin production increased as well, while concentration above 20 mg L^{-1} prevented their growth. The species *C. raciborskii* was more resistant to GBH, and this species uses the metabolite AMPA as a source of nitrogen for its growth. Considering that microalgae and cyanobacteria are the principal primary producers in aquatic ecosystems, use of the herbicide can stimulate the growth and production of toxins of certain groups. This affects water quality and modifies the functionality of the ecosystem of interest.

The effects of herbicides on nontarget aquatic plants are emerging as a major conservation issue in aquatic biodiversity [29]. *Ludwigia peploides*, an aquatic macrophyte, showed that glyphosate bioaccumulates in water surface and can, therefore, be used as a biomonitoring organism to evaluate glyphosate levels in freshwater. This is because it increases the concentration of the herbicide in the leaf, facilitating its detection in the biological matrix instead of the water. In the study,

DOI: http://dx.doi.org/10.5772/intechopen.85157

Species	Group	Chemical	Glyphosate concentration (μg L^{-1})	Effect	Reference
Amphora veneta	Catenulaceae	Roundup®	8456	Increases mortality	[36]
Anabaena sp.	Nostocaceae	Gly. (acid)	0.1–8.8 mM	Increases growth	[28]
Arthrospira fusiformis	Phormidiaceae	Gly. (acid)	0.005–0.048 mM	Increases growth	[2]
Chlorella vulgaris	Chlorellaceae	Gly. (acid)	293,000	Chlorophyll fluorescence/decreases PP	[35]
Gomphonema parvulum	Naviculaceae	Roundup®	1000–10,000	Increases mortality	[30]
Halophila ovalis	Hydrocharitaceae	DCMU Gly. (acid)	11,600	Decreases chlorophyll fluorescence	[31]
		Roundup®			[30]
Lemna gibba	Lemnaceae	Roundup®	2800	Increases growth	[2]
		Gly. (acid) Roundup®	46,900	Increases growth	[29]
Leptolyngbya boryana	Leptolyngbyaceae	Gly. (acid)	0.003–0.02 mM	Increases growth	[2]
Ludwigia peploides	Onagraceae	Gly. (acid)	4000 and 108,000	Bioaccumulation	[2]
Microcystis aeruginosa	Microcystaceae	Gly. (acid)	3–37	Increases growth and toxin production	[28]
					[18]
		Gly. (acid)	15,000	Increases growth and toxin production	[2]
Myriophyllum aquaticum	Haloragaceae	Gly. (acid) Roundup®	840	Decreases root	[30]
		Gly. (n.c.)	220	Chlorophyll fluorescence	[33]
Myriophyllum spicatum	Haloragaceae	Rodeo®	1000	Increases growth	[34]
Nostoc punctiforme	Nostocaceae	Gly. (acid)	>50 mM	Increases growth	[2]
Scenedesmus quadricauda	Chlorophyceae	Gly. (acid)	200,000	Chlorophyll fluorescence/decreases primary productivity (PP)	[2]
Spirulina platensis	Nostocaceae	Gly. (acid)	0.005–0.02 mM	Increases growth	[2]

Table 1.
Ecotoxicity of glyphosate-based herbicide (GBH) to aquatic plants worldwide.

surface water and sediment samples were collected at the same time to measure glyphosate and calculate both the bioconcentration factors (BCFs) and biota-sediment accumulation factors (BSAFs). Glyphosate was detected in 94.11% in the leaves, presenting concentrations between 4 and 108 mg kg^{-1}. In surface waters and sediments, it was detected in 75 and 100% of the samples at concentrations ranging from 0 to 1.7 mg L^{-1} and 5 and 10.50 mg kg^{-1} of dry weight, respectively. The mean BCF and BSAFs were 88.10 and 7.61 L kg^{-1}, respectively. These results indicate that *L. peploides* bioaccumulates glyphosate that is mainly bioavailable in surface waters. Thus, since the plant accumulates the herbicide, the high concentrations in the organisms are evidence of the trophic levels that will feed or interact with the plant [28]. The researchers also observed that only 0.5 mg L^{-1} glyphosate was sufficient to inhibit the growth of *Lemna gibba*, change its shape, and lower chlorophyll content, decreasing its photosynthetic rate and consequently its metabolism.

Another important community in aquatic ecosystems that is also affected by the use of glyphosate is the periphyton. In terms of primary production, the periphyton has a photosynthetic contribution 77% higher than that of phytoplankton [30]. Among the most common and potentially toxic outcrossing cyanobacteria, *M. aeruginosa* uses glyphosate as a source of phosphorus, growing uncontrollably and causing eutrophication of the aquatic ecosystem that modifies ecological conditions. As shown by Forlani and collaborators [31], there is a tolerance to glyphosate by cyanobacteria *Spirulina platensis*, *Nostoc punctiforme*, *Arthrospira fusiformis*, *Anabaena* sp., and *Leptolyngbya boryana*, and four of them were able to use phosphorus as the only source. *Anabaena* sp. presented the highest toxicity (C = 50 mg L^{-1}). Vera and collaborators [32] observed that the interaction of the periphyton with other communities and also with the abiotic environment was low when the mesocosms were treated with glyphosate, presenting an imbalance in the trophic webs of the ecosystem.

The exposure to GBH reduced 78% of the primary productivity of phytoplankton when used at low concentrations (0.125 mg L^{-1}) [33] and at high concentrations (3.8 mg L^{-1}) [34], causing a disturbance in the trophic levels. In freshwater systems, glyphosate at high levels stimulated eutrophication by increasing total phosphorus and favoring the growth of cyanobacteria on the periphyton, which altered the typology of the study ecosystem that was a mesocosm [32].

Species-based differences in sensitivity to GBH exposure may lead to decreased richness and abundance of ecosystem species [34]. Even though herbicides are thought to kill terrestrial plants, it can have an even more devastating effect in water, due to the imbalance that causes mortality of algae and aquatic plants. This causes an increase in decomposing organic matter in the water, which will reduce the concentrations of dissolved oxygen in the system and increase the stress of aquatic communities [35]. Thus, algae and aquatic plants are considered as nontarget organisms that are sensitive to the effects of glyphosate, and the damage to the balance of the aquatic environment is of concern. The damage of glyphosate on the aquatic plant community ranges from the death of the plant itself to the reduction of environmental heterogeneity promoted by the local plants. Consequently, this leads to the death of other aquatic species, causing an imbalance in the ecosystem.

2.2 Aquatic invertebrates

One of the pioneer studies of the effects of GBH on invertebrate organisms was carried out by Tsui and Chu [9] that studied the effects of this chemical on *Ceriodaphnia dubia* and *Acartia tonsa*, both crustaceans, in addition to other organisms such as algae, bacteria, and protozoans. They found the toxicity of this pesticide to these organisms and the most sensible was *A. tonsa* with a LC_{50} of 1.77 mg L^{-1}. There is a high variability of sensibility of invertebrate organisms to GBHs (**Table 2**).

Species	Chemical	Exposure time (h)	LC_{50} (μg L^{-1})	Reference
Acartia tonsa	Roundup®	48	1770 (1330–2340)	[38]
Burnupia stenochorias	Roundup®	96	4304 (2121–7902)	[44]
Caridina nilotica	Roundup®	96	2842 (2524–3190)	[44]
Ceriodaphnia dubia	Roundup®	48	5390 (4810–6050)	[38]
	Eskoba®, Panzer Gold®, Roundup Ultramax®, Sulfosato Touchdown®	48	250–16,770	[45]
Chironomus plumosus	Roundup®, POEAE, Glyphosate acid	96	18,000 (9400–32,000)	[46]
Chironomus riparius	Rodeo®, X-77 Spreader®, ChemTrol®	48	1,216,000 (996,000–1,566,000)	[47]
Daphnia magna	Eskoba®, Panzer Gold®, Roundup Ultramax®, Sulfosato Touchdown®	48	2670–15,430	[45]
	Roundup®, POEAE, Glyphosate acid	48	3000 (2600–3400)	[46]
	Eskoba®, Sulfosato Touchdown®	48	1620–31,410	[48]
	Rodeo®, X-77 Spreader®, ChemTrol®	48	218,000 (150,000–287,000)	[47]
Daphnia pulex	Roundup®	96	657 (472–914)	[44]
Gammarus pseudolimnaeus	Roundup®, POEAE, Glyphosate acid	48	62,000 (40,000–98,000)	[46]
	Roundup®, POEAE, Glyphosate acid	96	43,000 (28,000–66,000)	[46]
	Roundup®	96	340,000	[49]
Hyalella azteca	Rodeo®, X-77 Spreader®, ChemTrol®	96	720,000 (399,000–1,076,000)	[47]
Laeonereis acuta	Roundup®	96	8199 (6690–9580)	[50]
Nephelopsis obscura	Rodeo®, X-77 Spreader®, ChemTrol®	96	1,177,000 (941,000–1,415,000)	[47]
Notodiaptomus conifer	Eskoba®, Sulfosato Touchdown®	48	1220–1,282,000	[48]
Ruditapes decussatus	Roundup®	1440	2200	[51]
Tanytarsus flumineus	Roundup®	96	12,240 (9454–22,360	[44]
Utterbackia imbecillis	Roundup®	24	18.3 ± 12.9	[52]

Table 2.
Ecotoxicity of glyphosate-based herbicide (GBH) to aquatic invertebrates, exposure time, LC_{50} value (lower-upper values), and reference.

Specifically about microinvertebrates (<35 μm), these organisms persist within resting eggs (or egg banks) in lake sediments [36]. They represent a major source of regenerative potential in lake ecosystems near agricultural areas, and play a key role in influencing the active population and community dynamics, seasonal succession, biogeographic patterns, and the evolution of populations [36, 37]. Despite the widely accepted importance of resting egg banks in the ecology of aquatic micro-invertebrates' communities, recently, experimental studies have demonstrated that the extensive and inappropriate use of commercial GBH, associated with agricultural activities, may impair the hatching of resting eggs in the sediment of lakes [38, 39]. Gutierrez and collaborators [38] indicated that the GBHs (Sulfosato Touchdown®) affect the hatching dynamics of micro-invertebrates, and selectively alter the species richness and abundance of community hatched from lake sediment. Portinho and associates [39] extended these findings and indicated that commercial herbicides as Roundup® (a.i. glyphosate) separate or in combination with 2,4-dichlorophenoxyacetic acid (2,4-D) have the potential to suppress emergences of micro-invertebrates from resting egg banks from lake sediments.

The environmental implication of this scenario suggests that changes in micro-invertebrates' structure and composition induced by herbicides will occur, causing not only negative impacts on the process of recolonization from resting egg banks but also shifts in community composition. Recent attempts to develop guidelines for protecting aquatic organisms have focused on emergence from resting egg banks within the context of an ecological community [40], with potential implications for studies related to environmental risk to, and integrity assessment of, aquatic ecosystems.

2.3 Fish

Fish species are particularly vulnerable to GBH and their susceptibility depends on the commercial formulation, fish species, fish developmental stages, and exposure conditions, such as concentrations, exposure time, and route of exposure. Furthermore, gender-specific response of fish to GBH has been indicated in guppy *P. reticulata* exposed to glyphosate (50–73.2 mg L^{-1}) and their metabolite AMPA (86.8–180 mg L^{-1}) for 96 h [25], indicating the need for further studies about the molecular mechanisms of gender-specific effects.

In general, the surfactant and the commercial formulation showed higher toxicity to fish when compared to active ingredient (glyphosate pure) and their metabolite (AMPA). The 50% lethal concentration (i.e., LC_{50}) of GBHs for fish has high variability, ranging from 1000 to 9750 μg L^{-1} [6, 41]. Chandrasekera and Weeratunga [42] found a LC_{50} of 976 μg L^{-1} for 48 h of exposure in fries of *P. reticulata*, while Sadeghi and Hedayati [43] found a LC_{50} = 12,640 μg L^{-1} in adults for a 41% commercial formulation and Souza-Filho and collaborators [44] found 4212 μg L^{-1} for 48 h.

Glyphosate and formulation compounds can be taken by fish via gills and digestive tract through ingestion of contaminated food or water [6, 45]. Once inside the organisms, glyphosate is absorbed and distributed to the whole body through blood circuit, reaching several tissues. GBHs can affect fishes in different ways, affecting many organs and as well molecular levels. In liver, vacuolization process was reported in hepatocytes and nuclear pyknoses; in kidney, studies report Bowman capsule dilatation and accumulation of hyaline drops in tubular cells; and in gills, glyphosate causes hyperplasia, lamellar fusion and aneurism [46–50]. Besides that, Langiano and Martinez [49] showed activation of the stress axis, with increased blood glucose levels. Souza-Filho and collaborators [44] also showed genotoxic effects in fish cells. Concerning to enzymes, Sandrini and collaborators [17] showed that glyphosate impairs acetylcholinesterase activity in synapses, preventing detaching of acetylcholine from receptors, impairing electric transmission by neurons. This can impair muscle contraction and information transmittance. GBH in sub-lethal levels can also impair fish feeding behavior as shown by Giaquinto and collaborators [51]. Also, a recent *in vitro* study [52] showed that low concentrations of GBH, even those allowed by the USA, Canadian, and Brazilian laws (50 μg L^{-1}) kill yellowtail tetra fish (*Astyanax lacustris*) sperm cells, compromising fish reproduction and natural population persistence.

OMIC technologies, such as proteomics, transcriptomics, and metabolomics, have been applied to investigate the molecular mechanisms and toxicity of GBHs on fish. For example, proteomics-based methods (two-dimensional gel electrophoresis associated with mass spectrometry and bioinformatics) were used to complement the knowledge about the ecotoxicity of GBH on *P. reticulata* [53, 54]. The female guppy exposed to GBH (1.82 mg L^{-1}) for 24 h changed different cell processes in the gills (energy metabolism, regulation and maintenance of cytoskeleton, nucleic acid metabolism, and stress response) [53] and liver (cellular structure, motility and transport, energy metabolism, and apoptosis) [54], confirming tissue-specific responses at molecular levels.

2.4 Herpetofauna

The herpetofauna is composed of reptiles and amphibians, and due to the low mobility, physiological requirements, and habitat specificity, this group has become ideal models for environmental conservation studies [55]. Amphibians are sensitive to exposure to contaminants and are considered good bioindicators in monitoring water quality [56]. Characteristics such as permeable skin, reproduction, and larval stages dependent on the aquatic environment make anuran amphibians highly vulnerable to pesticide contamination [57]. Evidence suggests that anuran species decline is related to the intensive use of pesticides [58–60].

The decline of amphibian populations is related to the increase of environmental pollutants, the influence of climate change, habitat fragmentation, exposure to ultraviolet radiation, and human-induced environmental changes [61, 62]. Contamination of water bodies next to agricultural areas generally increases during the rainy season, that is, widely used to breed by most species of amphibians, and many species use temporary ponds and small streams adjacent to agricultural areas as part of their life cycle, harming the reproductive period and larval development [57, 58, 63]. During the rainy season, the agrochemical present in the soil are susceptible to be transported down the soil profiles and/or surfaces/underground water bodies and consequently affect the amphibian population [58] and other environmental (a) biotic elements [6, 64].

Herbicides may delay or inhibit the metamorphosis of amphibians directly impacting their reproduction [57]. According to Walker and collaborators [65], the main routes of herbicide absorption in anuran amphibians are through contaminated food ingestion and skin absorption of pollutants dissolved or suspended in water. After absorption, the substance is transported to different compartments of the body through blood. The effect of herbicides on tadpoles is less known when compared to adult amphibians, since the larvae of the anurans are less visible, and unlike adults, they do not have vocalization. Tadpoles of various species have not yet been described, which makes it even more difficult to study these organisms in depth [66].

The reduction in larval survival due to exposure to glyphosate was observed by Simioni and collaborators [67], Figueiredo and Rodrigues [68], and Costa and collaborators [69] in larvae of *Physalaemus albonotatus*, *Physalaemus centralis*, and *Physalaemus cuvieri* [70]. Rissoli and collaborators [71] also observed that the exposure of bullfrog tadpoles to Roundup Original® causes damage to the epithelium causing hypoxia in these animals. In the last 30 years, populations of amphibians have been suffering a great decline or even being extinct; almost half of the species are experiencing some population decline. On the basis of toxicity studies, sensitivity to glyphosate differs among species; however, there are several variations in experimental conditions and pesticide formula (different commercial formulations of glyphosate, different exposure times, different surfactant substances, number of replicates, abiotic conditions in the experiment, and stage of development) which make it difficult to compare and define which groups or species are more tolerant to contamination [67, 72, 73]. The LC_{50} values for the herpetofauna species are shown in **Table 3**.

Reptiles are extremely sensitive to herbicide formulations and may exhibit changes in their behavior after exposure of these xenobiotics [74]. This group is fairly uniform and exposure to GBHs may affect its energy storage process [75, 76]. Schaumburg and collaborators [77] found that exposure to sublethal concentrations of glyphosate during the embryonic phase of *Salvator merianae* may cause an increase in genetic damage. Therefore, it is assumed that glyphosate is capable of causing DNA damage, promoting chromatin fragmentation of epidermal cells, impairing cell division. Exposure to glyphosate does not alter the thermoregulatory behavior of lizards of the species *Oligosoma polychroma* [78]. Sub-lethal concentrations of the commercial glyphosate formulation (Roundup®) cause genotoxic damage and chromosome breaks in *Anguilla anguilla*. The increase in the damage index in this species can cause reproductive damage and adverse effects in the long term [79].

Currently in the Neotropical region, about 40 studies relate the indiscriminate use of herbicides based on glyphosate with the risk to biodiversity of herpetofauna. Schiesari and collaborators [80] reported that some species of amphibians, including tadpoles and adults and some reptiles are sensitive to exposure to formulations based on glyphosate. Exposure to sublethal concentrations of glyphosate is

Species	Chemical	Exposure time (h)	LC_{50} mg a.i./L	Reference
Anaxyrus americanus	Roundup®	384	0.55–2.52	[31]
	Roundup®	96	0.8–2.0	[80]
Anaxyrus boreas	Roundup®	96	0.8–2.0	[31]
Crinia insignifera	Roundup®	48	2.9–11.6	[31]
Dendropsophus minutus	Roundup®	96	0.28	[85]
Heleioporus eyrei	Roundup®	48	2.9–11.6	[31]
Hyla versicolor	Roundup®	384	0.55–2.52	[31]
	Roundup®	96	0.8–2.0	[31]
Litoria moorei	Roundup®	48	2.9–11.6	[31]
Lithobates sylvaticus	Roundup®	384	0.55–2.52	[31]
	Roundup®	96	0.8–2.0	[31]
Lithobates pipiens	Roundup®	384	0.55–2.52	[31]
	Roundup®	96	0.8–2.0	[31]
Lithobates clamitans	Roundup®	384	0.55–2.52	[31]
	Roundup®	96	0.8–2.0	[31]
Lithobates catesbeianus	Roundup®	384	0.55–2.52	[31]
	Roundup®	96	0.8–2.0	[31]
Limnodynastes dorsalis	Roundup®	48	2.9–11.6	[31]
Pseudacris crucifer	Roundup®	96	0.8–2.0	[31]
Rana cascadae	Roundup®	96	0.8–2.0	[31]
Rhinella arenarum	Roundup®	48	2.42	[83]
Scinax nasicus	Roundup®	48	1.74	[82]

Table 3.
Ecotoxicity of glyphosate-based herbicide (GBH) to herpetofauna, exposure time, and LC50 value.

sufficient to cause irreversible damage to the DNA of amphibians and reptiles, so the use of GBH should be controlled in arable areas avoiding the decline of species that make up the herpetofauna group.

2.5 Aquatic birds

Glyphosate when used in recommended rates is considered not bioaccumulative and of low toxicity in birds [81]. However, the present acquaintance is not enough to make affirmation about low toxicity risk and low exposure of birds to herbicide considering the possible complex process behind the movement and accumulation of glyphosate, additives, and waste in the environment. Moreover, even the few available studies [82–96] have found direct and indirect effects of glyphosate on bird species (**Figure 4**). Among those, only five studies along years 1994 and 2017 on Google Scholar database have analyzed effects on aquatic bird species. Direct effects have been analyzed on male ducks (*Anas platyrhynchos*) that receive two different concentrations of Roundup dissolved in distilled water according to the body weight (5 and 100 mg kg^{-1}). There was a decrease in testosterone level in blood plasma of about 90%. Moreover, anatomical and histological changes in seminiferous tubes and anatomical changes in the epididymis region have also been found [82].

Indirect effects have been found in wetlands where the glyphosate is used to control the increase of *Typha* spp. population [83–85]. Species of blackbirds and wren can be affected by habitat changes in target and nontarget plant communities that decrease available places to sheltering, nesting, and feeding. The lacks of those places lead birds to starvation, strong competition for resources, or leave the environment [84]. Part of control in coastal dunes of invasive species *Chrysanthemoides monilifera* ssp. *rotundata* is due to glyphosate. An 8-year study has found that a typical bird from coastal region, *Myzomela sanguinolenta,* was the rarest in places that receive the handling herbicide [86]. Environmental heterogeneity (e.g., microclimate and flora) and specific vegetation that is dead by glyphosate can be very important for conservation of some bird populations in the environment [85]. Sometimes, there is the increase of some bird populations after the

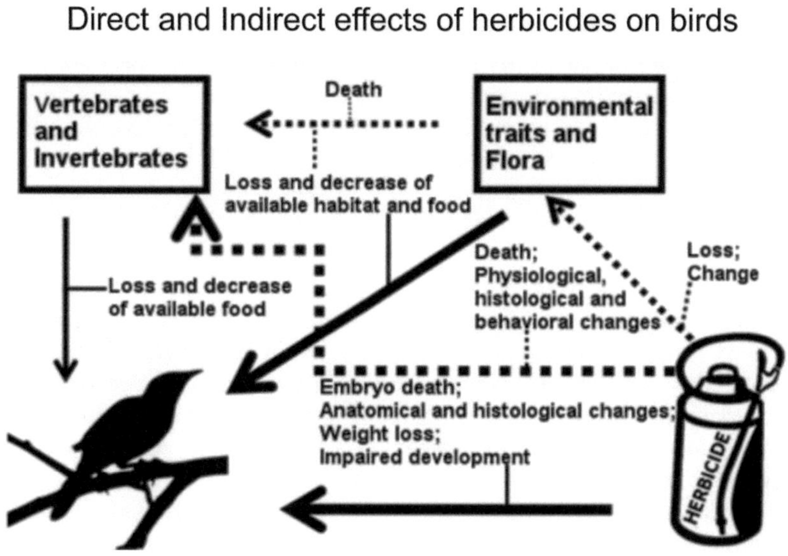

Figure 4.
Ecotoxicity of glyphosate-based herbicide (GBH) to aquatic birds. Direct (continuous arrows) and indirect (dashed arrows) effects of GBH on birds.

glyphosate application. However, it can be related with an immediate advantage due the removal of abundant plant species and other changes in the environment and in available food. Under those circumstances, other population traits, like reproductive success, could have been affected but not detected [83].

The direct effect of glyphosate on aquatic plants and macroalgae [87] can also affect aquatic birds once they make up the varied and plentiful diet of many of those birds. Changes in physiological, histological, and behavioral levels and lethal cases have been documented in fishes due to use of glyphosate [87, 88]. In this way, piscivorous birds can also be suffering indirect effects. In fact, all aquatic birds' food chain can be affected by glyphosate once effects on invertebrates [81, 87, 88], amphibians [89], and reptiles [90] have already been confirmed.

Birds are very similar in their physiology and anatomy. Then, studies that have tested direct and indirect effects of glyphosate on nonaquatic birds can be also considered here. In Japanese quails (*Coturnix japonica*), the low food consumption due to reduced palatability and the low absorption of nutrients in the digestive tract are responsible for body weight loss. Moreover, those birds have been fed with high glyphosate doses (250 and 500 mg kg^{-1} of food) and have exposed clinical symptoms of behavioral changes, malformed feathers, and slow development [91]. A total of 57.5% of dead embryos from chicken eggs have received glyphosate solution (0.1 ml with 2% Glialka Star) inside shell [92]. Herbicides can also act in synergy with other agrochemicals turning these toxic effects more complex. In this way, the combined effect between glyphosate and other chemicals on birds has been analyzed and all studies have demonstrated the increase of potential toxicological: 97.5% of dead embryos (0.1% of lead acetate plus 2% of glyphosate) [92] and decrease of hemoglobin and leucocytes (indoxacarb, an insecticide, plus glyphosate) [91]. Indirect effects on nonaquatic birds due the low vegetation complexity have also been reported: habitat loss replacing shrub by trees, for example, [93]; imbalance in the population structure (i.e., sex ratio) eliminating only habitats of one bird group [94, 95]; and changes in richness of the communities benefiting only birds related to sparse vegetation [96].

Therefore, the controlled and scaled use of glyphosate in large areas is necessary to contribute to conservation of environmental heterogeneity and biological diversity avoiding the plausible effects on bird communities [83–85, 94]. To know what plants are important to bird diet and to promote techniques that do not eliminate all of those plants from the place are important activities before glyphosate application [91]. More studies that aim to analyze the bird contamination by herbicides are also necessary [97]. Long-term studies that encourage collaborative work between ecologist, toxicologist, and chemist are more pertinent [98].

2.6 Aquatic mammals

For the best of our knowledge, GBH or glyphosate only was not tested in aquatic mammals. Searching on Web of Science website for the terms "Glyphosate AND mammal AND aquatic," there is no study reported to date. Despite that, mammals in general are considered less sensible to GBH damages than other groups due to reduced contact with the environment of mammals when compared to other groups as fishes, amphibians, or aquatic invertebrates [99]. The main way that GBH or the active ingredient glyphosate reaches mammals' bodies is through the digestive tract. However, it seems to be poorly absorbed and is excreted essentially nonmetabolized [100]. Essentially, mammals that were tested were rats, mice, and dogs [101], tested through injection or ingestion. Some studies report glyphosate in humans in medical case studies. Reported direct effects of GBH on mammals are described as a "wide range of clinical manifestations" such as skin and throat irritation, hypotension, or death [102] and include heart arrhythmias and atrioventricular block, cardiac electrophysiological changes and conduction blocks [103], pregnancy problems [104], disrupt transcriptional expression of the steroidogenic acute regulatory protein in testicle [105] and aromatase activity, alter mRNA levels, and interact with enzymes [106]. Indirect effects on mammals can be due to reduction of vegetation and animals that are a source of food such as invertebrates [101] and fishes. Although these mentioned studies were conducted in nonaquatic mammals, it is expected that aquatic mammals have similar or even more accentuated effect, since they have intense contact with water, and if it is contaminated, the exposure will be higher.

3. Regulations and perspectives

Despite the fact that GBHs were developed to control weeds, acting specifically in a restrict plan biochemical pathway, several studies demonstrated that there are many side effects on nontarget organisms in all great groups as reported extensively here. Looking to control these side effects, governments for many countries around the world established limits for usage and concentrations in water bodies. The USA, for example, allows 700 μg L^{-1} in water bodies, while Canada allows 280 μg L^{-1} in drink water. The Brazilian law is a little more restrictive, allowing 65 μg L^{-1} in water bodies class 2 that is used for crop and recreation of first degree (direct contact) [107]. However, we could check here that these maximum concentrations allowed are not safe for biodiversity conservation. Considering the Brazilian law, the more restrictive in American countries, populations of yellowtail tetra fish (*A. lacustris*) are not safe since sperm cells of this species are dead in lower concentrations than 65 μg L^{-1} [52]. In this way, European regulations are more plausible, because it is more restrictive (0.1 μg L^{-1}) [108] and can be more precise on conservation of aquatic biodiversity.

However, even with all those regulations, it is not being obeyed, since there is a large range of glyphosate and its metabolite (e.g., AMPA) concentrations in hydroresources [6, 64]. Therefore, another way of action for environment safety is preserving marginal forests of rivers, surveillance, and environment education. Another sustainable way to achieve this goal is changing the crop production matrix from large scale, that is, conventional-based production model to a smaller integrative-/organic-based production system, with controlled or restrictive usage of pesticides and other agrochemicals.

Acknowledgements

We are thankful to FAPEG (#201710267001261) for financial support.

Conflict of interest

The authors declare that there is no conflict of interest.

Author details

Bruno Bastos Gonçalves[1*], Percilia Cardoso Giaquinto[2],
Douglas dos Santos Silva[1], Carlos de Melo e Silva Neto[3],
Amanda Alves de Lima[4], Adriano Antonio Brito Darosci[5], Jorge Laço Portinho[6],
Wanessa Fernandes Carvalho[1] and Thiago Lopes Rocha[1]

1 Federal University of Goiás (UFG), Goiânia, GO, Brazil

2 Biosciences Institute, Universidade Estadual Paulista Júlio de Mesquita Filho, Botucatu, SP, Brazil

3 Federal Institute of Education, Science and Technology of Goiás, Cidade de Goiás, GO, Brazil

4 Goiás State University, Brazil

5 Federal Institute of Education, Science and Technology of Goiás, Formosa, GO, Brazil

6 Brazilian Company of Agriculture Research, Brazil

*Address all correspondence to: goncalves.b.b@gmail.com

References

[1] Brooker MP, Edwards RW. Aquatic herbicides and the control of water weeds. Water Research. 1975;**9**(1):1-15. Available from: https://www.sciencedirect.com/science/article/pii/0043135475901463 [Accessed: 04 February 2019]

[2] Cedergreen N, Streibig JC. The toxicity of herbicides to non-target aquatic plants and algae: Assessment of predictive factors and hazard. Pest Management Science. 2005;**61**(12): 1152-1160. DOI: 10.1002/ps.1117 [Accessed: 30 September 2018]

[3] Brown AA, Thompson AR. In: Brown AA, Thompson AR, editors. Ecology of Pesticides. 1st ed. Vol. 65. New York: John Wiley & Sons Inc; 1978. 536 p. DOI: 10.1002/iroh.19800650121 [Accessed: 29 August 2018]

[4] Edwards CA. In: Edwards CA, editor. Environmental Pollution by Pesticides. London: Springer US; 1973. 542 p

[5] Gilbert N. Case studies: A hard look at GM crops. Nature. 2013;**497**(7447):24-26. DOI: 10.1038/497024a [Accessed: 29 August 2018]

[6] Annett R, Habibi HR, Hontela A. Impact of glyphosate and glyphosate-based herbicides on the freshwater environment. Journal of Applied Toxicology. 2014;**34**(5):458-479. Available from: http://www.ncbi.nlm.nih.gov/pubmed/24615870 [Accessed: 18 September 2017]

[7] Glyphosate|C3H8NO5P—PubChem [Internet]. Available from: https://pubchem.ncbi.nlm.nih.gov/compound/glyphosate#section=3D-Conformer [Accessed: 29 August 2018]

[8] Steinrücken HC, Amrhein N. The herbicide glyphosate is a potent inhibitor of 5-enolpyruvylshikimic acid-3-phosphate synthase. Biochemical and Biophysical Research Communications. 1980;**94**(4):1207-1212. Available from: http://www.sciencedirect.com/science/article/pii/0006291X80905471

[9] Tsui MTK, Chu LM. Aquatic toxicity of glyphosate-based formulations: Comparison between different organisms and the effects of environmental factors. Chemosphere. 2003;**52**(7): 1189-1197. Available from: https://www.sciencedirect.com/science/article/pii/S0045653503003060?via%3Dihub [Accessed: 30 September 2018]

[10] Lajmanovich RC, Sandoval MT, Peltzer PM. Induction of mortality and malformation in *Scinax nasicus* tadpoles exposed to glyphosate formulations. Bulletin of Environmental Contamination and Toxicology. 2003;**70**(3):612-618. Available from: http://www.ncbi.nlm.nih.gov/pubmed/12592539 [Accessed: 18 September 2018]

[11] Costa R, Nomura F. Measuring the impacts of Roundup original® on fluctuating asymmetry and mortality in a neotropical tadpole. Hydrobiologia. 2015:1-12. DOI: 10.1007/s10750-015-2404-0

[12] Cattaneo R, Clasen B, Loro VL, de Menezes CC, Pretto A, Baldisserotto B, et al. Toxicological responses of *Cyprinus carpio* exposed to a commercial formulation containing glyphosate. Bulletin of Environmental Contamination and Toxicology. 2011;**87**(6):597-602. Available from: http://www.ncbi.nlm.nih.gov/pubmed/21931962 [Accessed: 18 September 2018]

[13] Glusczak L, dos Santos Miron D, Crestani M, Braga da Fonseca M, de Araújo Pedron F, Duarte MF, et al. Effect of glyphosate herbicide

on acetylcholinesterase activity and metabolic and hematological parameters in piava (*Leporinus obtusidens*). Ecotoxicology and Environmental Safety. 2006;**65**(2):237-241. Available from: http://www.ncbi.nlm.nih.gov/pubmed/16174533

[14] Menéndez-Helman RJ, Ferreyroa GV, Dos Santos Afonso M, Salibián A. Glyphosate as an acetylcholinesterase inhibitor in *Cnesterodon decemmaculatus*. Bulletin of Environmental Contamination and Toxicology. 2012;**88**(1):6-9. Available from: www.proquest.com [Accessed: 18 September 2018]

[15] Modesto KA, Martinez CB. Effects of roundup Transorb on fish: Hematology, antioxidant defenses and acetylcholinesterase activity. Chemosphere. 2010;**81**(6):781-787. Available from: http://www.ncbi.nlm.nih.gov/pubmed/20684975 [Accessed: 23 July 2012]

[16] Salbego J, Pretto A, Gioda CR, de Menezes CC, Lazzari R, Radünz Neto J, et al. Herbicide formulation with glyphosate affects growth, acetylcholinesterase activity, and metabolic and hematological parameters in piava (*Leporinus obtusidens*). Archives of Environmental Contamination and Toxicology. 2010;**58**(3):740-745. Available from: http://www.ncbi.nlm.nih.gov/pubmed/20112104

[17] Sandrini JZ, Rola RC, Lopes FM, Buffon HF, Freitas MM, Martins CDMG, et al. Effects of glyphosate on cholinesterase activity of the mussel Perna perna and the fish *Danio rerio* and *Jenynsia multidentata*: *In vitro* studies. Aquatic Toxicology. 2013;**130-131**:171-173. DOI: 10.1016/j.aquatox.2013.01.006

[18] Dörr F. Efeito Do Herbicida Glifosato Sobre o Crescimento e produção de metabólitos secundários Em Microcystis Aeruginosa e Cylindrospermopsis Raciborskii. São Paulo: Biblioteca Digital de Teses e Dissertações da Universidade de São Paulo; 2015. Available from: http://www.teses.usp.br/teses/disponiveis/9/9141/tde-10062015-171941/ [Accessed: 30 September 2018]

[19] Newton M, Howard KM, Kelpsas BR, Danhaus R, Lottman CM, Dubelman S. Fate of glyphosate in an Oregon forest ecosystem. Journal of Agricultural and Food Chemistry. 1984;**32**(5):1144-1151. DOI: 10.1021/jf00125a054 [Accessed: 30 September 2018]

[20] Newton M, Horner LM, Cowell JE, White DE, Cole EC. Dissipation of glyphosate and aminomethylphosphonic acid in North American forests. Journal of Agricultural and Food Chemistry. 1994;**42**(8):1795-1802. DOI: 10.1021/jf00044a043 [Accessed: 30 September 2018]

[21] Goldsborough LG, Brown DJ. Dissipation of glyphosate and aminomethylphosphonic acid in water and sediments of boreal forest ponds. Environmental Toxicology and Chemistry. 1993;**12**(7):1139-1147. DOI: 10.1002/etc.5620120702 [Accessed: 30 September 2018]

[22] Mackay D, Shiu WY, Ma KC. Illustrated Handbook of Physical-Chemical Properties and Environmental Fate for Organic Chemicals. Florida, USA: Lewis Publishers; 1992

[23] National Center for Biotechnology Information. Sarcosine [Internet]. Pubchem compound Database. 2018. Available from: https://pubchem.ncbi.nlm.nih.gov/compound/sarcosine#section=Top [Accessed: 17 October 2018]

[24] Giesy JP, Dobson S, Solomon KR. Ecotoxicological risk assessment for roundup® herbicide. Reviews of Environmental Contamination and Toxicology. 2000;**167**:35-120. DOI: 10.1007/978-1-4612-1156-3_2 [Accessed: 30 September 2018]

[25] Antunes AM, Rocha TL, Pires FS, de Freitas MA, Leite VRMC, Arana S, et al. Gender-specific histopathological response in guppies *Poecilia reticulata* exposed to glyphosate or its metabolite aminomethylphosphonic acid. Journal of Applied Toxicology. 2017;**37**(9): 1098-1107. Available from: http://www.ncbi.nlm.nih.gov/pubmed/28425566 [Accessed: 12 November 2018]

[26] Folmar LC, Sanders HO, Julin AM. Toxicity of the herbicide glyphosate and several of its formulations to fish and aquatic invertebrates. Archives of Environmental Contamination and Toxicology. 1979;**8**(3):269-278. DOI: 10.1007/BF01056243 [Accessed: 08 October 2018]

[27] Jeppesen E, Jensen JP, Søndergaard M, Lauridsen T, Pedersen LJ, Jensen L. Top-down control in freshwater lakes: The role of nutrient state, submerged macrophytes and water depth. Hydrobiologia. 1997;**342/343**(0):151-164. DOI: 10.1023/A:1017046130329 [Accessed: 30 September 2018]

[28] Sobrero C, Martin ML, Ronco A. Fitotoxicidad del herbicida roundup® max sobre la especie no blanco Lemna gibba en estudios de campo y laboratorio. Hidrobiológica. 2007;**17**(1):31-39. Available from: http://www.scielo.org.mx/scielo.php?pid=S0188-88972007000400004&script=sci_abstract [Accessed: 30 September 2018]

[29] Pérez DJ, Okada E, Menone ML, Costa JL. Can an aquatic macrophyte bioaccumulate glyphosate? Development of a new method of glyphosate extraction in *Ludwigia peploides* and watershed scale validation. Chemosphere. 2017;**185**: 975-982. Available from: https://www.sciencedirect.com/science/article/pii/S0045653517311451?via%3Dihub [Accessed: 30 September 2018]

[30] Saxton MA, Morrow EA, Bourbonniere RA, Wilhelm SW. Glyphosate influence on phytoplankton community structure in Lake Erie. Journal of Great Lakes Research. 2011;**37**(4):683-690. Available from: https://www.sciencedirect.com/science/article/pii/S0380133011001675 [Accessed: 30 September 2018]

[31] Forlani G, Pavan M, Gramek M, Kafarski P, Lipok J. Biochemical bases for a widespread tolerance of cyanobacteria to the phosphonate herbicide glyphosate. Plant & Cell Physiology. 2008;**49**(3):443-456. Available from: https://academic.oup.com/pcp/article-lookup/doi/10.1093/pcp/pcn021 [Accessed: 30 September 2018]

[32] Vera MS, Lagomarsino L, Sylvester M, Pérez GL, Rodríguez P, Mugni H, et al. New evidences of roundup® (glyphosate formulation) impact on the periphyton community and the water quality of freshwater ecosystems. Ecotoxicology. 2010;**19**(4):710-721. DOI: 10.1007/s10646-009-0446-7 [Accessed: 30 September 2018]

[33] Schaffer JD, Sebetich MJ. Effects of aquatic herbicides on primary productivity of phytoplankton in the laboratory. Bulletin of Environmental Contamination and Toxicology. 2004;**72**(5):1032-1037. Available from: http://www.ncbi.nlm.nih.gov/pubmed/15266702 [Accessed: 30 September 2018]

[34] Relyea RA. The impact of inseticides and herbicides on the biodiversity and productivity of aquatic communities. Ecological Applications. 2005;**15**(2): 618-627. DOI: 10.1890/03-5342 [Accessed: 30 September 2018]

[35] Mueller TC, Main CL, Thompson MA, Steckel LE. Comparison of glyphosate salts (isopropylamine, diammonium, and potassium) and calcium and magnesium concentrations on the control of various weeds. Weed Technology. 2006;**20**(01):164-171.

Available from: https://www.cambridge.org/core/product/identifier/S0890037X00018108/type/journal_article

[36] Gyllstrom M, Hansson L-A. Dormancy in freshwater zooplankton: Induction, termination and the importance of benthic-pelagic coupling. Aquatic Sciences. 2004;**66**(3):274-295. Available from: http://link.springer.com/10.1007/s00027-004-0712-y [Accessed: 06 October 2018]

[37] Ricci C. Dormancy patterns in rotifers. Hydrobiologia. 2001;**446/447**(1):1-11. DOI: 10.1023/A:1017548418201 [Accessed: 06 October 2018]

[38] Gutierrez MF, Battauz Y, Caisso B. Disruption of the hatching dynamics of zooplankton egg banks due to glyphosate application. Chemosphere. 2017;**171**:644-653. Available from: https://www.sciencedirect.com/science/article/pii/S0045653516318422 [Accessed: 06 October 2018]

[39] Portinho JL, Nielsen DL, Daré L, Henry R, Oliveira RC, Branco CCZ. Mixture of commercial herbicides based on 2,4-D and glyphosate mixture can suppress the emergence of zooplankton from sediments. Chemosphere. 2018;**203**:151-159. Available from: https://www.sciencedirect.com/science/article/pii/S0045653518305794 [Accessed: 06 October 2018]

[40] European food Safety Authority. Guidance on tiered risk assessment for plant protection products for aquatic organisms in edge-of-field surface waters. EFSA Journal. 2013;**11**(7):3290. DOI: 10.2903/j.efsa.2013.3290 [Accessed: 06 October 2018]

[41] Nwani CD, Ibiam UA, Ibiam OU, Nworie O, Onyishi G, Atama C. Investigation on acute toxicity and behavioral changes in *Tilapia zillii* due to glyphosate-based herbicide, Forceup. Journal of Animal and Plant Sciences. 2013;**23**(3):888-892

[42] Chandrasekera WU, Weeratunga NP. The lethal impacts of roundup ® (glyphosate) on the fingerlings of guppy, *Poecilia reticulata* Peters, 1859. Asian Fisheries Science. 2011;**24**:367-378

[43] Sadeghi A, Hedayati A. Investigation of LC_{50}, NOEC and LOEC of glyphosate, deltamethrin and pretilachlor in guppies (*Poecilia reticulata*). Iranian Journal of Toxicology. 2014;**8**(26):1124-1129

[44] De Souza Filho J, Sousa CCN, Da Silva CC, De Sabóia-Morais SMT, Grisolia CK. Mutagenicity and genotoxicity in gill erythrocyte cells of *Poecilia reticulata* exposed to a glyphosate formulation. Bulletin of Environmental Contamination and Toxicology. 2013;**91**:583-587. Available from: http://www.ncbi.nlm.nih.gov/pubmed/24042842 [Accessed: 09 October 2013]

[45] Hued AC, Oberhofer S, de los Ángeles Bistoni M. Exposure to a commercial glyphosate formulation (roundup®) alters normal gill and liver histology and affects male sexual activity of *Jenynsia multidentata* (Anablepidae, Cyprinodontiformes). Archives of Environmental Contamination and Toxicology. 2012;**62**(1):107-117. Available from: http://www.ncbi.nlm.nih.gov/pubmed/21643816 [Accessed: 15 August 2013]

[46] Ayoola SO. Histopathological effects of glyphosate on juvenile African catfish (*Clarias gariepinus*). American Journal of Environmental Science. 2008;**4**(3):362-367. Available from: http://citeseerx.ist.psu.edu/viewdoc/download?doi=10.1.1.328.8044&rep=rep1&type=pdf [Accessed: 18 September 2017]

[47] Harayashiki CAY, Junior ASV, Machado AADS, Cabrera LDC, Primel

EG, Bianchini A, et al. Toxic effects of the herbicide roundup in the guppy *Poecilia vivipara* acclimated to fresh water. Aquatic Toxicology. 2013;**142-143**:176-184. Available from: http://linkinghub.elsevier.com/retrieve/pii/S0166445X13002130 [Accessed: 05 September 2013]

[48] Jiraungkoorskul W, Upatham ES, Kruatrachue M, Sahaphong S, Vichasri-Grams S, Pokethitiyook P. Biochemical and histopathological effects of glyphosate herbicide on Nile tilapia (*Oreochromis niloticus*). Environmental Toxicology. 2003;**18**(4):260-267. Available from: http://www.ncbi.nlm.nih.gov/pubmed/12900945 [Accessed: 18 September 2017]

[49] Langiano VDC, Martinez CBR. Toxicity and effects of a glyphosate-based herbicide on the neotropical fish *Prochilodus lineatus*. Comparative Biochemistry and Physiology, Part C: Toxicology & Pharmacology. 2008;**147**(2):222-231. Available from: http://www.ncbi.nlm.nih.gov/pubmed/17933590 [Accessed: 23 July 2012]

[50] Nesković NK, Poleksić V, Elezovíc I, Karan V, Budimir M. Biochemical and histopathological effects of glyphosate on carp, *Cyprinus carpio* L. Bulletin of Environmental Contamination and Toxicology. 1996;**56**(2):295-302. Available from: http://www.ncbi.nlm.nih.gov/pubmed/8720103 [Accessed: 18 September 2017]

[51] Giaquinto PC, de Sá MB, Sugihara VS, Gonçalves BB, Delício HC, Barki A. Effects of glyphosate-based herbicide sub-lethal concentrations on fish feeding behavior. Bulletin of Environmental Contamination and Toxicology. 2017;**98**(4):460-464

[52] Gonçalves BB, Nascimento NF, Santos MP, Bertolini RM, Yasui GS, Giaquinto PC. Low concentrations of glyphosate-based herbicide cause complete loss of sperm motility of yellowtail tetra fish *Astyanax lacustris*. Journal of Fish Biology. 2018;**92**(4):1218-1224

[53] Rocha TL, Santos AP, Yamada ÁT, Soares CM, Borges CL, Bailão AM, et al. Proteomic and histopathological response in the gills of *Poecilia reticulata* exposed to glyphosate-based herbicide. Environmental Toxicology and Pharmacology. 2015;**40**(1):175-186. DOI: 10.1016/j.etap.2015.04.016

[54] Santos AP, Rocha TL, Borges CL, Bailão AM, de Almeida Soares CM, de Sabóia-Morais SMT. A glyphosate-based herbicide induces histomorphological and protein expression changes in the liver of the female guppy *Poecilia reticulata*. Chemosphere. 2017;**168**:933-943

[55] Silvano DL, Segalla MV. Conservação de anfíbios no Brasil. In: Megadiversidade [Internet]. 1st ed. Belo Horizonte: Conservação internacional; 2005. pp. 79-86. Available from: https://books.google.com.br/books?id=nGCySCIb3eIC&pg=PA84&lpg=PA84&dq=.+Conservação+de+anfíbios+no+Brasil+Megadiversidade&source=bl&ots=fgsM9Mn_Ap&sig=GTTGyuhtXffw4CbzCDuFtFevuek&hl=pt-BR&sa=X&ved=2ahUKEwj8y6PZ3oPeAhUChZAKHWztB1w4ChDoATAEeg

[56] den Besten PJ, Munawar M, Suter G. Ecotoxicological testing of marine and freshwater ecosystems: Emerging techniques, trends and strategies. Integrated Environmental Assessment and Management. 2007;(2):3, 305-306. DOI: 10.1002/ieam.5630030221 [Accessed: 13 October 2018]

[57] Hayes TB, Falso P, Gallipeau S, Stice M. The cause of global amphibian declines: A developmental endocrinologist's perspective. The Journal of Experimental Biology. 2010;**213**(6):921-933. Available from: http://www.ncbi.nlm.nih.gov/pubmed/20190117

[58] David M, Marigoudar SR, Patil VK, Halappa R. Behavioral, morphological deformities and biomarkers of oxidative damage as indicators of sublethal cypermethrin intoxication on the tadpoles of *D. melanostictus* (Schneider, 1799). Pesticide Biochemistry and Physiology. 2012;**103**(2):127-134. Available from: https://www.sciencedirect.com/science/article/pii/S0048357512000582 [Accessed: 13 October 2018]

[59] Freire C, Koifman RJ, Sarcinelli PN, Simões Rosa AC, Clapauch R, Koifman S. Long-term exposure to organochlorine pesticides and thyroid status in adults in a heavily contaminated area in Brazil. Environmental Research. 2013;**127**: 7-15. Available from: https://www.sciencedirect.com/science/article/pii/S0013935113001552 [Accessed: 13 October 2018]

[60] Relyea RA. Amphibians are not ready for roundup®. In: Elliott JE, Bishop CA, Morrissey C, editors. Wildlife Ecotoxicology: Forensic Approaches. 3rd ed. New York: Springer; 2011. pp. 267-300. Available from: http://link.springer.com/10.1007/978-0-387-89432-4_9 [Accessed: 13 October 2018]

[61] Davidson C, Shaffer HB, Jennings MR. Declines of the California red-legged frog: Climate, UV-B, habitat, and pesticides hypotheses. Ecological Applications. 2001;**11**(2):464-479. Available from: https://esajournals.onlinelibrary.wiley.com/doi/full/10.1890/1051-0761%282001%29011%5B0464%3ADOTCRL%5D2.0.CO%3B2 [Accessed: 13 October 2018]

[62] Woehl G Jr, Woehl EN. In: Woehl G Jr, Woehl EN, editors. Anfíbios da Mata Atlântica. 1st ed. Jaraguá do Sul: Instituto Rã-Bugio para conservação da biodiversidade; 2008. 32 p. Available from: www.ra-bugio.org.br [Accessed: 13 October 2018]

[63] Howe CM, Berrill M, Pauli BD, Helbing CC, Werry K, Veldhoen N. Toxicity of glyphosate-based pesticides to four North American frog species. Environmental Toxicology and Chemistry. 2004;**23**(8):1928. DOI: 10.1897/03-71

[64] Ondrasek G. Introductory chapter: Irrigation after millennia—Still one of the most effective strategies for sustainable management of water footprint in agricultural crops. In: Ondrasek G, editor. Irrigation in Agroecosystems. Zagreb, Croatia: Intech Open; 2019. pp. 1-3. Available from: https://www.intechopen.com/books/irrigation-in-agroecosystems/introductory-chapter-irrigation-after-millennia-still-one-of-the-most-effective-strategies-for-susta [Accessed: 05 February 2019]

[65] Walker CH, Colin H, Sibly RM, Hopkin SP, Peakall DB. In: Walker CH, Colin H, Sibly RM, Hopkin SP, Peakall DB, editors. Principles of Ecotoxicology. 3rd ed. Florida, USA: CRC Press; 2012. 381 p

[66] McDiarmid RW, Altig R. In: McDiarmid RW, Altig R, editors. Tadpoles: The Biology of Anuran Larvae. Chicago and London: University of Chicago Press; 1999. 444 p

[67] Simioni F, da Silva DFN, Mott T. Toxicity of glyphosate on *Physalaemus albonotatus* (Steindachner, 1864) from Western Brazil. Ecotoxicology and Environmental Contamination. 2013;**8**(1):55-58. Available from: https://siaiap32.univali.br/seer/index.php/eec/article/view/3356 [Accessed: 13 October 2018]

[68] Figueiredo J, de Jesus Rodrigues D. Effects of four types of pesticides on survival, time and size to metamorphosis of two species of tadpoles (*Rhinella marina* and *Physalaemus centralis*) from the southern Amazon, Brazil. Herpetological

Journal. 2014;**24**:65-68. Available from: https://ppbio.inpa.gov.br/sites/default/files/10.0000%40ingentaconnect.com%40content%40bhs%40thj%402014%4000000024%4000000001%40art00003.pdf [Accessed: 13 October 2018]

[69] Costa RN, Nomura F. Measuring the impacts of roundup original® on fluctuating asymmetry and mortality in a neotropical tadpole. Hydrobiologia. 2016;**765**(1):85-96. DOI: 10.1007/s10750-015-2404-0 [Accessed: 13 October 2018]

[70] Blaustein AR, Kiesecker JM. Complexity in conservation: Lessons from the global decline of amphibian populations. Ecology Letters. 2002;**5**(4):597-608. DOI: 10.1046/j.1461-0248.2002.00352.x [Accessed: 13 October 2018]

[71] Rissoli RZ, Abdalla FC, Costa MJ, Rantin FT, McKenzie DJ, Kalinin AL. Effects of glyphosate and the glyphosate based herbicides roundup original® and roundup Transorb® on respiratory morphophysiology of bullfrog tadpoles. Chemosphere. 2016;**156**:37-44. Available from: https://www.sciencedirect.com/science/article/pii/S0045653516305690 [Accessed: 13 October 2018]

[72] Relyea RA, Jones DK. The toxicity of roundup original max® to 13 species of larval amphibians. Environmental Toxicology and Chemistry. 2009;**28**(9):2004. DOI: 10.1897/09-021.1 [Accessed: 13 October 2018]

[73] Mann RM, Bidwell JR. The toxicity of glyphosate and several glyphosate formulations to four species of southwestern Australian frogs. Archives of Environmental Contamination and Toxicology. 1999;**36**(2):193-199. Available from: http://www.ncbi.nlm.nih.gov/pubmed/9888965 [Accessed: 13 October 2018]

[74] Angilletta MJ, Niewiarowski PH, Navas CA. The evolution of thermal physiology in ectotherms. Journal of Thermal Biology. 2002;**27**(4):249-268. Available from: https://www.sciencedirect.com/science/article/pii/S0306456501000948 [Accessed: 13 October 2018]

[75] Peixoto F. Comparative effects of the roundup and glyphosate on mitochondrial oxidative phosphorylation. Chemosphere. 2005;**61**(8):1115-1122. Available from: https://www.sciencedirect.com/science/article/pii/S0045653505004558?via%3Dihub [Accessed: 13 October 2018]

[76] Pianka ER, Vitt LJ, Greene HW. In: Pianka ER, Vitt LJ, Greene HW, editors. Lizards: Windows to the Evolution of Diversity. Berkeley: University of California Press; 2003. 333 p. Available from: https://www.jstor.org/stable/10.1525/j.ctt1pp0q8 [Accessed: 13 October 2018]

[77] Schaumburg LG, Siroski PA, Poletta GL, Mudry MD. Genotoxicity induced by roundup® (glyphosate) in tegu lizard (Salvator merianae) embryos. Pesticide Biochemistry and Physiology. 2016;**130**:71-78. Available from: https://www.sciencedirect.com/science/article/pii/S0048357515300699 [Accessed: 13 October 2018]

[78] Carpenter JK, Monks JM, Nelson N. The effect of two glyphosate formulations on a small, diurnal lizard (*Oligosoma polychroma*). Ecotoxicology. 2016;**25**(3):548-554. DOI: 10.1007/s10646-016-1613-2 [Accessed: 13 October 2018]

[79] Guilherme S, Gaivao I, Santos MA, Pacheco M. European eel (*Anguilla anguilla*) genotoxic and pro-oxidant responses following short-term exposure to roundup(R)—A glyphosate-based herbicide. Mutagenesis. 2010;**25**(5):523-530. Available from: https://academic.oup.com/mutage/article-lookup/doi/10.1093/mutage/geq038 [Accessed: 13 October 2018]

[80] Schiesari L, Waichman A, Brock T, Adams C, Grillitsch B. Pesticide use and biodiversity conservation in the Amazonian agricultural frontier. Philosophical Transactions of the Royal Society of London. Series B, Biological Sciences. 2013;**368**(1619):20120378. Available from: http://www.ncbi.nlm.nih.gov/pubmed/23610177 [Accessed: 13 October 2018]

[81] Sullivan TP, Sullivan DS. Vegetation management and ecosystem disturbance: Impact of glyphosate herbicide on plant and animal diversity in terrestrial systems. Environmental Reviews. 2003;**11**(1):37-59. Available from: http://www.nrcresearchpress.com/doi/10.1139/a03-005 [Accessed: 01 October 2018]

[82] Oliveira AG, Telles LF, Hess RA, Mahecha GAB, Oliveira CA. Effects of the herbicide roundup on the epididymal region of drakes Anas platyrhynchos. Reproductive Toxicology. 2007;**23**(2):182-191. Available from: https://www.sciencedirect.com/science/article/pii/S0890623806002711 [Accessed: 01 October 2018]

[83] Linz GM, Bergman DL, Blixt DC, Bleier WJ. Response of black terns (*Chlidonias niger*) to glyphosate-induced habitat alterations on wetlands. Colonial Waterbirds. 1994;**17**(2):160. Available from: https://www.jstor.org/stable/1521294?origin=crossref [Accessed: 01 October 2018]

[84] Linz GM, Blixt DC, Hall S, Bergman DL, Bleier WJ. Responses of red-winged blackbirds, yellow-headed blackbirds and marsh wrens to glyphosate induced alterations in cattail density. Journal of Field Ornithology. 1996;**67**(1):167-176. Available from: https://sora.unm.edu/sites/default/files/journals/jfo/v067n01/p0167-p0176.pdf [Accessed: 01 October 2018]

[85] Linz GM, Homan HJ. Use of glyphosate for managing invasive cattail (*Typha* spp.) to disperse blackbird (Icteridae) roosts. Crop Protection. 2011;**30**(2):98-104. Available from: https://www.sciencedirect.com/science/article/pii/S0261219410003005 [Accessed: 01 October 2018]

[86] Lindenmayer DB, Wood J, Macgregor C, Hobbs RJ, Catford JA, Lindenmayer C, et al. Non-target impacts of weed control on birds, mammals, and reptiles. Ecosphere. 2017;**8**(5):1-19. Available from: www.esajournals.org [Accessed: 01 October 2018]

[87] Gill JPK, Sethi N, Mohan A, Datta S, Girdhar M. Glyphosate toxicity for animals. Environmental Chemistry Letters. 2018;**16**(2):401-426. Available from: http://link.springer.com/10.1007/s10311-017-0689-0 [Accessed: 01 October 2018]

[88] Carlisle SM, Trevors JT. Glyphosate in the environment. Water, Air, and Soil Pollution. 1988;**39**(3-4):409-420. DOI: 10.1007/BF00279485 [Accessed: 01 October 2018]

[89] Wagner N, Reichenbecher W, Teichmann H, Tappeser B, Lötters S. Questions concerning the potential impact of glyphosate-based herbicides on amphibians. Environmental Toxicology and Chemistry. 2013;**32**(8):1688-1700. DOI: 10.1002/etc.2268 [Accessed: 01 October 2018]

[90] Siroski PA, Poletta GL, Latorre MA, Merchant ME, Ortega HH, Mudry MD. Immunotoxicity of commercial-mixed glyphosate in broad snouted caiman (*Caiman latirostris*). Chemico-Biological Interactions. 2016;**244**: 64-70. Available from: https://www.sciencedirect.com/science/article/pii/S0009279715301332 [Accessed: 01 October 2018]

[91] Bhojane N, Ingole R, Hajare S, Kuralkar S, Manwar S, Waghmare S. Individual and combined toxicity

effect of indoxacarb and glyphosate on general performance and hematological parameters in Japanese quails. Journal of Entomology and Zoology Studies. 2018;**6**(2):1212-1216. Available from: http://www.entomoljournal.com/archives/?year=2018&vol=6&issue=2&ArticleId=3326 [Accessed: 01 October 2018]

[92] Szemerédy G, Szabó R, Kormos É, Szalai C, Lehel J, Budai P. Model study to investigate the toxic interaction between tebuconazole fungicide and lead acetate on chicken embryos. Columella-Journal of Agricultural and Environmental Sciences. 2017;**4**(1):15-19. Available from: https://www.cabdirect.org/cabdirect/abstract/20183050312 [Accessed: 01 October 2018]

[93] Morrison ML, Meslow EC. Effects of the herbicide glyphosate on avian community structure in the Oregon coast range. Forest Science. 1984;**30**(1):95-106. Available from: https://pubs.er.usgs.gov/publication/5221931 [Accessed: 01 October 2018]

[94] Santillo DJ, Brown PW, Leslie DM. Response of songbirds to glyphosate-induced habitat changes on clearcuts. Journal of Wildlife Management. 1989;**53**(1):64. Available from: https://www.jstor.org/stable/3801307?origin=crossref [Accessed: 01 October 2018]

[95] Eggestad M, Enge E, Hjeljord O, Sahlgaard V. Glyphosate application in forest—Ecological aspects. Scandinavian Journal of Forest Research. 1988;**3**(1-4):129-135. DOI: 10.1080/02827588809382503 [Accessed: 01 October 2018]

[96] Schulz CA, Leslie DM, Lochmiller RL, Engle DM, Engle DM. Herbicide effects on cross timbers breeding birds. Journal of Range Management. 1992;**45**(4):407. Available from: https://www.jstor.org/stable/4003093?origin=crossref [Accessed: 01 October 2018]

[97] EFSA. Conclusion on the peer review of the pesticide risk assessment of the active substance glyphosate. EFSA Journal. 2015;**13**(11):1-107. Available from: http://enfo.agt.bme.hu/drupal/sites/default/files/(EFSA)-2015-EFSA_Journal.pdf [Accessed: 01 October 2018]

[98] Kissane Z, Shephard JM. The rise of glyphosate and new opportunities for biosentinel early-warning studies. Conservation Biology. 2017;**31**(6): 1293-1300. DOI: 10.1111/cobi.12955 [Accessed: 01 October 2018]

[99] Zaranyika MF, Nyandoro MG. Degradation of glyphosate in the aquatic environment: An enzymatic kinetic model that takes into account microbial degradation of both free and colloidal (or sediment) particle adsorbed glyphosate. Journal of Agricultural and Food Chemistry. 1993;**41**:838-842. Available from: https://pubs.acs.org/sharingguidelines [Accessed: 03 October 2018]

[100] Williams GM, Kroes R, Munro IC. Safety evaluation and risk assessment of the herbicide roundup and its active ingredient, glyphosate, for humans. Regulatory Toxicology and Pharmacology. 2000;**31**(2):117-165. Available from: https://www.sciencedirect.com/science/article/pii/S0273230099913715 [Accessed: 03 October 2018]

[101] Freedman B. Controversy over the use of herbicides in forestry, with particular reference to glyphosate usage. Journal of Environmental Carcinogenesis Reviews. 1990;**8**(2):277-286. DOI: 10.1080/10590509009373384 [Accessed: 03 October 2018]

[102] Mahendrakar K, Venkategowda PM, Rao SM, Mutkule DP. Glyphosate surfactant herbicide poisoning and management. Indian Journal of Critical Care Medicine. 2014;**18**(5):328-330. Available from: http://www.ncbi.nlm.

nih.gov/pubmed/24914265 [Accessed: 03 October 2018]

[103] Gress S, Lemoine S, Séralini G-E, Puddu PE. Glyphosate-based herbicides potently affect cardiovascular system in mammals: Review of the literature. Cardiovascular Toxicology. 2015;**15**(2):117-126. DOI: 10.1007/s12012-014-9282-y [Accessed: 03 October 2018]

[104] Savitz DA, Arbuckle T, Kaczor D, Curtis KM. Male pesticide exposure and pregnancy outcome. American Journal of Epidemiology. 1997;**146**(12): 1025-1036. Available from: http://www.ncbi.nlm.nih.gov/pubmed/9420527 [Accessed: 03 October 2018]

[105] Walsh LP, McCormick C, Martin C, Stocco DM. Roundup inhibits steroidogenesis by disrupting steroidogenic acute regulatory (StAR) protein expression. Environmental Health Perspectives. 2000;**108**(8): 769-776. Available from: http://www.ncbi.nlm.nih.gov/pubmed/10964798 [Accessed: 03 October 2018]

[106] Richard S, Moslemi S, Sipahutar H, Benachour N, Seralini G-E. Differential effects of glyphosate and roundup on human placental cells and aromatase. Environmental Health Perspectives. 2005;**113**(6):716-720. Available from: http://www.ncbi.nlm.nih.gov/pubmed/15929894 [Accessed: 18 September 2018]

[107] Brasil. Resolução no 357 de 17 de março de 2005 [Internet]. Diário Oficial da União, 357 CONAMA; 2005. pp. 58-63. Available from: http://www.mma.gov.br/port/conama/res/res05/res35705.pdf

[108] EPA. European Communities (Drinking Water) (No. 2) Regulations. Wexford, Ireland: Environmental Protection Agency; 2010. p. 327. Available from: http://www.wsntg.ie [Accessed: 01 October 2018]

Chapter 3

Water Resource Pollution by Herbicide Residues

Kassio Ferreira Mendes, Ana Paula Justiniano Régo, Vanessa Takeshita and Valdemar Luiz Tornisielo

Abstract

Herbicides are frequently used in the chemical control of weeds in various crops in Brazil and worldwide, so they are more frequently detected outside the application areas, contributing to the risk of environmental contamination. The importance of knowledge of the physicochemical properties of the environment and the pesticide used in the agricultural area is in order to understand its effects on terrestrial and aquatic ecosystems and the search for the prevention of future bioaccumulation potentials (bioconcentration and/or biomagnification) of molecules of pesticides in living nontarget organisms, minimizing their negative effects on the environment. The understanding of analytical techniques for measuring the quality of water resources as well as techniques for the remediation of contaminated water is essential to minimize the possible impacts caused by the application of pesticides to the environment.

Keywords: contamination, leaching, runoff, volatilization

1. Introduction

The fate of herbicides in the environment contributes to the contamination of water resources and is governed by retention (adsorption, absorption, and precipitation), transformation (decomposition or degradation) and transport (drift, volatilization, leaching, and runoff), and by the interactions of these processes [1]. The problem of contamination is higher mainly with herbicides that are applied directly on the soil in pre-emergence or pre-planting (PPI) in relation to other forms of applications.

Leaching is indicated as the main cause of groundwater contamination by herbicides [2]. This process is the main form of transport in the soil of nonvolatile and water-soluble herbicides [3]. It is of great importance to point out that leaching is essential for the incorporation of herbicides in the soil profile in order to reach the soil seed bank, contributing to the efficiency of the products in weed control [4]. However, negatively, herbicides can be transported to deeper layers of the soil profile until they reach sites less exploited by the roots, contaminating the groundwater table [5].

Water contamination is not only related to the proximity of the water resources of the treated agricultural areas, the physical and chemical characteristics of the products, the climate, the topography, and the management of the area, but also technical application characteristics such as water use, inventory, handling, and packaging [6].

IntechOpen

Thus, monitoring practices of water resources and the safe use of herbicides should be applied. According to Santos et al. [6], chromatography is the most used technique for identification and quantification of herbicides and, in general, pesticides and contaminants of the water bodies. However, in addition to the detection of contaminants, adequate control is necessary before and in the moment of application to generate the minimum residues as possible in the environment.

In this chapter, we will discuss the main factors that affect water pollution by herbicides, exemplifying herbicides' potential to contaminate water resources, emphasizing the effects, monitoring, and detection of herbicides in water resources, and finalizing strategies to minimize contamination and herbicide removal techniques in contaminated drinking water.

2. Factors affecting water pollution by herbicides

Several factors affect the pollution of water resources by herbicides, and were listed in the base Safe Drinking Water Foundation (SDWF) [7]. The factors are related with soil, herbicides, and environment.

In soil, drainage affects herbicides because it contributes to leaching. Agricultural soils are often well drained, as are natural soil drainage associated with excess rainwater, and irrigation can increase transport herbicides to groundwater and freshwater. This transport occurs in the water path in the soil profile and rapidly reaching a large geographical area. Thereby, the herbicide mobility in soil is coordinated by the movement of water in different directions, being vertical (leaching) and horizontal (runoff and/or run-in). In soil, temperature also affects the fate of herbicides, for the reason that it interferes in microbiology activity. This fact can promote the less biodegradation of herbicides, a process that results in a product formation, frequently, less toxic for the environment. Besides, the chemical degradation and photochemical degradation also reduce the toxicity of herbicides in soil.

With regard to the herbicides, the physicochemical properties are responsible for their behavior in soil, as well as the risks of contamination. Firstly, the solubility in water (S_w) indicates the possible herbicide leaching with water flux in soil, as also the disponibility of the molecule for other processes of dissipation in soil. The Sw is necessary for many herbicides, because it needs to be applied with water and to be absorbed by the target plant. The higher the solubility of the herbicide, the greater the risk of leaching. When herbicide no leaching, that is, it has your persistence for more time in soil, the sorption is controlling your behavior. The sorption coefficient (K_d) normalized for the organic carbon of soil (K_{oc}) indicates this affinity from molecule to soil sorption. This situation reduces the contamination of groundwater by leaching, but increases surface water contamination by runoff on slopes and high rainfall.

The more sorbed the herbicide in soil, will more persistence have this molecule in environment. The persistence can be measured by means of the half-life ($t_{1/2}$). In terms of half-life, the longer the degradation takes, the greater is its persistence. The half-life is unique for individual herbicides, but variable depending on application factors and specific environmental conditions, mainly of microbial activity in soil.

Still, about physical chemical properties of herbicides, the same authors indicate the vapor pressure (VP) as interfering in herbicide behavior in the environment. It is directly related to the volatilization of the herbicides, which is the other form of transport of these molecules to the atmosphere and these can be carried by the wind and reach the soil again in the form of precipitation. The formulations are forms for reducing this effect, besides additives used in mixtures (wetting agents, solvents, extenders, adhesives, buffers, preservatives, and emulsifiers) to improve absorption and decrease losses for the environment. However, much this formulation can contain environmental contaminants also.

Treatment of herbicides in nonagricultural areas can be a cause of environmental pollution. In many areas, such as paved roads, carriers, and sidewalks, among others (rigid surfaces), have nothing to absorb and are particularly vulnerable to transport into watercourses and nontarget areas, especially after precipitation. Thus, herbicides found in water can often be the result of nonagricultural use. In addition, independent of the application area, applying high rates of products can increase the concentration in the environment.

Another factor that affects water pollution by herbicides is precipitation, because high levels of precipitation increase the risk of herbicide contamination. The movement of herbicides in watercourses occurs directly by applying these products to target areas in drains after precipitation. It may also occur within the soil structure by displacement of the herbicides from the absorption sites by the water and the treated soil that has moved into the water by soil erosion. The greater distances of the water resources and the place of application of the herbicides are also crucial to minimize the impacts of the residues in the aquatic system [7].

Persistent herbicides in the environment which have high solubility, mobility, and sorption capacity to soil particles and/or volatilization can present great potential for contamination of water if not used properly. Before carrying out the herbicide application in weed management, checking the risk of each product to the environment is essential. From these data, it is possible to make a decision about the mode of application, season, area, dose, and measures that minimize the impacts.

3. Herbicides with potential for contamination of the environment, ecology, and human health

3.1 Potential for contamination of the environment

For the evaluation of the herbicide runoff, Goss [8] considered the herbicide half-life ($t_{1/2}$) in the soil and the soil sorption potential (K_{oc}) of the herbicide by soil particles when in soil transport as criteria, as presented in **Table 1**. For Leonard [9], the solubility (S_w) of the herbicide is relevant, since it determines the runoff in the soil solution, considering also the intensity and occurrence of rainfall in this process.

In relation to the transport potential associated with sediment, to be will high potential when $t_{1/2} \geq 40$ days and $K_{oc} \geq 1000$ L Kg^{-1}; $t_{1/2} \geq 40$ days, $K_{oc} \geq 500$ L Kg^{-1} and $S_w \leq 0.5$ mg L^{-1}. The potential will low when $t_{1/2} < 1$ day, $t_{1/2} \leq 2$ days and $K_{oc} \leq 500$ L Kg^{-1}, $t1_{/2} \leq 4$ days, $K_{oc} \leq 900$ L Kg^{-1} and $S_w \geq 0.5$ mg L^{-1}, $t1_{/2} \leq 40$ days, $K_{oc} \leq 500$ L Kg^{-1} and $S_w \geq 0{,}5$ mg L^{-1}; $t1_{/2} \leq 40$ days, $K_{oc} \leq 900$ L Kg^{-1} and $S_w \geq 2$ mg L^{-1} [8].

The transport potential dissolved in water will be high potential when: $t_{1/2} > 35$ days, $K_{oc} < 100{,}000$ L Kg^{-1} and $S_w \geq 1$ mg L^{-1}; $t_{1/2} < 35$ days, $K_{oc} \leq 700$ L Kg^{-1}, and $S_w \geq 10$ e ≤ 100 mg L^{-1} and low potential when $K_{oc} \geq 100{,}000$ L Kg^{-1}; $t1_{/2} \leq 1$ day and $K_{oc} \geq 1000$ L Kg^{-1}; $t_{1/2} < 35$ days, and $S_w < 0.5$ mg L^{-1} [8]. The solubility in water will be influenced, when it rains soon after application, $S_w > 30$ mg L^{-1}, and "free" transport in solution (in water) [9].

Table 1 shows the indexes for evaluating the surface runoff of some herbicides, of the relationship between sorption potential and mobility.

To evaluate the potential risk of herbicide leaching, three theoretical indexes (GUS, CDFA, and Cohen) were used according to Inoue et al. [5]. The physicochemical properties of the herbicides were used to calculate the proposed indexes, compiled from the European database [11], according to **Table 2**.

Herbicide	K_{oc} (L Kg^{-1})	$t_{1/2}$ (days)	S_w (mg L^{-1})	Goss[1]	Goss[2]	Mobility[3]
Cloransulam-methyl	30	11	184	LPC	—	M
Diuron	813	75.5	35.5	PC	PC	LM
Glyphosate	1424	15	10,500	—	—	LM
Sodium hydrogen methyl arsonate (MSMA)	1680[4]	200	580,000	PC	PC	—
Paraquat	10,000,000	3000	620,000	PC	LPC	NM
Trifluralin	15,800	181	0.221	PC	PC	NM

[1]*Transport potential associated with sediment: PC = potential for contamination of surface waters and LPC = low potential for contamination of surface waters.*

[2]*Transport potential dissolved in water: PC = potential for contamination of surface water and LPC = low potential for contamination of surface water.*

[3]*LM = slightly mobile; M = mobile; and NM = not mobile.*

[4]*Kegley et al. [10].*
Source: PPDB [11].

Table 1.
Indexes for evaluating the runoff of herbicides on the potential for surface water contamination (Goss).

Herbicide	K_{oc} (L Kg^{-1})	$t_{1/2}$ (days)	GUS[1]	CDFA	Cohen
Ametryn	316	37	0.52 (LL)	L	L
Aminocyclopyrachlor	24	31	3.19 (HL)	L	L
Atrazine	100	75	3.20 (HL)	L	L
Bentazone	55.3	20	2.89 (HL)	L	L
Comazone	300	83	3.00 (HL)	L	L
Imazaquin	18[1]	60	5.42 (HL)	L	L
Imazethapyr	52	90	6.29 (HL)	L	L
Metolachlor	120	90	2.10 (IN)	L	L
Nicosulfuron	30	26	3.25 (HL)	L	L
Picloram	13	82.8	6.03 (HL)	L	L
Simazine	130	60	2.00 (IN)	L	L
Sulfentrazone	43	541	6.16 (HL)	L	L
Sulfometuron-methyl	85	24	2.86 (HL)	L	L
Tebuthiuron	80	400	5.36 (HL)	L	L

[1]*HL = highly leachable, L = leachable, IN = intermediary, LL = low leaching, and NL = non-leachable. Kegley et al. [10].*
Source: PPDB [11].

Table 2.
Indexes for evaluating herbicide leaching for potential groundwater contamination (GUS, CDFA, and Cohen).

The Groundwater Ubiquity Score (GUS) is like log $t_{1/2}$ (4 - log K_{oc}). GUS < 1.8 is nonleachable, GUS > 2.8 is leachable, and –1.8 < GUS < 2.8 is intermediary [12]. The California Department of Food and Agriculture (CDFA) [13] classifies K_{oc} < 512 L kg^{-1} and $t_{1/2}$ > 11 days as leachable. According to Cohen et al. [14], the criterion of the *Environmental Protection Agency* (EPA) classifies K_{oc} < 300 L kg^{-1} and $t_{1/2}$ > 21 days as leachable and K_{oc} > 500 L kg^{-1} and $t_{1/2}$ < 14 days as nonleachable.

Even the theoretical criteria, taking into account the characteristics of each herbicide molecule, distinguish each other. This can be seen in **Table 2**, where herbicide properties are directly related to leaching and classification according to the theoretical criteria. On the other hand, these criteria can help in the chemical management with the herbicides, allowing a correct decision-making based on one of the factors that most influence the behavior of the herbicide molecule in the environment.

For the volatilization, estimation proposed by Lyman et al. [15] is considered only the constant of Henry's Law (H), which represents the concentration of the solute in the air in relation to the concentration in the water, being exemplified in **Table 3**. However, the VP is a property that can also contribute to the evaluation of the volatility of the herbicide, as it demonstrates the potential for evaporation of a molecule in relation to temperature.

Lyman et al. [15] classified $H > 10^{-5}$ as highly volatile, $H < 10^{-7}$ as low volatility, and $10^{-7} > H < 10^{-5}$ as moderately volatile.

3.2 Potential for ecological contamination

The ecotoxicology is the science that studies the effects of physical and chemical agents on organisms, populations, and environment of communities, whether terrestrial or aquatic [16–19]. Aquatic ecotoxicology aims to evaluate the effect of toxic chemicals on organisms representative of the aquatic ecosystem. The toxic effects can manifest themselves at different levels of organization, from cellular structures to individuals, populations, and communities [18, 20, 21].

Environmental monitoring through ecotoxicological studies integrates important parameters, since it uses organisms' representative of aquatic environments for the quality of the environment under study. The main advantage of using ecotoxicological studies on the physicochemical approach is that organisms interact with the ambient conditions for a time, while the chemical data are measured instantly in nature, and therefore, require a large number of measurements to obtain greater precision in the results.

Ecotoxicological tests may be classified according to their time available for evaluation of acute and chronic effects. These tests differ in duration and final responses are measured and are a necessary tool for ecotoxicological characterization of environmental samples, both the potential risk assessment as the establishment of maximum permissible limits for the protection of aquatic life [22]. **Table 4** shows definitions of terms commonly used in toxicity tests.

Herbicide	H	Lyman	Volatilization based on constant H	VP	Volatilization based on VP
Atrazine	1.50×10^{-04}	HV	NV	0.039	LV
Clomazone	4.20×10^{-3}	HV	NV	19.2	HV
Dicamba	1.0×10^{-04}	HV	NV	1.67	LV
Linuron	2.00×10^{-04}	HV	NV	0.051	LV
Metsulfuron	2.87×10^{-06}	MV	NV	1.40×10^{-08}	LV
Trifluralin	6.13×10^{-3}	HV	MV	9.5	MV
2.4-D	4.0×10^{-06}	MV	NV	0.009	LV

HV = highly volatile, MV = moderately volatile, LV = low volatility, and NV = nonvolatile.
Source: PPDB [11].

Table 3.
Indexes for evaluating the volatilization of herbicides on the potential for rainwater contamination.

Acute toxicity tests are used to measure the effects of toxic agents on aquatic species over a short period of time over the life span of the organism, while chronic toxicity tests are performed to measure the effects of chemicals on species for a period which may cover part or all of the life cycle of the test organism. The acute toxicity study is important to predict more immediate impacts to ecosystems, while the study of chronic toxicity is important in cases where organisms are continually exposed to toxic substances at lower concentrations.

The toxicological effects of herbicides on aquatic organisms have been studied to determine, mainly, the effect of herbicides on the different trophic levels that surround this environment. Aquatic toxicology contributes to the determination of the maximum concentration of herbicide that can be considered tolerable in an environment without causing significant damage to biota. You also study the quantitative and qualitative effects of these contaminants on aquatic organisms. **Table 5** shows the toxicological effect of herbicides on the major aquatic organisms.

According to FAO [24], herbicides are included in a wide range of organic micro-pollutants that have ecological impacts. Different groups of herbicides have different types of data on the living body, so a generalization is difficult. Water can be contaminated by runoff of herbicides. Contamination can occur directly through pesticide applications in growing areas or indirectly by exposing pesticide residues to the environment. Contamination can occur directly through pesticide applications in growing areas or indirectly by exposing pesticide residues to the environment.

The mechanisms are bioaccumulation, bioconcentration, and biomagnification. The bioaccumulation of substances in organisms, according to their trophic level of the food chain, can be divided into:

- **Bioconcentration**: the direct capture of pollutants present in water, through the gills, skin, and oral route;

- **Biomagnification**: consumption of contaminated prey, associated with different trophic levels.

The bioaccumulation process refers to the entry of xenobiotic molecules into organs of living organisms, over the time of exposure. Now the rate of excretion of

Parameter	Definition	Exposure time
LD_{50}	Average lethal dose: dose of sample causing mortality of 50% of organisms at the time of exposure and test conditions.	24 to 96 h
LC_{50}	Medium lethal concentration: concentration of sample that causes an acute effect (death, for example) to 50% of organisms at the time of exposure and under test conditions.	24 to 96 h
EC_{50}	Average effective concentration: concentration of sample causing an acute effect (immobility, for example) to 50% of organisms at the time of exposure and under test conditions.	24 or 48 h
CENO	Unobserved effect concentration: higher concentration of toxic agent that does not cause statistically significant deleterious effect on organisms at the time of exposure and test conditions.	7 days
CEO	Observed effect concentration: lower concentration of toxic agent causing statistically significant deleterious effect on organisms at time of exposure and test conditions.	7 days

Source: Espíndola et al. [23].

Table 4.
Definition of some terms used in toxicity tests.

Herbicide	Toxicological test	Value (mg L^{-1})	Water agencies	Classification
2.4-D	Fish—Sharp 96 h LC50	100.00	*Pimephales promelas*	Moderate
	Fish—Chronic 21 days CENO	27.20	*Oncorhynchus mykiss*	Low
	Aquatic invertebrates—Acute 48 h EC50	134.20	*Daphnia magna*	Low
	Aquatic invertebrates—Chronic 21 days CENO	46.20	*Daphnia magna*	Low
	Aquatic plants (biomass)—Acute 7 days EC50	2.70	*Lemna perpusilla*	Moderate
	Algae—Acute 72 h EC50	24.20	*Raphidocelis subcapitata*	Low
	Algae—Chromatic 96 h CENO	100.00	*Chlorella vulgaris*	Low
Ametryn	Fish—Sharp 96 h LC50	5.00	*Oncorhynchus mykiss*	Moderate
	Aquatic invertebrates—Acute 48 h EC50	28.00	*Daphnia magna*	Moderate
	Aquatic invertebrates—Chronic 21 days CENO	0.32	*Daphnia magna*	Moderate
	Aquatic crustaceans—Acute 96 h EC50	1.70	*Americamysis bahia*	Moderate
	Aquatic plants (biomass)—Acute 7 days EC50	0.10	*Lemna perpusilla*	Moderate
	Algae—Acute 72 h EC50	0.0036	*Raphidocelis subcapitata*	High
Atrazine	Fish—Sharp 96 h LC50	4.50	*Oncorhynchus mykiss*	Moderate
	Fish—Chronic 21 days CENO	2.00	*Oncorhynchus mykiss*	Low
	Aquatic invertebrates—Acute 48 h EC50	8.50	*Daphnia magna*	Moderate
	Aquatic invertebrates—Chronic 21 days CENO	1.00	*Daphnia magna*	Moderate
	Aquatic crustaceans—Acute 96 h EC50	1.00	*Americamysis bahia*	Moderate
	Sediment Organisms—96 h acute LC50	1.00	*Chironomus riparius*	Moderate
	Aquatic plants (biomass)—Acute 7 days EC50	0.10	*Lemna perpusilla*	Moderate
	Algae—Acute 72 h EC50	0.0036	*Raphidocelis subcapitata*	Moderate
Diuron	Fish—Sharp 96 h LC50	6.70	*Cyprinodon variegatus*	Moderate
	Fish—Chronic 21 days CENO	0.41	*Oncorhynchus mykiss*	Low
	Aquatic invertebrates—Acute 48 h EC50	5.70	*Daphnia magna*	Moderate
	Aquatic invertebrates—Chronic 21 days CENO	0.096	*Daphnia magna*	Moderate
	Crustáceos aquáticos—Agudo 96 h CE_{50}	1.10	*Americamysis bahia*	Moderate
	Aquatic plants (biomass)—Acute 7 days EC50	0.0183	*Lemna perpusilla*	Moderate
	Algae—Acute 72 h EC50	0.0027	*Scenedesmus agricauda*	High

Herbicide	Toxicological test	Value (mg L^{-1})	Water agencies	Classification
Glyphosate	Fish—Sharp 96 h LC50	38.00	*Oncorhynchus mykiss*	Moderate
	Fish—Chronic 21 days CENO	25.00	*Oncorhynchus mykiss*	Low
	Aquatic invertebrates—Acute 48 h EC50	40.00	*Daphnia magnmagnaa*	Moderate
	Aquatic invertebrates—Chronic 21 days CENO	30.00	*Daphnia magna*	Low
	Aquatic crustaceans—Acute 96 h EC50	40.,00	*Americamysis bahia*	Moderate
	Aquatic plants (biomass)—Acute 7 days EC50	12.00	*Lemma perpusilla*	Low
	Algae—Acute 72 h EC50	4.40	*Scenedesmus agricauda*	Moderate
	Algae—Chromatic 96 h CENO	2.00	—	Low
Simazine	Fish—Sharp 96 h LC50	90.00	*Lepomis macrochirus*	Moderate
	Fish—Chronic 21 days CENO	0.70	—	Moderate
	Aquatic invertebrates—Acute 48 h EC50	1.10	*Daphnia magna*	Moderate
	Aquatic invertebrates—Chronic 21 days CENO	25.00	*Daphnia magma*	Moderate
	Aquatic plants (biomass)—Acute 7 days EC50	3.00	*Lemma perpusilla*	Moderate
	Algae—Acute 72 h EC50	0.04	*Scenedesmus agricauda*	Moderate
	Algae—Chromatic 96 h CENO	0.60	—	Moderate
Trifluralin	Fish—Sharp 96 h LC50	0,088	*Oncorhynchus mykiss*	High
	Fish—Chronic 21 days CENO	10.00	*Pimephales promelas*	Moderate
	Aquatic invertebrates—Acute 48 h EC50	0.245	*Daphnia magna*	Moderate
	Aquatic invertebrates—Chronic 21 days CENO	0.051	*Daphnia magna*	Moderate
	Aquatic crustaceans—Acute 96 h EC50	0.074	*Americamysis bahia*	High
	Sediment Organisms—96 h acute LC50	1.00	*Chironomus riparius*	Moderate
	Sediment Organisms—Chronic 21 days CENO—water	0.25	*Chironomus riparius*	Moderate
	Sediment Organisms—Chronic 21 days CENO—sediment	810.00	*Chironomus riparius*	Low
	Aquatic plants (biomass)—Acute 7 days EC50	0.0122	*Lemma perpusilla*	Moderate
	Algae—Acute 72 h EC50	0.0036	*Raphidocelis subcapitata*	Moderate
	Algae—Chromatic 96 h CENO	0.60	—	Moderate

Source: PPDB [11].

Table 5.
Toxicological effects of herbicides detected in different water resources in Brazil on the main aquatic organisms.

the substances present in the organism and/or their metabolism is low; besides the sorption of the molecules of the substances to the constituents of the body, there will be an increase of the concentration in the organisms, exceeding the values of the medium. The mechanism of bioconcentration is the direct transfer of a molecule of xenobiotic into the body, in its tissues and/or organs [25].

The environment is formed by different phases, such as terrestrial, aquatic, atmospheric, and biota, and the xenobiotic when introduced in this system is distributed according to its physicochemical properties. The sediment has particles and colloids from the soil, serving as a reservoir of xenobiotic molecules, being a source of accumulation of pollutants. Thus, there may be higher concentrations of persistent toxic pollutants in the sediments relative to water, and aquatic biota may metabolize significant amounts of pollutants over time, but these concentrations may be below the detection limits of traditional analytical techniques.

The indicator used to measure the bioaccumulation potential of pollutants in living organisms is the octanol/water partition coefficient (K_{ow}). Thus, K_{ow} (**Table 6**) is the measure of the affinity of the molecule for the apolar phase (1-octanol = lipophilicity) and polar (water = hydrophilicity). Therefore, the higher the K_{ow} value, the greater the lipophilicity (**Table 7**), that is, the higher the bioaccumulation potential [26].

Some herbicides such as diclofop-methyl, fluazifop-P-butyl, atrazine, and oxyfluorfen are lipophilic, which means that they are soluble and accumulated in adipose tissue, such as edible fish tissue and human adipose tissue. Other herbicides with low K_{ow}, such as glyphosate, are metabolized and excreted.

The term biomagnification refers to the increasing concentration of a chemical as food energy is transformed within the food chain. As larger organisms consume smaller organisms, the concentration of herbicides and other pesticides is increasing in tissues and other organs. Very high concentrations can be observed in higher predators, including man.

The ecological effects of herbicides are varied and are often interrelated. The effects on the organism or the ecological level are generally considered as an indicator of early warning of possible impacts on human health. The main types of effects are listed below and vary depending on the organism studied and the type of herbicide. The important point is that many of these effects are chronic (nonfatal) and often not observed by casual observers, but have consequences for the entire food chain, as described below, according to FAO [24]:

- Death of the organism;
- Cancers, tumors, and lesions in fish and animals;
- Inhibition or reproduction failure;
- Suppression of the immune system;
- Endocrine (hormonal) disturbance;
- Cell and DNA damage;
- Teratogenic effects (physical deformities such as curved beaks in birds);
- Weakened health of fish marked by a low proportion of red to white blood cells, excessive slime in fish scales, and gills, among others;
- Inter inter-generational effects (effects are not evident until subsequent generations of the organism); and
- Other physiological effects, such as the thinning of eggshell.

$LogK_{ow}$	K_{ow}	Lipophilicity
<0.1	<1	Hydrophilic
0.1–1	1–10	Moderately liposoluble
1–2	10–100	Lipophilic
2–3	100–1000	Very lipophilic
3	>1000	Extremely lipophilic

Source: Christoffoleti and López-Ovejero [26].

Table 6.
Classification of lipophilicity of herbicides.

Herbicide	Log K_{ow}	Potential to bioaccumulate
Alachlor	3.09	High
Atrazine	2.70	Moderate
Glyphosate	−3.2	Low
Imazapyr	1.34	Low
Mesotrione	0.11	Low
Paraquat	−4.5	Low
Pendimethalin	5.4	High
Tebuthiuron	1.79	Low

Source: PPDB [11].

Table 7.
Bioaccumulation potential of herbicides.

Herbicide	Effects on human health
2.4-D	Effects on the kidney (pigmentation of tubular cells)
Atrazine	Developmental effects (reduction of children's body weight) Other: increased potential risk of ovarian cancer or lymphomas (classified as possible carcinogen)
Dicamba	Liver effects (vacuolation, necrosis, fatty deposits, and changes in liver weight)
Diclofop-methyl	Liver effects (enlargements and enzymatic changes)
Diquat	Cataract formation
Diuron	Weight loss, increased liver weight, and blood effects
Glyphosate	Reduced body weight gain
MCPA	Effects on the kidney (increase of absolute and relative weight, urinary bilirubin, crystals, and pH) Others: systemic, hepatic, testicular, reproductive, and developmental effects, and effect on the nervous system
Metolac3hlor	Liver lesions and tumors in the nasal cavity
Metribuzin	Liver effects (increased incidence and severity of mucopolysaccharide droplets)
Paraquat	Various effects on body weight, spleen, testis, liver, lung, kidney, thyroid, heart, and adrenal gland
Picloram	Changes in body and liver weights and clinical chemistry parameters Others: effects on kidney (ratio of liver weight and body weight, and histopathology)
Simazine	Changes in body weight and effects on serum and thyroid gland
Trifluralin	Changes in liver and spleen weights and serum chemistry

Source: Health Canada [27].

Table 8.
Effects on human health from exposure to herbicides based on the acceptable maximum residue limit (MRL).

These effects are not necessarily caused solely by exposure to herbicides or other organic contaminants, but may be associated with a combination of environmental stresses such as eutrophication and pathogens. These associated stresses need not be large to have a synergistic effect with organic micro pollutants. The ecological effects of herbicides extend beyond individual organisms and can extend to ecosystems, affecting biodiversity.

3.3 Potential for contamination to human health

The effects of herbicides on human health generally affect the rural worker who, in some way, has exposure to these compounds. Problems are often associated with factors such as inappropriate substance use, high toxicity of certain products, lack of health and safety information, and lack of vigilance. In addition to occupational exposure, food and environmental contamination places other groups of people at risk, including families of farmers, the surrounding population of the production unit, and the general population, through the consumption of contaminated food or water. The effects of some herbicides on human health are reported in **Table 8**.

4. Some of the techniques for removal from water resources

To remove herbicides from drinking water, various strategies involving, for example, adsorption, photocatalysis, and/or advanced oxidation processes were used. Regarding adsorption, adsorbents of natural origin (for example, plant biomass) have become attractive in view of the availability of abundant supplies, high adsorption capacity, and low cost. This is a remarkable aspect, especially if the regional biomass is used. The use of agricultural residues follows well the strategies of treatment of effluents with high efficiency and economic viability; for example, Silva et al. [28] reported that dry banana peel was efficient in removing atrazine and ametryn in drinking water and rivers.

In order to mitigate pesticide leaching contamination in surface and groundwater with practices within agricultural properties, the biobed system, created in 1993 in Sweden, has been developed and studied [29]. This system consists of a tank excavated at 60 cm depth covered with impermeable material or not, containing a straw, soil, and peat biomass (50:25:25% volume), covered by a layer of grass. It is used to deposit water from the washes of the containers and sprayers, in order to retain the pesticides, promoting the sorption and biodegradation of the product by the microbial stimulus that occurs with the use of the organic materials in the soil. The substrate is used for 12 months without the need of renewal, and at the end of the use, this material should be stored in the form of composting for 6 months and later distributed in the agricultural areas. Sannino et al. [30] verified in a sorption cycle the total removal of paraquat and partial 2.4-D with the use of a polymeric substance, a polymer of humic acid recovered from the waste water of olive oil mill, presenting potential for use in biomechanics of biobeds, as well as in biofilters. However, there is a need for further research into the efficacy of other biosorbents that may assist in this system.

The use of bovine bone char (bone charcoal) is an alternative for the removal of hexazinone, diuron, ametryn, and sulfometuron methyl in drinking water [31]. In general, the authors stated that herbicide removal in contaminated drinking water samples was in the following descending order: diuron > ametryn > sulfometuron methyl > hexazinone. After 7 days of the application of the bone char treatment, no herbicide desorbed the material, remaining strongly retained. For all herbicides, the removal of about 100% was obtained with the highest dose of bone char (1 g) added to the water samples. The bovine bone char presented a great herbicide removal potential for use in contaminated drinking water. Depending on each geographical region, the water samples are contaminated with different herbicides. Thus, this bone char can be tested more specifically for each region and potentially can represent a low-cost method to be used in water treatment plants or household filters.

Hexazinone and diuron are often found as micro-contaminants of soil and water resources located near agricultural sites where they are constantly applied [32–35]. In addition, the concentrations of both herbicides found in water resources ranged from 15.0 ng L^{-1} to 408.0 μg L^{-1}.

Conventional techniques applied in water treatment systems do not exhibit great efficiency in the removal of organic micro contaminants, such as herbicides, and it is necessary to add suitable pre- or post-treatments for the removal of these undesirable compounds [36]. Due to this, currently, we are looking for technologies that are environmentally and economically feasible in the removal of these micro contaminants.

In order to obtain high quality water, membrane technologies that include reverse osmosis [37] are used. This technique is used in water desalination and demineralization [38] whose principle is to apply a force higher than the osmotic pressure in the concentrated solution compartment, causing the inversion of flow, forcing the passage of solvent, and retaining the solvent and solute [39]. Reverse osmosis has been widely applied as an important option for wastewater recovery because it can achieve high efficiency of removal of microorganisms, colloidal matter, dissolved solids, and organic and inorganic materials present in water [40].

Several technologies have been studied and developed with the aim of minimizing the impacts generated by the use of herbicides and pesticides in general in the environment. Many of the techniques are extremely costly; however, it is up to the organs and professionals of the different regions to adapt and implement them, in order to serve the population with regard to the supply of drinking water.

5. Final considerations

Highly water-soluble herbicides should be applied exclusively during the dry season so that impacts on water resources are minimized. In addition, establishing regulatory limits for the maximum amount of herbicide residues in the water is complex worldwide. First, the type of water is relevant to the proposed limit, for example, drinking water, reservoir water, lakes and streams, groundwater, aquaculture water, irrigation water, and drinking water for farm animals. A limit based on a risk to human health or the environment could allow much higher levels of herbicide residues in waters than would ever occur in practice.

Also, regarding the preservation of water resources, small actions that contribute to the noncontamination of the water, such as the proper handling of herbicide packaging and agronomic management techniques that avoid the loss of products, be it by volatilization, runoff and/or leaching, are essential. Preventing the arrival of herbicide residues from water sources reduces the need for remediation practices, which are often extremely costly and ineffective for a range of herbicides.

Author details

Kassio Ferreira Mendes*, Ana Paula Justiniano Régo, Vanessa Takeshita
and Valdemar Luiz Tornisielo
Center of Nuclear Energy in Agriculture, University of São Paulo, Brazil

*Address all correspondence to: kassio_mendes_06@hotmail.com

References

[1] Queiroz SDN, Ferracini VL, Gomes MA, Rosa MA. Comportamento do herbicida hexazinone em área de recarga do Aqüífero Guarani cultivada com cana-de-açúcar. Química Nova. 2009;**32**:378-381

[2] Flury M. Experimental evidence of transport of pesticides through field soils—A review. Journal of Environmental Quality. 1996;**25**:25-45. DOI: 10.2134/jeq1996.00472425002500010005x

[3] Monquero PA, Amaral LR, Binha DP, Silva AC, Silva PV. Potencial de lixiviação de herbicidas no solo submetidos a diferentes simulações de precipitação. Planta Daninha. 2008;**26**:403-409. DOI: 10.1590/S0100-83582008000200017

[4] Oliveira MF. Behavior of herbicides in the environment. In: Oliveira RS Jr, Constantin J, editors. Plantas Daninhas e seu Manejo. Guaíba: Agropecuária; 2001. pp. 315-362. ISBN: 85-85347-80-5

[5] Inoue MH, Santana DC, Oliveira RS Jr, Clemente RA, Dallacort R, Possamai ACS, et al. Potencial de lixiviação de herbicidas utilizados na cultura do algodão em colunas de solo. Planta Daninha. 2010;**28**:825-833. DOI: 10.1590/S0100-83582010000400016

[6] Santos EA, Correia NM, Botelho RG. Resíduos de herbicidas em corpos hídricos—Uma revisão. Revista Brasileira de Herbicidas. 2013;**12**: 188-201. DOI: 10.7824/rbh.v12i2.245

[7] SDWF—Safe Drinking Water Foundation. Pesticides and Water Pollution. 2017. Available from: https://www.safewater.org/fact-sheets-1/2017/1/23/pesticides [Accessed: 16 February 2018]

[8] Goss DW. Screening procedure for soils and pesticides for potential water quality impacts. Weed Technology. 1992;**6**:701-708. Available from: https://www.jstor.org/stable/3987238 [Accessed: 17 February 2018]

[9] Leonard LA. Movement of pesticides into surface waters. In: Cheng HH, editor. Pesticides in the Soil Environment: Processes, Impacts, and Modeling. Madison, USA: Soil Science Society of America; 1990. pp. 303-350. ISBN: 089118791X

[10] Kegley SE, Hill BR, Orme S, Choi AH. PAN-Pesticide Database. Oakland, CA: Pesticide Action Network, North America; 2016. Available from: http://www.pesticideinfo.org/ [Accessed: 01 March 2018]

[11] PPDB—Pesticide Properties DataBase. List of Pesticide Active Ingredients. University of Hertfordshire. Available from: https://sitem.herts.ac.uk/aeru/ppdb/en/atoz.htm [Accessed: 18 February 2018]

[12] Gustafson DI. Groudwater ubiquity score: A simple method for assessing pesticide leachibility. Environmental Toxicology and Chemistry. 1989;**8**: 339-357. DOI: 10.1002/etc.5620080411

[13] Widerson MR, Kim KD. The Pesticide Contamination Prevention Act: Setting Specific Numerical Values. Sacramento, USA: California Department of Food and Agriculture, Environmental Monitoring and Pest Management; 1986. DOI: 10.1.1.588.9546. 287p

[14] Lyman WJ, Reehl WF, Rosenblatt DH. Handbook of Chemical Property Estimation Methods: Environmental Behavior of Organic Compounds. New York: McGraw-Hill/American Chemical Society; 1990. DOI: 10.1002/recl.19911100212. 977p

[15] Cohen SZ, Creeger SM, Carsel RF, Enfield CG. Potential pesticide

contamination of groundwater from agricultural uses. In: Kruger RF, Seiber JN, editors. Treatment and Disposal of Pesticide Wastes. Washington, DC: American Chemistry Society; 1984. pp. 297-325. DOI: 10.1021/bk-1984-0259.ch018

[16] Rand GM, Wells PG, Mccarty LS. Introduction to aquatic toxicology. In: Rand GM, editor. Fundamentals of Aquatic Toxicology: Effects, Environmental Fate and Risk Assessment. 2nd ed. Washington, DC: Taylor Francis; 1995. pp. 3-67. ISBN: 9781560320913

[17] Kendall RJ, Anderson TA, Baker RJ, Bens CM, Carr JA, Chiodo LA, et al. In: Klaassen CD, editor. Em Casarett and Doull's Toxicology—The Basis Science of Poisons. New York: McGraw-Hill; 2001. p. 1454. ISBN: 9780071769235

[18] Ronco A, Báez MCD, Granados YP. In: Morales GC, editor. Ensayos Toxicológicos y Métodos de Evaluación de Calidad de Águas—Estandarizacíon, Intercalibración, Resultados y Aplicaciones. Ottawa: Centro Internacional de Investigaciones para El Desarrollo; 2004. ISBN: 968-5536-33-3

[19] Araújo RPA, Zagatto PA, Bertoletti E. Ecotoxicologia aquática—Princípios e aplicações. In: Avaliação da Qualidade de Sedimentos. São Carlos: RiMa; 2006. pp. 269-286

[20] Adams WJ, Rowland CD. Aquatic toxicology test methods. In: Hoffman DJ, Rattner BA, Burton GA, Cairns J, editors. Handbook of Ecotoxicology. 2nd ed. Boca Raton: Lewis Publishers; 2003

[21] Costa CR, Olivi P, Botta CMR, Espindola ELG. A toxicidade em ambientes aquáticos: Discussão e métodos de avaliação. Química Nova. 2008;**31**:1820-1830

[22] Zagatto PA, Bertoletti E. Ecotoxicologia Aquática—Princípios e Aplicações. 2nd ed. São Carlos: Editora Rima; 2008. p. 472

[23] Espíndola ELG, Neto ALO, Paschoal CMRB. Estudo de avaliação e identificação da toxicidade aquática nos efluentes hídricos da RPBC e no Rio Cubatão; Consultoria; Avaliar e identificar a toxicidade dos efluentes lançados pela Empresa PETROBRÁS no Rio Cubatão; 52; 210; Restrita; PETROBRÁS; Cubatão; BR; Impresso; 2004

[24] Health Canada. Guidelines for Canadian Drinking Water Quality. Summary Table. Ottawa, Ontario: Water and Air Quality Bureau, Healthy Environments and Consumer Safety Branch, Health Canada; 2017. Available from: https://www.canada.ca/content/dam/hc-sc/migration/hc-sc/ewh-semt/alt_formats/pdf/pubs/water-eau/sum_guide-res_recom/sum_guide-res_recom-eng.pdf [Accessed: 12 March 2018]

[25] FAO—Food and Agriculture Organization of the United Nations. Chapter 4: Natural resources management and environment department. In: Pesticides as Water Pollutants. Rome: FAO; 1996. Available from: http:// www.fao.org/docrep/w2598e/w2598e07.htm#TopOfPage [Accessed: 18 February 2018]

[26] Melo IS, Azevedo JL. Microbiologia Ambiental. Jaguariúna: Embrapa; 1997. 438p

[27] Christoffoleti PJ, López-Ovejero RF. Comportamento dos Herbicidas Aplicados ao Solo na Cultura da Cana-de-Açúcar. 2008. 90p. Available from: https://edisciplinas.usp.br/pluginfile.php/3825040/mod_resource/content/1/Livro%20Herbicidas%20no%20Solo.pdf [Accessed: 18 February 2018]

[28] Silva CR, Gomes TF, Andrade GCRM, Monteiro SH, Dias ACR, Zagatto EAG, et al. Banana peel as an adsorbent for removing atrazine and ametryne from waters. Journal of Agricultural and Food Chemistry. 2013;**61**:2358-2363. DOI: 10.1021/jf304742h

[29] Castillo MDP, Torstensson L, Stenström J. Biobeds for environmental protection from pesticide use—A review. Journal of Agricultural and Food Chemistry. 2008;**56**:6206-6219. DOI: 10.1021/jf800844x

[30] Sannino F, Lorio M, Martino A, Pucci M, Brown CD, Capasso R. Remediation of waters contaminated with ionic herbicides by sorption on polymerin. Water Research. 2008;**42**:643-652. DOI: 10.1016/j.watres.2007.08.015

[31] Mendes KF, Freguglia RMO, Martins BAB, Dias RC, Pimpinato RF, Tornisielo VL. Cow bonechar for pesticide removal from drinking water. Scholars Journal of Agriculture and Veterinary Sciences. 2017;**4**:504-512. DOI: 10.21276/sjavs.2017.4.11.11

[32] Davis A, Lewis S, Bainbridge Z, Brodie J, Shannon E. Pesticide residues in waterways of the lower Burdekin region: Challenges in ecotoxicological interpretation of monitoring data. Australasian Journal of Ecotoxicology. 2008;**14**:89-108. Available from: http://www.leusch.info/ecotox/aje/archives/vol14p89.pdf [Accessed: 05 March 2018]

[33] Pascholato CFPR, Dantas AB, Rosa IDA, Faleiros RJR, Bernardo L. Uso de carvão ativado para remoção dos herbicidas diuron e hexazinone de água. Revista DAE. 2009;**179**:34-41. DOI: 10.4322/dae.2014.026

[34] Ferreira LR, Ferreira FA, Machado AFL. Tecnologia de aplicação de herbicidas. In: Silva AA, Silva JF, editors. Tópicos em Manejo de Plantas Daninhas. Viçosa: Universidade Federal de Viçosa; 2007. pp. 326-367. ISBN: 9788572692755

[35] Metcalfe CD, Sultana T, Li H, Helm PA. Current-use pesticides in urban watersheds and receiving waters of western Lake Ontario measured using polar organic chemical integrative samplers (POCIS). Journal of Great Lakes Research. 2016;**42**:1432-1442. DOI: 10.1016/j.jglr.2016.08.004

[36] Voltan PEN, Dantas AB Paschoalato CFR, Bernardo L. Predição da performance de carvão ativado granular para remoção de herbicidas com ensaios em coluna de escala reduzida. Engenharia Sanitária e Ambiental. 2016;**21**:241-250. DOI: 10.1590/S1413-41522016138649

[37] ANA—Agency National Water. Quality Indicators—Water Quality Index (IQA). 2007. Available from: http://portalpnqa.ana.gov.br/indicadores-indice-aguas.aspx [Accessed: 18 February 2018]

[38] Bitaw TN, Park K, Yang DR. Optimization on a new hybrid forward osmosis-electrodialysis-reverse osmosis seawater desalination process. Desalination. 2016;**398**:265-281. DOI: 10.1016/j.desal.2016.07.032

[39] Gouvêa CAK, Hurtado ALB, Borzio RF, Folletto MA. Use of water processed by reverse osmosis for vapor generation in tobacco industry. Revista Científica Eletrônica de Engenharia de Produção Online. 2012;**12**:522-536. ISSN: 1676-1901

[40] Tang F, Hu HH, Sun LJ, Sun YX, Shi N, Crittenden JC. Fouling characteristics of reverse osmosis membranes at different positions of a full-scale plant for municipal wastewater reclamation. Water Research. 2016;**90**:329-336. DOI: 10.1016/j.watres.2015.12.028

Chapter 4

Challenges for Assessing Toxicity of Nanomaterials

Akanksha Gupta, Sanjay Kumar and Vinod Kumar

Abstract

On the development of nano-world, nanotechnology provides enormous opportunities in daily routine products and further future sustainable innovations. The nanotechnology extends its benefits to various fields such as engineering, medical, biological, environmental, and communication. However, the exponential growth of nanomaterials production would lead to severe complications related to their hazardous effects to the human health and environment. Moreover, negative impact of nanomaterials toxicity on human health is one of the significant issues on exhausting nano-products. The most vulnerable situation is associated with the use of nanomaterials in the biomedical application. The several efforts have been ongoing to study the nanotoxicity and its interaction with the biomolecules. Nevertheless, it is hard to assess and validate the nanotoxicity in a biological system. This chapter aims to study the challenges in determining the toxicity of nanomaterials. The toxicity assessment and hurdles in determining the impact on biological systems are epoch making. *In-vitro*, *in-vivo*, and *in-silico* studies are summarized in this chapter in assessing the toxicity of engineered nanomaterials. The different approaches of toxicity assessment have their difficulties faced by researchers while characterizing nanomaterials in powder form, solution-based, and interacting with biological systems. The assessment tools and characterization techniques play a vital role in overcoming the challenges, while the cytotoxic assays involve nanoparticle shape, morphology, and size consideration.

Keywords: nanotechnology, nanoparticles, characterization, *in-vitro*, *in-vivo*, *in-silico*

1. Introduction

In today's high-tech world, nanotechnology has become so much popular in various fields due to its unique and beneficial physicochemical properties [1]. Some of the essential applications in multiple areas have been mentioned in **Table 1**. Bringing the materials to nanoscale level helps in improving mechanical, optical and electrical properties. It can be explained due to the increase in surface area to volume ratio and hence, surface-related properties become more significant.

The small size and higher specific surface area of NMs furnishes the distinctive properties and leads to unpredicted biological response on interaction with biological system. Further, they also impart different biokinetic behavior and capabilities to reach farther in body as compared with their larger counterparts.

Applications	Usage	Ref.
Nanomedicine	Fluorescence and multiphoton bioimaging, *in vitro* diagnostics, *in vivo* fluorescence imaging, drug delivery, photodynamic therapy, Photothermal-controlled drug delivery and cancer treatment, drug release, bioimaging, Tissue engineering, gene therapy, regenerative medicine, MRI, magnetically guided control drug delivery, magnetic biosensing, Drug release and gene delivery, gene material and vaccines	[2]
Health sector	Therapeutic targets in chemotherapy; bio-nanosensors; nanocoatings; nanocarrier for vaccination; antimicrobial activities; nanophotothermolysis for cancer, nanofilter, cosmetic products,	[3–6]
Food and agriculture	Nanofertilizers, nanofungicides, nanopesticides, engineered nanomaterials, CNT (carbon nanotube), nanoporous membrane, food-based nanodelivery vehicles, food storage and packaging, functional foods, bio-actives, nutraceutical systems, and pharma foods	[7–11]
Energy and environment	Wastewater treatment, adsorption and degradation of organic/inorganic pollutant, nanofilters/membranes, Solar energy, energy storage, H_2 generation, Li-ion battery	[12–20]
Defense and security	Smart materials, fuel additives, modern weapon, nanocoatings, nanocomposites, night vision camera, sensors and electronics, and energy devices, robotics	[21–24]
Automobile	Nanomaterials in paints, nanocoatings, catalyst as additives, nano-based lubricants, fuel cells, composite fillers, smart lights	[25–27]
Building	Pigment in Interior and exterior paints, as a thin film on glass windows, photocatalyst, adsorbent, as a membrane, hydrophilicity, climate control, sensors, Rheological behavior under uniaxial extensional flow, improved mechanical properties, fire retardant and insulation, cement composite	[28]
Electronics device	LED, OLED, nanotransitor, nano-based memory device, opto-magnetic, spintronics, electrochromic device, nanogenerator	[29–31]
Textiles	Smart fibers, stain repellence, wrinkle-freeness, nanocoatings, high absorbency, softness and breathability, military applications	[32, 33]
Sports	Nanofibers, ball coatings, CNT based sports items	[34, 35]

Table 1.
List of numerous applications of nanomaterials in different area.

With the increasing use and production of nanomaterials (NMs), occupational exposure is also growing. Other concern is related to environment and ecosystem disturbance. Some of these apprehensions have forced scientist to investigate and understand the potential adverse effects of engineered nanomaterials on health and environment and also, explore the challenges to assess the toxicity of these materials. Several reports on toxicity assessment of NMs published in the last few decades. However, still it is a challenging task to investigate the interactions of nanoparticles (NPs) with biological systems. One of the probable reasons could be due to experimental methods and precise characterization involving toxicological assessment of NMs. Although, human health is at considerable risk because of toxicity of these nanotechnology-based goods on exposure/intake by several routes (**Figure 1** and **Table 2**) [36].

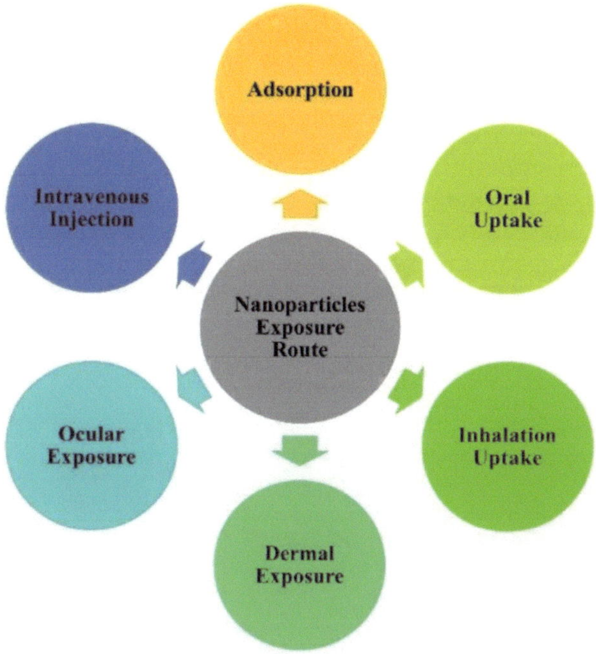

Figure 1.
Exposure pathways of nanoparticles.

Nanomaterials	Possible risks
Carbon, silver and gold NPs	Affect the central nervous system, respiratory toxicity, liver toxicity
Carbon NPs	Pulmonary inflammation, granulomas, and fibrosis, inhibition of DNA enzymes, enhanced cytotoxicity, pulmonary toxicity
Cd-based compounds	Nephrotoxic potential, cell and DNA damage, lungs and liver toxicity, fetus malformation, hampered growth, enhanced cytotoxicity
CuO NPs	Suppress immune system, cell and DNA damage, toxic to aquatic organisms
Ceria NPs	Reactive Oxygen Species (ROS) production, decreased lifespan, cell membrane and DNA damage, lipid peroxidation
TiO_2 NPs	Genotoxicity, metabolic change, neurotoxicity, skin penetration, cell damage, ROS production, reproductive toxicity
ZnO NPs	Hepatic oxidative stress, severe liver damage, reproductive toxicity on earthworms
QDs (Quantum Dots)	Lung infection and inflammation, fetus malformation, hampered growth, sperm count and quality decreases, cell damage
SiO_2 NPs	Chronic obstructive pulmonary disease, tuberculosis. Lipid peroxidation and membrane damage, mitochondrial dysfunction, lung cancer, cell death (necrosis)
Nano-MOFs	Reproductive and respiratory toxicity, immunotoxicity, neurotoxicity, carcinogenicity

Table 2.
List of nanoparticles causes possible toxicity to the human body [2].

2. Challenges in characterization

To study the toxicity of any chemical substances, characterization of materials plays a significant role. There are several techniques available these days which can be used to characterize nanomaterials in powder form, film as well as in solution and further its interaction with biomolecules can be studied (**Figure 2**). Although, it becomes much more imperative and extensive in case of nanomaterials due to the different shapes and sizes with variable surface area, charge and chemistry, crystallinity, porosity, agglomeration, solubility, etc., (**Figure 3**). Further, the nanomaterials generated from experiments must ensure reproducibility of

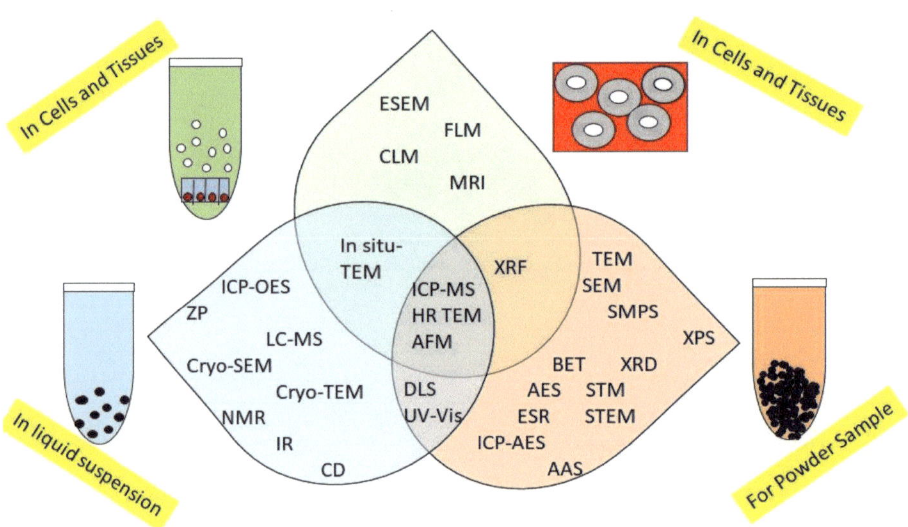

Figure 2.
Characterization of nanoparticles in different media [37].

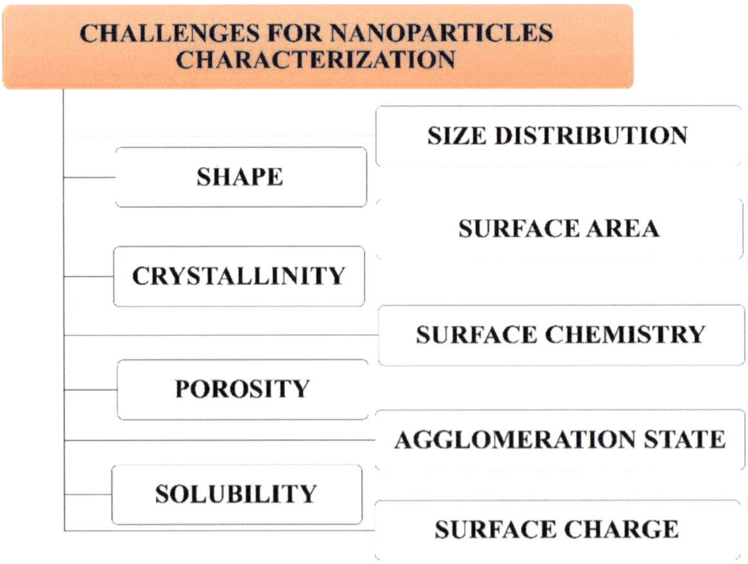

Figure 3.
Challenges of characterization of nanoparticles.

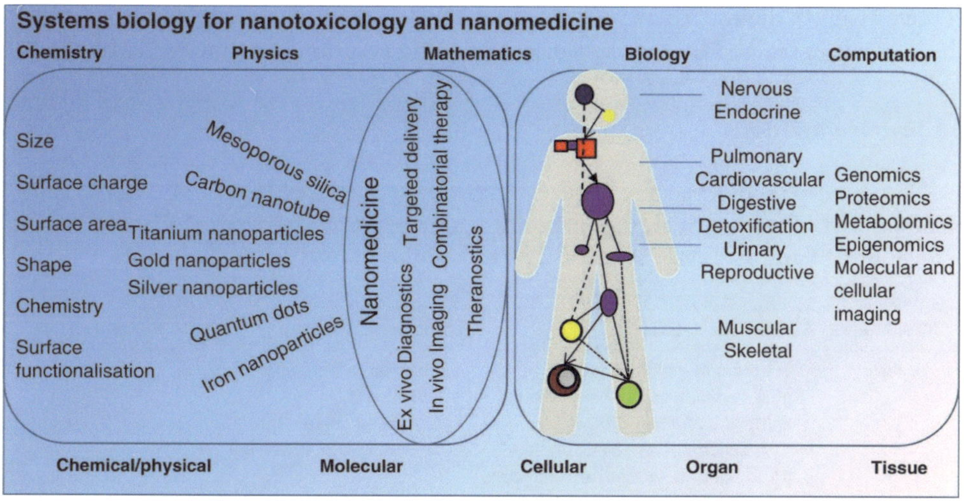

Figure 4.
Safe application of nanomaterials in therapeutics requires a deeper understanding of the material properties and behaviors at different levels of biological organization; increasing insight necessitates cross-disciplinary research collaborations (©2017 her majesty the queen in right of Canada. WIREs Nanomedicine and Nanobiotechnology published by Wiley periodicals, Inc.) [38].

nanomaterials and thus higher reliability of the results. Characterization of nanomaterials requires highly sophisticated instruments and skilled human resources to study them. The precise properties of nanoparticles and their toxicity details are poorly understood. Thus, a more wide-ranging and comprehensive characterization, including size distribution, shape, surface area, surface chemistry, crystallinity, porosity, agglomeration state, surface charge, solubility, etc., is suggested for nanomaterials in order to determine the perfect connection between their physicochemical properties and the biological effects they produce [37]. However, due to limited facilities in lab, scientists are bound to utilize the techniques available to them. Therefore, characterization techniques plays crucial role in experimental findings of nanomaterials.

On account of toxicity assessment, size is one of the crucial factors which alter the functionality of nanomaterial along with diversified interaction with living system. Size of nanoparticles can be determined by several techniques such as Brunauer–Emmett–Teller (BET), dynamic light scattering (DLS) and transmission electron microscopy (TEM). Nevertheless, further challenge is to find out accurate average sizes and size distribution which are in fact different provided by different methods. It is due to different principles involved in the several techniques. Additionally, measurement differences can also be explained based on sample preparation methods and instrument functioning procedures. However, this may generate misperception to find out the correct nanoparticle size and size distribution; therefore, one has to be well competent in the principles and technical details of the measurement methods involved. However, a deep understanding needed of NMs toxicity and their interactions with biological system **Figure 4**.

3. Assessment of nanomaterial toxicity via *in-vivo, in-vitro*, and *in-silico* approaches

The route followed by nanomaterials inside the organisms and their persistence as well as their assimilation pathways determined with a deeper understanding of the nature and interactions of NPs. There are numerous pathways to find out NPs route as well as their affirmative parameters inside the body of organisms. Broadly, these analyses framed under *in-vivo, in-vitro*, and *in-silico* assessment (**Table 3**).

3.1 *In-vitro* methods

The *in-vitro* techniques for toxicity assessment are considered to be the most reliable, cost-effective, wider applicability, a broad range of accessibility, and more ethical due to animal fewer studies. The techniques based on the principle of

Technique	Assessment details	Instrumentation	References
In-vitro	• Selection of cell lines such as phagocytes, hepatic, hematologic, epithelial, and tumorous, etc. • Cytotoxicity assays based on ROS production, detection, and effector, etc. • Cell viability assays • Cell stress assays such as gene expression, an inflammatory marker, cell visualization, etc. • Disadvantages like lack of secondary inferences of NMs and unrevealed physiological pathways.	• Electron microscopy (SEM, TEM, etc.) • Optical spectroscopy • Dynamic light scattering	[39–43]
In-vivo	• Intracellular behavior of NMs is different and may affect various organs which mainly include: hematological toxicity, nephrotoxicity, hepatotoxicity, pulmonary toxicity, and splenic toxicity. • Studies crucially dependent upon size, surface charge, surface coating, and shape of nanoparticles. • Model living animals such as mice, zebrafish, rodents, and non-human primates • Disadvantages include non-ethical nature and a more extended assessment period	• Electron and optical microscopy • Magnetic resonance imaging • Atomic force microscopy	[41, 44–47]
In-silico	• Computational simulation and assessment of the relationship between physicochemical properties and nanotoxicity • Models illustrating nano-bio interfaces • Hazard control and risk assessment of NMs. • Development of High throughput screening (HTS) data and Quantitative structure–activity relationship (QSAR) models. • Generated data set depend upon reliable experimental toxicity results obtained through in vitro and in vivo studies.	• Theoretical calculations and computational simulations are needed to generate reliable data sets for comparative studies	[48–52]

Table 3.
Summarizes the assessment of nanomaterial toxicity via three different approaches in-vivo, in-vitro *and* in-silico.

mimicking cellular components and predicting results concerning the body of an organism [53]. The reviews are extremely helpful in regulating the dosage limits and fate of xenobiotic exposed. The different cell lines in a suitable environment exposed to nanomaterials and after incubation, the proliferation and metabolism of an exposed component are assessed with the help of different assays [54, 55]. However, physiological outcomes and prediction of results of xenobiotics are very critical. Still, primary assessment follows *in-vitro* procedures because of minor hurdles and easy availability.

Fast and comprehensive detection using in vitro technique (**Figure 5**) is proved to be the most widely accepted methodologies and various assays used in cytotoxicity investigation. The assays are different only in their mechanism of cell death and detection methodology [53, 57].

3.2 Common assays for *in-vitro* toxicity assessment

3.2.1 MTT assay

Viable and non-viable cells due to their metabolic activities releases enzymes which can further form complexes with dye molecules are the basis of colorimetric determination of cytotoxicity caused by nanoparticles [58]. The cytotoxicity assessment by analyzing the mitochondrial activity performed using MTT assay. MTT is (3-[4,5-dimethylthiazol-2-yl]-2,5-diphenyltetrazolium) cation (MTT+) an useful redox indicator in pharmacology [59]. The colorimetric assay based on metabolic activities of viable cells [60]. Along with mitochondrial activity, MTT assay also applicable to non-mitochondrial enzymes and endosomes, etc. The MTT tetrazolium salt crosses the membrane of active cells and reduces to formazan (1-[4,5-dimethylthiazol-2-yl]-3,5-diphenylformazan) which is a purple-colored product. The colored solution further analyzed with the help of spectrophotometry.

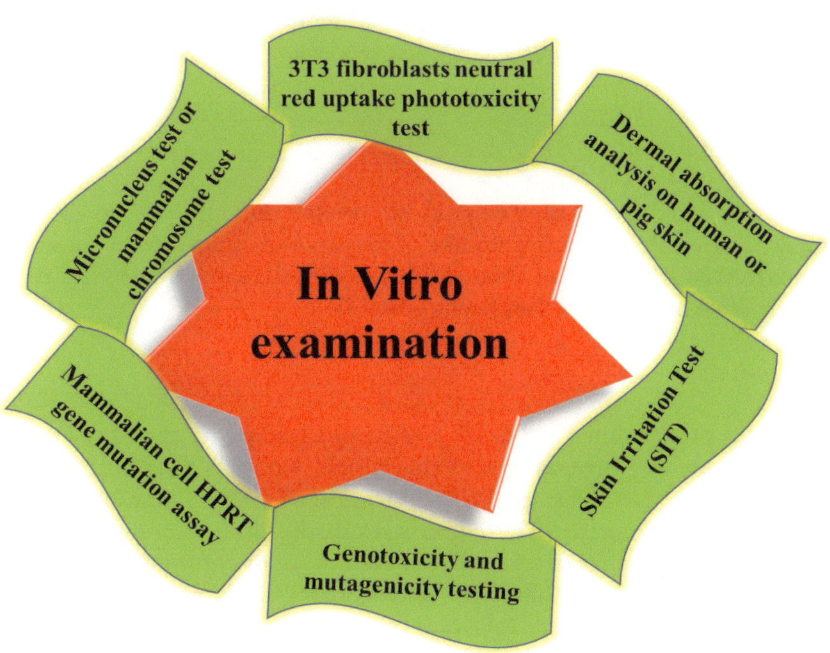

Figure 5.
Validated in-vitro *techniques used [56].*

The color intensity is proportional to the concentration of living cells; hence, the quantitative determination of viable cells can be completed with the help of this assay [61]. Further modification of this test leads to formation of tetrazolium derivatives such as 3-(4,5-dimethyl-2-thiazolyl)-2,5-diphenyl-2H-tetrazolium bromide (MTT), salt (WST-1), 2-(2-methoxy-4-nitrophenyl)-3-(4-nitrophenyl)-5-(2,4-disulfophenyl)-2H-tetrazolium, monosodium salt (WST-8) which form water-soluble formazan while interacting with cells [62–64]. However, the reports show some unmatched results such as more viable cell count even at high exposure of toxic nanomaterials. Braun et al. [61] reported the overestimation of cytotoxicity at a moderate concentration of mesoporous silica nanoparticles with MTT assay when compared with ATP based assay.

3.2.2 LDH leakage assay

Lactate dehydrogenase (LDH) is a cytosolic enzyme present in all living cells. When a breakdown of the cellular membrane occurs due to nanoparticle toxicity, LDH oozes out to extracellular space where it can indicate the cytotoxicity. The free LDH in extracellular space catalyzes the interconversion of pyruvate to lactase and β-nicotinamide adenine dinucleotide (NADH) to NAD^+. Since NADH has absorbance at 340 nm, the concentration of LDH level can be determined by decreased concentration of known initial concentration of NADH and lactate [65]. Also, enzyme diaphorase utilizes NADH and H^+ for catalyzing the reductive conversion of tetrazolium salt to a highly colored formazan salt which can be measured spectrophotometrically. Wang et al. [66] reported the LDH assay for cytotoxicity determination of single-walled carbon nanotubes (SWCNTs) and oxidized SWCNTs. The formazan concentration decreases with increasing concentration of SWCNTs elucidated from spectrophotometric determination, where absorbance at 490 nm. Each cell type has specific LDH pool and passage; therefore, test measurements were first standardized with purified LDH and then LDH derived from lysed DH-82 cells were tested. Nanoparticle toxicity can affect the activity of LDH by dynamic adsorption of LDH on nanoparticle surface leading to inactivation. Also, NPs can generate free radicals or metal catalyzed oxidation processes for inactivation of LDH.

3.2.3 Trypan blue dye +assay

Trypan is an azo dye and used to stain non-viable cells and used in the cytotoxic assessment. The viable cell resists uptake of trypan and cytoplasm of these cells remain unaffected while trypan treated non-viable cells show blue cytoplasm and colorimetric determination of these cells possible.

3.2.4 Apoptosis assay

Apoptosis is programmed cell death and categorized under type-I cell death. The cell death controlled by various type of cell signals, where, a sudden stop of these signals triggers cell death. The apoptosis activation starts the initiation of extracellular proteases called caspases. These proteases further initiate activities leading to cell death. Apoptosis is characterized by condensation of chromatin and nucleus as well as DNA fragmentation. There are various assays for determining apoptosis such as TUNEL, Lamina-B, and, Apostain techniques. TUNEL is terminal deoxynucleotidyl transferase dUTP nick end labeling technique which detects the fragments of DNA which produce in the final step of apoptosis. Mechanism of the TUNEL technique involves the fluorescent dye coupling with dUTP nucleotide present in assay, which further fastens with fragmented DNA. The quantitative analysis with the help of fluorescent microscopy or immunohistochemical staining can be done. Despite being a cost-effective and smooth operation of this technique, this technique does not distinguish necrosis and apoptosis while observing only the end stage result of the process. Apostain technique is associated with early detection of caspase-3 in the cytoplasm and does not rely on fragments of DNA. Hence, this technique is useful in early detection where activation of apoptosis and release of specific protease lead to brown coloration, and healthy cells remain blue when observed under the light microscope. This technique is particular, sensitive, and remains one of the most used methods in apoptosis analysis. Unlike apostain, Lamina-B is also an early-stage assessment technique. The nuclear lamina is the structures responsible for DNA replication, even for the reorganization of chromatin, and present in nuclear membrane. This lamina is of two type lemin-A (acidic or neutral) and lemin-B (neutral). The release of caspase −6 during apoptosis leads to lemin cleavage, which further triggers the chromatin condensation. Immunohistochemistry antigens markers are used to identify lemin-B.

3.2.5 2′, 7′-dichlorofluorescein diacetate (DCFH-DA) assay

Reactive oxidative species (ROS)induces the oxidative stress to the living cells due to internalization. The Injured cells membrane is porous for entry of non-polar dye 2,7-dichlorofluorescin diacetate (DCFH-DA) and converts into non-fluorescent DCFH due to hydrolyzation of intracellular esterase. The DCFH oxidized to fluorescent dichlorofluorescein in the presence of ROS. Thus, the quantification of ROS can be measured with fluorescence intensity measurements.

3.2.6 Comet assay

This assay named after its visual appearance, which looks like a comet, consist of single-cell gel electrophoresis technique (SCGE). This assay is widely used in vitro analysis technique, which is most reliable and inexpensive. The DNA damage during nanoparticle toxicity analyzed in this technique, whereas negatively charged DNA fragments separated using gel electrophoresis. Cells with toxicity encapsulated in agarose gel further lysed with salts and detergents which digest cytoplasm and other cell components except for nucleoids. Further electrophoresis at high pH results into a comet-like structure where the head of the comet represents intact DNA and tail comprises of the fragmented portion. Hence, the fluorescent marking and intensity of the tail show the damaged part of DNA leading to the estimation of toxicity.

3.3 *In-vivo* methods

These methods retain their most favorable and primary standards for assessment of toxicity. These studies based on the use of living animal, which is considered a little less ethical. The mode of in vivo studies involves the administration of nanomaterial into the body of testing animal and monitoring the signs of progress through different techniques. Since this procedure requires real-time analysis, and result obtained are more coherent with human body functioning, minimizing the impact of time and cost.

The *in-vivo* results for toxicity assessment are different from in vitro counterparts because of various crucial factors, which cannot involve in *in-vitro* assessment. The impact of hormonal changes, cell–cell and cell-matrix interactions add on *in-vivo* assessment. The long-term chronic effects are not possible *in-vitro* studies; hence, some impacts are missing during *in-vitro* analysis. The in vivo studies, however, carried out with more considerable precautions because they are interlaced with many challenges. *In-vivo* dose is determined based on actual exposure of nanomaterial to the body, which is a technical challenge because of minimal size and peculiar properties in the biological system. During *in-vivo* experiments, the vehicle to carry out nanoparticle dose must be non-reactive, and NPs must disperse appropriately in it. Since NPs are very susceptible to agglomeration due to their larger surface area. Agglomeration and poor dispersion lead to improper biological distribution and unwanted results. Once the nanomaterial inside the body, they can interact with protein counterpart leading to the formation of the protein corona. These lead to alteration in the properties of NPs, their interaction, and biodistribution. Protein structure further undergoes conformational changes and leads to modified biological functions as well as altered signaling pathways. Hence before assessing the toxicity of NPs in a biological system, one must also consider the various interferences of NPs with another substrate [67].

Chen et al. [68] investigated gold nanoparticles (AuNPs) of size 21 nm on male C57BL/6 mice by collecting the tissues after 1, 24, and 72 h post injecting the 7.85 μg AuNPs/g solution of AuNPs. Further analysis was done using Scanning Electron Microscopy (SEM) and proinflammatory cytokine expression, as well as macrophage counting, was done with real-time PCR. The results show the compatible nature of AuNPs with living tissues and not observed a significant change in the number of macrophages. However, the reported results show an accumulation of AuNPs in abdominal fat, and some quantity also found in the liver, leading to a reduction of fat in AuNPs treated mice. Rizzo et al. [69] used zebrafish embryo for correlating the results obtained from in vitro analysis with in vivo studies. Authors used different NMs for toxicity assessment both in vitro assays. The coating on nanomaterials with biocompatible polymers shows a significant decrease in the toxicity. The results for pristine ultra-small superparamagnetic iron oxide (USPIO) and flavin mononucleotide coated USPIO (FLUSPIO) and sineram tested in vitro on HeLa (human cervical carcinoma), HUVEC (human umbilical vein endothelial) and SMC (ovine smooth muscle) and in vivo studies carried out on zebrafish embryo assay. The in vitro studies do not show any cytotoxic effect on different cell lines up to concentration 10 mg/mL, on the other hand in vivo studies for toxicity analysis on zebrafish embryo assay show different results as compare with in vivo. The similar dose of NP causes lethal effect on embryo. The toxicity of pristine USPIO greater than coated counterparts, FLUSPIO and sineram. Even the lethal effect not observed for coated nanoparticles at high exposure time up to 72 and 168 h. The probable reason for cytotoxic effects given by authors was aggregation of uncoated nanoparticles and further due to larger hydrodynamic size lead to blockage of egg chorion pores [70]. In another study based on zebrafish embryo shows stage-dependent toxicity and specific phenotype with AgNPs (97 ± 13 nm). Different developmental stages of embryos have different critical concentration of nanoparticles such as Cleavage stage (3.5pM), Gastrula stage (4pM), Segmentation stage (6pM), Hatching stage (8pM) [71]. The maximum number of abnormalities found in deformed zebrafish developed from cleavage and gastrula stage of embryos. However, the later stages do not show significant deformities. The early-stage embryos show head and eyes deformities which are not present in later-stage embryos. The cleavage stage and gastrula stage abnormalities are more prominent and also increases with increase in concentration of AgNPs owing to their impact on early determinative events like cell signaling and gene transcription. The AgNPs stays inside embryos throughout their development. The longitudinal thin layer sections with all deformities shown in **Figure 6**. The observed NPs found embedded in eye, pericardial space, and in tail which are characterized by LSPR spectra of individual AgNPs.

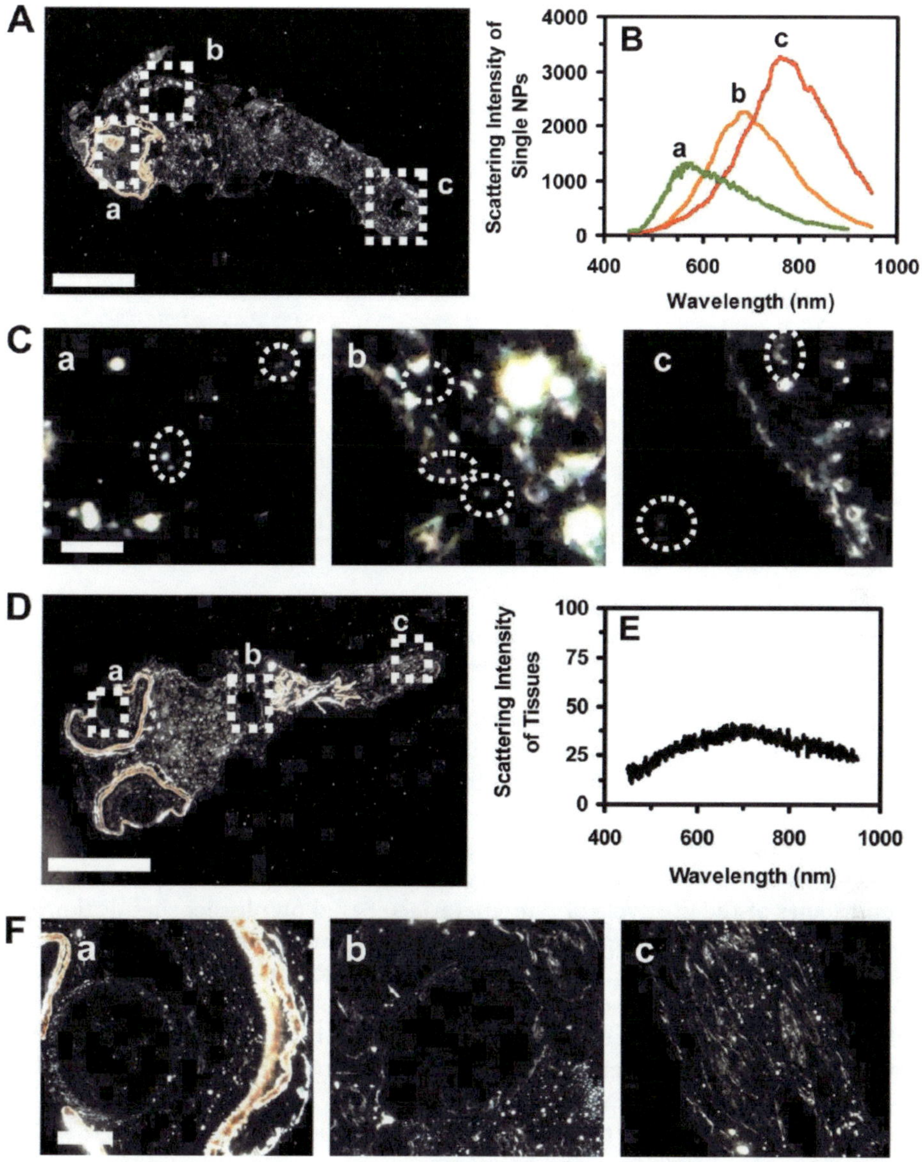

Figure 6.
Imaging and characterization of individual Ag NPs embedded in the tissues of (a − C) deformed zebrafish and (D − F) normal zebrafish (control) using DFOMS-MSIS. Optical image of thin-layer longitudinal section of fixed (a) deformed zebrafish with five types of deformities and (D) normal zebrafish. (C) and (F) zoom-in optical images of the tissue sections of (a − c) as highlighted in (a) and (D), respectively: (a) eye (retina), (b) pericardial space, and (c) tail. (B) LSPR spectra of individual Ag NPs as circled in (C) show distinctive λ_{max} (fwhm): (a) 567 (176), (b) 688 (185), and (c) 759 (179) nm. (E) Scattering intensity of the tissues of normal zebrafish in (F) shows the background (nondistinctive plasmonic colors). Scale bars in (a) and (D) are 250 μm and in (C) and (F) are 5 and 30 μm, respectively. "Reprinted with permission from [71] (2013) American Chemical Society.

3.4 *In-silico* assay

Considering the time requirement, ethical standards, and reliable results, scientist prompted to use alternative ways for analyzing the toxicity of materials. The *in-silico* analysis one of the novel approaches as compared with general studies. The procedure is based on the principle of theoretical modeling and simulation of results for various physicochemical properties of molecules (**Figure 7**). The available data

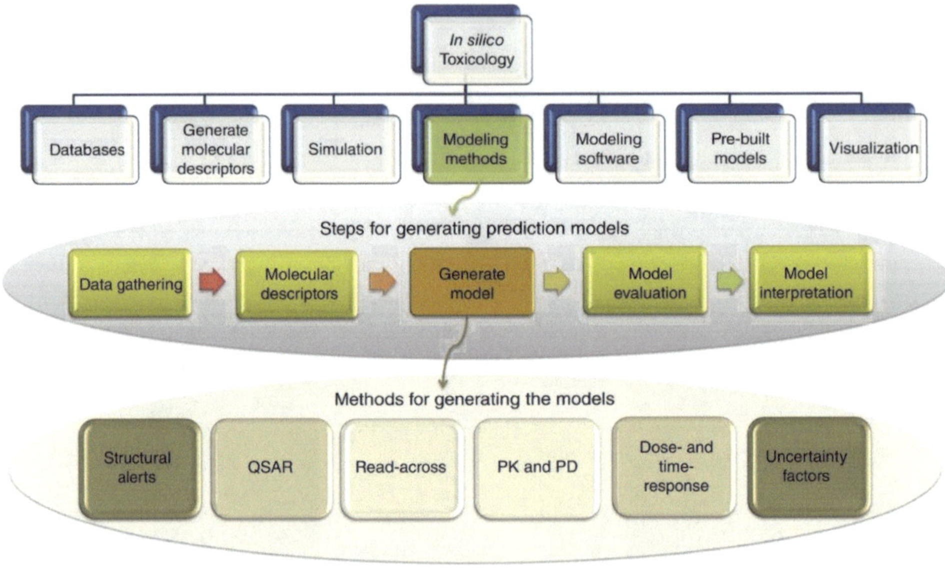

Figure 7.
In-silico *toxicology tools, steps to generate prediction models, and categories of prediction models (copyright © 2016 the authors. WIREs computational molecular science published by John Wiley & Sons, Ltd. [73]).*

of toxicity of material and their interpolation using multiple mathematical models, in silico studies owes many advantages still there are limitations because experimental verification needed additionally to prove the toxicological effects. Also, due to the data gap, the quantitative risk assessment of nanomaterials on web-based tools has not much explored. Current methodologies based on exposure assessment in production and manufacturing life stages while ignoring the exposure during use and end stages of the life cycle of nanomaterials. Based on physicochemical properties and their descriptions, computational chemistry methods has been modified to nano-based models such as nano quantitative structure–activity relationship (nano-QSAR) or quantitative nanostructure activity relationship (QNAR) [73].

In-silico methodology selects the models that have historical development or represent state-of-the-art methods for assessment of toxicity. Structural alerts and rule-based models are used for evaluation of toxicity. The structural alerts are chemical structures representing the toxicity while rule-based models are derived either from human knowledge and literature (Human-based Rules) or from computational simulations of data (Induction-based Rules), which rely on probabilities [72, 74].

Two European projects named GUIDEnano tools and SUN Decision Support System (SUNDS) provides valuable information about the implementation of tools for assessment of nano-enabled products in their whole life cycle [75, 76]. These web-based tools create a sustainable portfolio for production, handling, and end cycles of engineered nanomaterials. It also needs the exploited data about physicochemical, toxicological, and exposure of nanomaterials. Life cycle analysis approach critically required for assessing the impact of nanomaterials on the environment. The collection of data, transfer, and transformations of nanomaterials, Leading to toxicological effects to humans and environment can be predicted through risk assessment tools.

The above-discussed assays, however, experience production of erroneous results due to interference arising due to NPs solubility, agglomeration, particle sedimentation, and, the formation of the protein corona. The problem can be appropriately acknowledged by designing and establishing a standard set of essays which need to be following particular nanotoxicological standards and uniform applicability. The generation of standardized protocol further faces the challenge of different nature of nanomaterials to be assessed since metallic NPs, and carbon-based nanotubes have different physicochemical characteristics in physiological conditions. The metallic NPs and CNTs show different physical traits at nano-cellular interface leading to altering the biological response. CNTs and metallic NPs both produce ROS species but follows different pathways where metal NMs causes apoptosis, while CNT leads to fibrosis and inflammation [77]. CNTs and metallic NPs are also different in their assimilation pathways in the biological system. CNTs found to be less biodegradable and persisting in system for a longer duration while, metallic NPs undergo dissolution into ions further disrupting the biological pathways [78, 79].

3.5 Physicochemical parameters for toxicity assessment

Cellular responses are directly linked to physicochemical parameters of nanomaterials. The advancement in material science has achieved a precise synthesis of nanomaterials with adjustable target and specific action. There are various morphological factors on which nanotoxicological response depend such as size, surface morphology, charge and, composition, etc.

3.5.1 Size of NMs

Size of the NMs are a primary factor for determination of cytotoxic response. It affects the internalization process into cells and endocytosis process, which ultimately altering the intracellular fate of nanomaterials. Most of the studies conclude that smaller the size of NPs, higher the degree of cytotoxicity [80, 81]. Bharadwaj et al. [82] reported the assessment of variable sized nanoparticles ranging from 20 to 500 nm in processed brain tissue sections with the help of confocal microscopy. Maximum accumulation was observed for 1 hour and it was found that 500 nm particles accumulated the most. However, NPs shows selective accumulation behavior. In the case of quantum dots (QDs), the cytotoxicity and size depend upon the method of preparation. QDs produced by using ligands like trioctylphosphine lead to hydrophobic nature and further converted to hydrophilic, leading to an increase in hydrodynamic radius of NMs [83].

3.5.2 Surface

Cellular uptake mechanism and cytotoxicity relies on the morphology of NPs. NMs have different kind of shapes, which includes spheres, needles, cubes, tubes, rods, etc. Membrane interactions during internalization of NPs affect the nature of barriers. Researchers reported the formation of pores in cell membranes due to interactions of NPs, leading to an imbalance in an ionic concentration outside and inside of the cell [84]. Chithrani et al. [85] reported the effect of size and shape of AuNPs in internalization and concluded that when morphology changes from rod shape to spherical, there is an increase in uptake up to 500%. Recently, Maysinger et al. [86] also studied the gold nanourchins whose surface morphology has an irregular shape. The functionalization with polyethylene glycol (PEG) on AuNPs did not show any significant alteration in viability and morphology while cetyltrimethylammonium bromide (CTAB) modification showed adverse effects on filamentous actin and, nuclear lamina.

3.5.3 Surface coating and charge on NMs

Surface coating on the nanoparticles surface act as a connecting link between nano-cellular interfaces. Coating affects the interparticle interactions, cellular contacts, internalization, and cytotoxicity of material [87]. Surface coating possesses distinct charges which can alter the cytotoxicity of materials. Various studies show that positively charged NMs internalized more effectively and also result in more toxic effects than neutral or with negatively charged particles [88, 89]. Coatings broadly divided based on interactions into three types by Richards et al. [90]. These are covalent coatings having covalent bonding, the electrostatic surface coating having electrostatic interactions, and atomic layer deposition where chemical bond formed between molecule and coating material. Coating plays a crucial role in various nanomaterial application in drug delivery, imaging, and cancer treatment [91, 92]. Coating of chitosan reduces the production of ROS species in different CuNPs and Fe_2O_3 NPs and reduces the inflammatory response and overall toxicity of nanomaterials [93, 94]. Yin et al. [95] studied nickel ferrite NPs and explained their toxicity through their surface coating with oleic acid. The toxicity with coated nickel ferrite NPs depends upon the dose of material. The coating also shows significant effects when changed from single layer to double layer by changing hydrophobic and hydrophilic, respectively. It was observed that hydrophobic coating impart a high level of toxicity than the hydrophilic counterpart. Nanomaterials are internalized through lipid bilayer membrane structure where the charge on the membrane is negative. Hence, opposite charged NPs pass through effectively due to electrostatic interactions while negatively charged bound less efficiently. The acid treatment of carbon nanotubes (CNTs) leads to high toxicity due to surface functionalization. The negative charge introduced due to hydroxyl (—OH) and carboxylic acid (—COOH) contribute to more toxicity [96].

4. Future prospective and conclusion remarks

Nanotechnology exhibit excellent potential in developing new materials every day; hence, nanomaterial safety also deserves much attention for their safer use. Therefore, understanding the environmental fate and biological impact is highly desired for designing biocompatible materials in place of abandoning nanomaterials. There are numerous techniques to date for analyzing the toxicity caused by nanomaterials. Still, diversified nanoparticles, different behavioral impacts and variegate incubation protocols have rendered it and impossible to draw the conclusion regarding toxicity. Nanotoxicity assessment broadly carried out in two concerning fields; biological and environmental. The environmental factors such as temperature, ionic strength and transformation of NMs inside biological system regulate the toxicity. The properties of agglomeration, physicochemical changes, and nano-bio interface interactions needs pharmacokinetic studies of NMs. Most of the studies carried out with pristine NPs for toxicity assessment; however, product or degradation product of NMs enter into environment and should be encountered instead of pristine NMs. The transformed or degraded materials in environment remain major challenge toward assessing toxicity specially in case of carbon-based nanomaterials on biological substrates.

Biological fate of nanoparticle toxicity is the second major field where high-quality instrumentation, sophisticated culture medium, and reliable in vitro and in vivo assays are needed. Many recent studies accentuate in the present perspective and put forward some model system to address the critical issues and dealing with the impediment of assessment of nanotoxicity. Apart from standard viability tests, other parameters need to be considered such as intracellular stability, degradation potential, and excretion pathways. There is a dire need for collaborative approach and multidisciplinary aspect to analyze the broad field of NPs and cell interactions. The major challenge in intracellular molecular events where relationship among biological functions need to be addressed. The recent development in assessment of toxicity include the adverse outcome pathways that include more proficient, predictive mechanistically approaches. This conceptual framework links the biological event with molecular initiating event at earlier stages [97]. Advanced electroanalytical methods can be used to monitor these events and play determinant role in assessment. In silico approach for nanotoxicity determination has also emerged out as an alternative to in vivo and in vitro analysis. The computational simulation of data, however, relies on experimental findings but more ethical mean for toxicity assessment. The characterization of nanomaterials plays substantial role in computation of engineered NMs along with establishing the relationship between biological activity and nanostructure [98]. Hence, programmatically executed reliable experimental data can be utilized to predict the nanotoxicity before their manufacture and use. In upcoming decade, Qiu et al. [99] presumed four basic predictive models for nanomaterial properties and biological effects. These analytical challenges include nanotoxicological mechanism changed from correlative to causative aspect, to conquer nanoparticle interferences for explicit in vitro analysis, establishing single-cell level cellular response for nanoparticle interaction, and understanding kinetic parameters of nano-bio interfaces.

Author details

Akanksha Gupta[1], Sanjay Kumar[2] and Vinod Kumar[3]*

1 Department of Chemistry, Sri Venkateswara College, University of Delhi, India

2 Department of Chemistry, Deshbandhu College, University of Delhi, India

3 Department of Chemistry, Kirori Mal College, University of Delhi, India

*Address all correspondence to: vinod7674@gmail.com; vinodkumar@kmc.du.ac.in

References

[1] Dutta J. Nanotechnology in the Developing World: 2015

[2] Kumar V et al. Nanotechnology: Nanomedicine, nanotoxicity and future challenges. Nanoscience & Nanotechnology. 2019;**9**(1):64-78

[3] Parhizkar M et al. Latest developments in innovative manufacturing to combine nanotechnology with healthcare. Nanomedicine. 2018;**13**(1):5-8

[4] Vance ME et al. Nanotechnology in the real world: Redeveloping the nanomaterial consumer products inventory. Beilstein Journal of Nanotechnology. 2015;**6**(1):1769-1780

[5] Koopaei NN, Abdollahi M. Opportunities and obstacles to the development of nanopharmaceuticals for human use. BioMed Central. 2016; **23**:24(1-6). Available from: https://doi.org/10.1186/s40199-016-0163-8

[6] Carvalho IT, Estevinho BN, Santos L. Application of microencapsulated essential oils in cosmetic and personal healthcare products–a review. International Journal of Cosmetic Science. 2016;**38**(2):109-119

[7] He X, Hwang H-M. Nanotechnology in food science: Functionality, applicability, and safety assessment. Journal of Food and Drug Analysis. 2016;**24**(4):671-681

[8] Singh H. Nanotechnology applications in functional foods; opportunities and challenges. Preventive Nutrition and Food Science. 2016;**21**(1):1

[9] Yu H et al. An overview of nanotechnology in food science: Preparative methods, practical applications, and safety. Journal of Chemistry. 2018;**2018**:5427978

[10] Cerqueira MA, Vicente AA, Pastrana LM. Nanotechnology in food packaging: Opportunities and challenges. In: Nanomaterials for Food Packaging. Elsevier; 2018. pp. 1-11

[11] Sundarraj AA. Nano-agriculture in the food industry. In: Plant Nanobionics. Springer; 2019. pp. 183-200

[12] Dasgupta N, Ranjan S, Lichtfouse E. Environmental Nanotechnology. Vol. 1. Springer; 2018

[13] Andrews D, Nann T, Lipson RH. Comprehensive Nanoscience and Nanotechnology. Academic Press; 2019

[14] Hess DJ, Lamprou A. Nanotechnology and the environment. In: Nanotechnology and Global Sustainability. CRC Press; 2018. pp. 50-73

[15] Ahmadi MH et al. Renewable energy harvesting with the application of nanotechnology: A review. International Journal of Energy Research. 2019;**43**(4): 1387-1410

[16] Ramsden J. Applied Nanotechnology: The Conversion of Research Results to Products. William Andrew; 2018

[17] Kumar V et al. Facile synthesis of Ce–doped SnO2 nanoparticles: A promising Photocatalyst for hydrogen evolution and dyes degradation. ChemistrySelect. 2019;**4**(13):3722-3729

[18] Kumar V et al. Novel lithium-containing honeycomb structures. Inorganic Chemistry. 2012;**51**(20): 10471-10473

[19] Kumar V, Govind A, Nagarajan R. Optical and photocatalytic properties of heavily F−-doped SnO2 nanocrystals by a novel single-source precursor

approach. Inorganic Chemistry. 2011; **50**(12):5637-5645

[20] Kumar V, Uma S. Investigation of cation (Sn2+) and anion (N3−) substitution in favor of visible light photocatalytic activity in the layered perovskite K2La2Ti3O10. Journal of Hazardous Materials. 2011;**189**(1–2): 502-508

[21] Petkov P et al. Advanced Nanotechnologies for Detection and Defence against CBRN Agents. Springer; 2018

[22] Johny J et al. Waveguide-based machine readable fluorescence security feature for border control and security applications. In: Counterterrorism, Crime Fighting, Forensics, and Surveillance Technologies II. International Society for Optics and Photonics; 2018

[23] Burmaoglu S, Saritas O, Yalcin H. Defense 4.0: Internet of things in military. In: Emerging Technologies for Economic Development. Springer; 2019. pp. 303-320

[24] Mulhall D. Our Molecular Future: How Nanotechnology, Robotics, Genetics and Artificial Intelligence Will Transfor M our World. Prometheus Books; 2010

[25] Werner M, Wondrak W, Johnston C. Nanotechnology and transport: Applications in the automotive industry. In: Nanoscience and Nanotechnology: Advances and Developments in Nano-Sized Materials. Walter de Gruyter GmbH; 2018. p. 260

[26] Mathew J, Joy J, George SC. Potential applications of nanotechnology in transportation: A review. Journal of King Saud University. 2018;**31**:586-594

[27] Banerjee B. Rubber Nanocomposites and Nanotextiles: Perspectives in Automobile Technologies. Walter de Gruyter GmbH & Co KG; 2019

[28] Sobolev K et al. Nanomaterials and nanotechnology for high-performance cement composites. In: Proceedings of ACI Session on Nanotechnology of Concrete: Recent Developments and Future Perspectives. Pennsylvania State University, USA; 2006. pp. 91-118

[29] Deleonibus S. Electronic Devices Architectures for the NANO-CMOS Era. CRC Press; 2019

[30] Verma A, Urbani F, Stollberg DW. Electronic device with microfilm antenna and related methods, Google Patents: 2018

[31] Yuan H et al. Flexible electronic skins based on piezoelectric nanogenerators and piezotronics. Nano Energy. 2019;**59**:84-90

[32] Yetisen AK et al. Nanotechnology in textiles. ACS Nano. 2016;**10**(3): 3042-3068

[33] Afroj S et al. Engineering graphene flakes for wearable textile sensors via highly scalable and ultrafast yarn dyeing technique. ACS Nano. 2019;**13**(4): 3847-3857

[34] Subic A. Materials in Sports Equipment. Woodhead Publishing; 2019

[35] Harifi T, Montazer M. Application of nanotechnology in sports clothing and flooring for enhanced sport activities, performance, efficiency and comfort: A review. Journal of Industrial Textiles. 2017;**46**(5):1147-1169

[36] Warheit DB, Sayes CM. Routes of exposure to nanoparticles: Hazard tests related to portal entries. In: Nanoengineering. Elsevier; 2015. pp. 41-54

[37] Ribeiro A et al. Challenges on the toxicological predictions of engineered nanoparticles. NanoImpact. 2017;**8**:59-72

[38] Halappanavar S et al. Promise and peril in nanomedicine: The challenges and needs for integrated systems biology approaches to define health risk. Wiley Interdisciplinary Reviews: Nanomedicine and Nanobiotechnology. 2018;**10**(1):e1465

[39] Cohen JM, DeLoid GM, Demokritou P. A critical review of in vitro dosimetry for engineered nanomaterials. Nanomedicine. 2015; **10**(19):3015-3032

[40] Hillegass JM et al. Assessing nanotoxicity in cells in vitro. Wiley Interdisciplinary Reviews: Nanomedicine and Nanobiotechnology. 2010;**2**(3):219-231

[41] Ajdary M et al. Health concerns of various nanoparticles: A review of their in vitro and in vivo toxicity. Nanomaterials. 2018;**8**(9):634

[42] Jones CF, Grainger DW. In vitro assessments of nanomaterial toxicity. Advanced Drug Delivery Reviews. 2009;**61**(6):438-456

[43] Arora S, Rajwade JM, Paknikar KM. Nanotoxicology and in vitro studies: The need of the hour. Toxicology and Applied Pharmacology. 2012;**258**(2): 151-165

[44] Aillon KL et al. Effects of nanomaterial physicochemical properties on in vivo toxicity. Advanced Drug Delivery Reviews. 2009;**61**(6): 457-466

[45] Menard A, Drobne D, Jemec A. Ecotoxicity of nanosized TiO2. Review of in vivo data. Environmental Pollution. 2011;**159**(3):677-684

[46] Zhu X et al. Developmental toxicity in zebrafish (Danio rerio) embryos after exposure to manufactured nanomaterials: Buckminsterfullerene aggregates (nC60) and fullerol. Environmental Toxicology and Chemistry. 2007;**26**(5):976-979

[47] Ema M, Gamo M, Honda K. A review of toxicity studies on graphene-based nanomaterials in laboratory animals. Regulatory Toxicology and Pharmacology. 2017;**85**:7-24

[48] Landvik NE et al. Criteria for grouping of manufactured nanomaterials to facilitate hazard and risk assessment, a systematic review of expert opinions. Regulatory Toxicology and Pharmacology. 2018;**95**: 270-279

[49] Basei G et al. Making use of available and emerging data to predict the hazards of engineered nanomaterials by means of in silico tools: A critical review. NanoImpact. 2019;**13**:76-99

[50] Oksel C et al. SAR modelling of nanomaterial toxicity: A critical review. Particuology. 2015;**21**:1-19

[51] Oksel C et al. Literature review of (Q) SAR modelling of nanomaterial toxicity. In: Modelling the Toxicity of Nanoparticles. Springer; 2017. pp. 103-142

[52] Sizochenko N et al. In silico methods for nanotoxicity evaluation: Opportunities and challenges. In: Nanotoxicology. CRC Press; 2018. pp. 527-557

[53] Fard JK, Jafari S, Eghbal MA. A review of molecular mechanisms involved in toxicity of nanoparticles. Advanced Pharmaceutical Bulletin. 2015;**5**(4):447

[54] León-Silva S, Fernández-Luqueño F, López-Valdez F. Silver nanoparticles (AgNP) in the environment: a review of potential risks on human and environmental health.

Water. Water, Air, & Soil Pollution. 2016;**227**(9):306

[55] Liu R et al. Evaluation of toxicity ranking for metal oxide nanoparticles via an in vitro dosimetry model. ACS Nano. 2015;**9**(9):9303-9313

[56] Raj S et al. Nanotechnology in cosmetics: Opportunities and challenges. Journal of Pharmacy & Bioallied Sciences. 2012;**4**(3):186

[57] Fotakis G, Timbrell JA. In vitro cytotoxicity assays: Comparison of LDH, neutral red, MTT and protein assay in hepatoma cell lines following exposure to cadmium chloride. Toxicology Letters. 2006;**160**(2):171-177

[58] Bahadar H et al. Toxicity of nanoparticles and an overview of current experimental models. Iranian Biomedical Journal. 2016;**20**(1):1

[59] Lison D et al. Nominal and effective dosimetry of silica nanoparticles in cytotoxicity assays. Toxicological Sciences. 2008;**104**(1):155-162

[60] Hussain S et al. In vitro toxicity of nanoparticles in BRL 3A rat liver cells. Toxicology In Vitro. 2005;**19**(7):975-983

[61] Braun K et al. Comparison of different cytotoxicity assays for in vitro evaluation of mesoporous silica nanoparticles. Toxicology In Vitro. 2018;**52**:214-221

[62] Almutary A, Sanderson B. The MTT and crystal violet assays: Potential confounders in nanoparticle toxicity testing. International Journal of Toxicology. 2016;**35**(4):454-462

[63] Jiang Q et al. Combined effects of low levels of palmitate on toxicity of ZnO nanoparticles to THP-1 macrophages. Environmental Toxicology and Pharmacology. 2016;**48**: 103-109

[64] Chng ELK, Pumera M. Toxicity of graphene related materials and transition metal dichalcogenides. RSC Advances. 2015;**5**(4):3074-3080

[65] Han X et al. Validation of an LDH assay for assessing nanoparticle toxicity. Toxicology. 2011;**287**(1):99-104

[66] Wang J et al. Oxygen vacancy induced band-gap narrowing and enhanced visible light Photocatalytic activity of ZnO. ACS Applied Materials & Interfaces. 2012;**4**(8):4024-4030

[67] Guadagnini R et al. Toxicity screenings of nanomaterials: Challenges due to interference with assay processes and components of classic in vitro tests. Nanotoxicology. 2015;**9**(sup1):13-24

[68] Chen H et al. In vivo study of spherical gold nanoparticles: Inflammatory effects and distribution in mice. PLoS One. 2013;**8**(2):e58208

[69] Rizzo LY, et al. In vivo nanotoxicity testing using the zebrafish embryo assay. Journal of Materials Chemistry B. 2013;**1**(32):3918-3925

[70] Bai W et al. Toxicity of zinc oxide nanoparticles to zebrafish embryo: A physicochemical study of toxicity mechanism. Journal of Nanoparticle Research. 2010;**12**(5):1645-1654

[71] Browning LM et al. Silver nanoparticles incite size- and dose-dependent developmental phenotypes and Nanotoxicity in Zebrafish embryos. Chemical Research in Toxicology. 2013; **26**(10):1503-1513

[72] Raies AB, Bajic VB. In silico toxicology: Computational methods for the prediction of chemical toxicity. Wiley Interdisciplinary Reviews: Computational Molecular Science. 2016; **6**(2):147-172

[73] Fourches D, Pu D, Tropsha A. Exploring quantitative nanostructure-

activity relationships (QNAR) modeling as a tool for predicting biological effects of manufactured nanoparticles. Combinatorial Chemistry & High Throughput Screening. 2011;**14**(3): 217-225

[74] Venkatapathy R, Wang NCY. Developmental toxicity prediction. In: Computational Toxicology. Springer; 2013. pp. 305-340

[75] Park M et al. Hazard evaluation in GUIDEnano: A web-based guidance tool for risk assessment and mitigation of nano-enabled products. In: New Tools and Approaches for Nanomaterial Safety Assessment. Malaga, Spain: DiVA; 2017

[76] Fadeel B et al. Advanced tools for the safety assessment of nanomaterials. Nature Nanotechnology. 2018;**13**(7):537

[77] Manke A, Wang L, Rojanasakul Y. Mechanisms of nanoparticle-induced oxidative stress and toxicity. BioMed Research International. 2013; **2013**:15

[78] Khalid P et al. Toxicology of carbon nanotubes-a review. International Journal of Applied Engineering Research. 2016;**11**(1):148-157

[79] Li X, Lenhart JJ, Walker HW. Aggregation kinetics and dissolution of coated silver nanoparticles. Langmuir. 2011;**28**(2):1095-1104

[80] Kim I-Y et al. Toxicity of silica nanoparticles depends on size, dose, and cell type. Nanomedicine: Nanotechnology, Biology and Medicine. 2015;**11**(6):1407-1416

[81] Hao N, Li L, Tang F. Roles of particle size, shape and surface chemistry of mesoporous silica nanomaterials on biological systems. International Materials Reviews. 2017; **62**(2):57-77

[82] Bharadwaj VN et al. Temporal assessment of nanoparticle accumulation after experimental brain injury: Effect of particle size. Scientific Reports. 2016;**6**:29988

[83] Chen N et al. The cytotoxicity of cadmium-based quantum dots. Biomaterials. 2012;**33**(5):1238-1244

[84] Salatin S, Maleki Dizaj S, Yari Khosroushahi A. Effect of the surface modification, size, and shape on cellular uptake of nanoparticles. Cell Biology International. 2015;**39**(8):881-890

[85] Chithrani BD, Ghazani AA, Chan WCW. Determining the size and shape dependence of gold nanoparticle uptake into mammalian cells. Nano Letters. 2006;**6**(4):662-668

[86] Maysinger D et al. Gold nanourchins and celastrol reorganize the nucleo-and cytoskeleton of glioblastoma cells. Nanoscale. 2018;**10**(4):1716-1726

[87] Albanese A, Tang PS, Chan WC. The effect of nanoparticle size, shape, and surface chemistry on biological systems. Annual Review of Biomedical Engineering. 2012;**14**:1-16

[88] Pozzi D et al. Effect of polyethyleneglycol (PEG) chain length on the bio–nano-interactions between PEGylated lipid nanoparticles and biological fluids: From nanostructure to uptake in cancer cells. Nanoscale. 2014; **6**(5):2782-2792

[89] Stark WJ. Nanoparticles in biological systems. Angewandte Chemie International Edition. 2011;**50**(6): 1242-1258

[90] Richards D, Ivanisevic A. Inorganic material coatings and their effect on cytotoxicity. Chemical Society Reviews. 2012;**41**(6):2052-2060

[91] Karimi Z, Karimi L, Shokrollahi H. Nano-magnetic particles used in

biomedicine: Core and coating materials. Materials Science and Engineering: C. 2013;**33**(5):2465-2475

[92] Avcu E et al. Electrophoretic deposition of chitosan-based composite coatings for biomedical applications: A review. Progress in Materials Science. 2019;**103**:69-108

[93] Worthington KL et al. Chitosan coating of copper nanoparticles reduces in vitro toxicity and increases inflammation in the lung. Nanotechnology. 2013;**24**(39):395101

[94] Shukla S et al. In vitro toxicity assessment of chitosan oligosaccharide coated iron oxide nanoparticles. Toxicology Reports. 2015;**2**:27-39

[95] Yin H, Too H, Chow G. The effects of particle size and surface coating on the cytotoxicity of nickel ferrite. Biomaterials. 2005;**26**(29):5818-5826

[96] Magrez A et al. Cellular toxicity of carbon-based nanomaterials. Nano Letters. 2006;**6**(6):1121-1125

[97] Bal-Price A, Meek MEB. Adverse outcome pathways: Application to enhance mechanistic understanding of neurotoxicity. Pharmacology & Therapeutics. 2017;**179**:84-95

[98] Saini B, Srivastava S. Nanotoxicity prediction using computational modelling - review and future directions. IOP Conference Series: Materials Science and Engineering. 2018;**348**:012005

[99] Qiu TA, Clement PL, Haynes CL. Linking nanomaterial properties to biological outcomes: Analytical chemistry challenges in nanotoxicology for the next decade. Chemical Communications. 2018;**54**(91): 12787-12803

Chapter 5

Residue of Selected Persistent Organic Pollutants (POPs) in Soil of Some Areas in Vietnam

Toan Vu Duc, Chi Do Thi Lan and Mai Ngo Tra

Abstract

This chapter evaluates the contamination of selected persistent organic pollutants (S-POPs) in soil of some typical areas in Vietnam (mangrove forest, industrial, and urban areas in northern part). S-POPs are composed of polychlorinated biphenyls (PCBs) and polyaromatic hydrocarbons (PAHs). The collected data and analyzed results indicated the wide occurrence of significant S-POPs residues in study areas. The main sources of S-POPs are discussed by using composition analyses and diagnostic ratios of S-POPs indicator. Risk assessment of S-POPs in soil is assessed by using the guidance of the US Environmental Protection Agency. The obtained results have contributed to assess the S-POPs fate in the soil environment in Vietnam.

Keywords: soil, PCBs, PAHs, residues

1. Introduction

Of all the persistent organic pollutants (POPs) with a potential environmental and human health impacts, polychlorinated biphenyls (PCBs) and polyaromatic hydrocarbons (PAHs) have received a lot of attention. Concern over the toxicology of these compounds (S-POPs) has led to international efforts to research on their contamination and fate in the environment. S-POPs are distributed into every compositions of environment and seriously affected public health.

PAHs are a group of organic compounds containing only carbon and hydrogen, constituted by two or more fused-benzene rings. They are a ubiquitous group of several hundred chemically related compounds, environmentally persistent with various structures and varied toxicity. PAHs have low polarization, solubility, and volatility change and accumulate in organisms from low molecular weights to high molecular weights [1]. With low-molecular-weighted PAHs, the solubility is high while accumulating in low organisms with high volatility. In contrast, with high-molecular-weighted PAHs (four or more rings), the solubility is low, and accumulation in the organism is high with low volatility. The amount of benzene rings in the chemical structure of the PAHs determines the solubility in water. As the number of benzene rings increases, the hydrophobicity of the PAHs increases. PAHs are relatively inert chemical compounds. Since they are composed of benzene rings, PAHs have the properties of aromatic hydrocarbons, which can participate in substitution and addition reactions. The low solubility of PAHs in water will lead to PAHs that tend to adsorb in soil and sediment, thus greatly affecting their ability to be biodegradable by microorganisms. PAHs interact strongly with sediment organic carbon, which have relatively low volatility, resulting in bioaccumulation and toxicities in some aquatic organisms [2, 3]. International researches often concentrated on 16 representative PAHs including naphthalene (Nap), acenaphthylene (Acey), acenaphthene (Ace), fluorene (Flu), phenanthrene (Phe), anthracene (Ant), fluoranthene (Flt), pyrene (Pyr), chrysene (Chr), benzo[a]anthracene (BaA), benzo[b]fluoranthene (BbF), benzo[k]fluoranthene (BkF), benzo[a]pyrene (BaP), indeno[1,2,3-cd]pyrene (IcdP), dibenzo[a,h]anthracene (DahA), and benzo [g,h,i]pyrene (BghiP) (**Figure 1**).

PAHs are formed from two sources: natural and man-made sources. Some PAHs in the environment originate from natural sources such as combustion (natural forest fires, volcanic eruptions), rock formation processes, sedimentation processes, oil leaks, or coal mines (this is human activities) [4, 5]. However, natural sources are not the main source. In terms of human activities, PAHs are formed by incomplete combustion of raw materials, such as coal, oil, gas, wood, grass, and waste, or the process of smoking, grilling, or frying food. Almost all sectors (industrial production, agriculture, livelihoods, transport, and other activities) can generate PAHs [3, 6]. PAHs generated from different sources have different characteristics. In the environment, PAHs can be found everywhere: air, water, sediment, soil, and organisms [7]. The existence of PAHs in many environmental components is due to the PAHs spread and deposition process. Initially, PAHs are discharged into the air, which exists in either gaseous form or are adsorbed onto the dust. Under normal conditions, the amount of PAHs contained in the dust can account for up to 90% [8, 9]. By the spreading process, PAHs can be transported in long distance in the air, which then condense and accumulate in soil, water, sediment, and organisms. Studies on PAHs in soils are prevalent because of PAHs' high accumulation

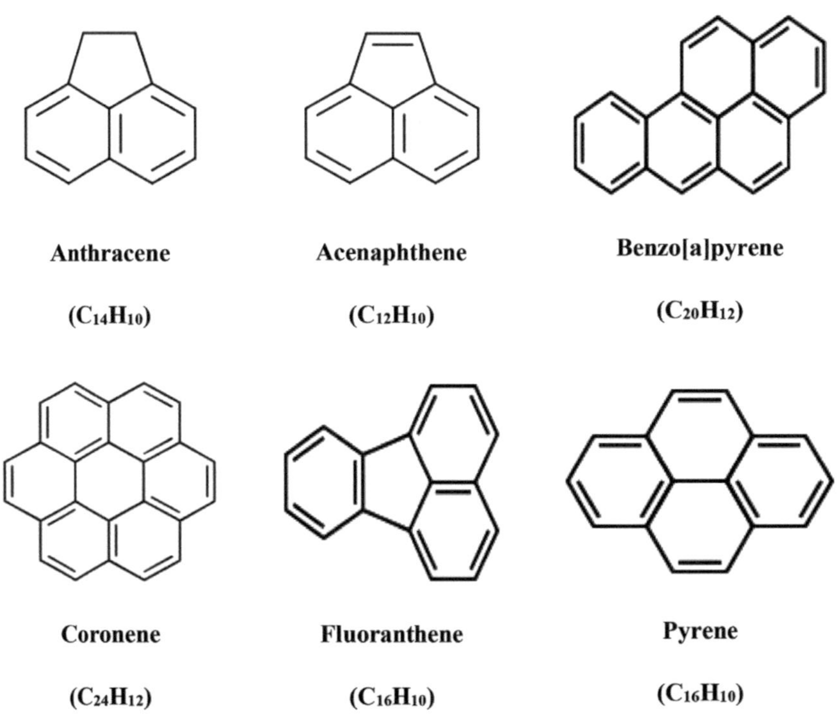

Figure 1.
Structure of some typical PAHs.

potential, and traceability in soil is easier to detect than in other component environments.

There are many types of PAHs that cause cancer and gene mutations [1, 10, 11]. Human are exposed to PAHs through food, water, breathing air, or direct contact with materials containing PAHs. Scientists have now discovered hundred types of PAHs. Most studies focus on a number of characteristic of PAHs, which most significantly are health damage (cancer and genetic mutations) and volatility in the environment.

PCBs are chemical industrial products which have a global environmental health hazard. PCBs groups have 209 isomers and congeners with 1 to 10 chlorine atoms attached to the biphenyl molecule (**Figure 2**). The physical and chemical properties of PCBs are important in studying their fate and their transformation in the environment. PCBs vary from colorless for the lower chlorinated compounds to yellow for the most highly chlorinated types. They exhibit low water solubility (from 1.2.10 to 6.5.5 g/m^3), low Henry constant (from $0.3.10^{-4}$ to $8.97.10^{-4}$ atm^3/mole), and low electrical conductivity. In contrast, PCBs have high boiling point (from 285 to 456°C) and high value of lgKow (from 4.3 to 8.3). PCBs with fewer chlorine atoms are, in general, less persistent, more water soluble, and more flammable than PCBs with more chlorine atoms. PCBs are very resistant to decomposition and are also non-corrosive as well as relatively non-flammable. Due to these properties, PCBs can be distributed in many places in the environment, into the food chain and accumulated in the human body and other organisms.

Physical and chemical properties of PCBs made them useful in industrial. Of the 209 possible PCB congeners, about 100 compounds are recovered in industrial mixtures. PCBs have an excellent insulating property as well as a high heat capacity [1]. Their properties have led to many industrial applications such as insulator in transformers and capacitors, plasticizers, surface coatings, additives in paints, flame retardants, etc.

The industrial application of PCBs started in the early 1939. The following countries have been the main manufacturers of PCBs: Austria, China, Czechoslovakia, France, Germany, Italy, Japan, Russia, Spain, the United Kingdom, and the United States. PCBs mixtures have been marketed under variety of trade names such as Aroclor (the United States, the United Kingdom, Canada, and Australia), Phenochlor and Pyralene (France), Clophen (Germany), Fenoclor (Italy), Chlofen (Poland), Sovol (Soviet Union), Kanechlor (Japan), and Derlor (Czecchoslovakia). Between 1929 and 1989, the total world production of PCBs was 1,5 million tons, an average of about 26,000 tons per year. Since 1940, Vietnam has imported between 27,000 and 30,000 tons of PCBs from Russia, China, and Romania, mainly as insulator in transformers.

Since early 1960, scientists discovered that PCBs are toxic, affecting human health. PCB poisoning has occurred, including Yusho in Japan in 1968 and Yucheng in Taiwan in 1979, causing hundreds of deaths and thousands of people suffering from various effects.

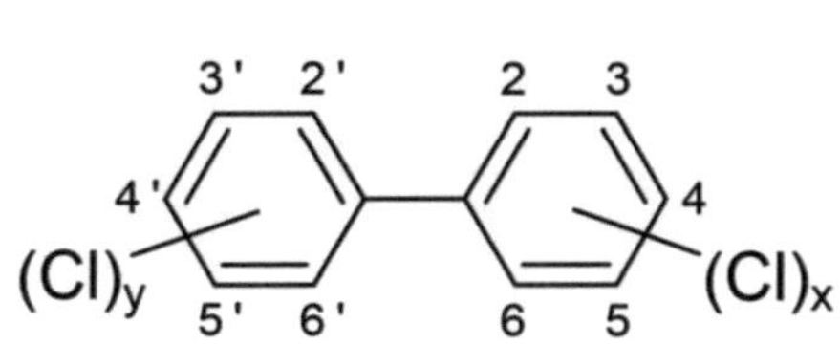

Figure 2.
Structure of PCBs (x + y ≤ 10).

PCBs have been demonstrated to cause cancer and a number of serious non-cancer health effects in animals, including effects on the immune system, reproductive system, nervous system, and endocrine system and other health effects. Studies in humans provide supportive evidence for potential carcinogenic and non-carcinogenic effects of PCBs. The degree of impact depends on the substance in the PCB group.

PCBs enter the environment in three main ways: by disposing of PCB-containing waste in landfills, and from which PCBs enter the groundwater, into the river, into the sea; incorrect combustion of PCB waste causes PCBs to disperse into the atmosphere; and due to PCB leakage from electrical appliances such as transformers and capacitors. The transport of PCBs in the environment is due to the effects of air, water, animals, and some other pathways. PCBs can accumulate in the fat, milk, brain, serum, liver, and muscles of the human body and can be excreted from the body through urine and breast milk. After detecting the toxicity of PCBs, many countries around the world have in turn prohibited the production and use of PCB. In Vietnam, PCB has been restricted since 1992.

2. Residue of PAHs in mangrove forest soil in Northern Vietnam

2.1 Contamination status of PAHs

Mangrove forests are important habitats and are of high economic value. Mangroves in Vietnam are severely damaged by a variety of causes, including pollutants. Mangroves of Dong Rui, Tien Yen, Quang Ninh, situated in Northern Vietnam, are a unique ecosystem, close to Vietnam's largest coal mining area and thermal power plants. The research has found that PAHs in soil of Dong Rui mangrove are present with significant concentrations.

Studies of PAHs in soil are quite diverse and show that concentration of PAHs accumulated from region to region, ranging from mild to very severe. The concentration of PAHs in mangrove forests around the world fluctuates in a large range from a few hundred μg/kg to thousands of μg/kg, some places even higher concentration than the accumulation in industrial land.

Our studies of PAHs in mangrove forest soil are implemented in Dong Rui area from August 2014 to January 2017. Comparison of PAH concentrations in Dong Rui mangroves with other places showed that PAHs in Dong Rui mangrove at the lowest value are still higher than those in mangroves in the Sundarbans, India. However, since the highest value in Dong Rui is smaller than in India, Hong Kong, so it can be said that the level concentration of PAHs of mangrove in Dong Rui is average (**Table 1**).

Among 16 PAHs (classified by the US Environmental Protection Agency) studied at Dong Rui mangroves, Vietnam from August 2014 to January 2017, there were

Place	Min values	Max values	Mean values
Mangroves: Dong Rui, Vietnam (this study)	312.5	1407.0	692.6
Mangroves: the Sundarbans, India	132	2938	634
Four wetlands mangroves: Hong Kong	356	11098	1142
Mangroves: Ho Chung, Hong Kong	1162	3322	2202

Source: [5, 14, 15].

Table 1.
Concentrations of Σ_{16} PAHs (μg/kg) in soil in some mangrove areas in the world.

8 PAHs (BaA, Chr, BbF, BkF, BaP, Ind, BghiP, DahA) identified as potentially carcinogenic. Those PAHs are composed of four or more benzene rings, which are highly durable in the environment, less degradable, and have high accumulation in soil [12, 13]. Considering the ratio of Σ_8PAHs to Σ_{16}PAHs at the sampling sites, most Σ_8PAHs were found to be high compared to Σ_{16}PAHs. The percentage of Σ_8PAHs/Σ_{16}PAHs ranged from 50.2% to 71.4% with an average of 59.6%. This is also consistent with studies by Hussein et al. (2016) on PAHs in soils with an average of Σ_8PAHs/Σ_{16}PAHs of 67.1% [4] (**Figure 3**).

Of the 16 typical PAHs, PAHs can be represented from two benzene rings to six benzene rings. Two-ring PAHs are Nap; three-ring PAHs include Acy, Ace, Flu, Phe, and Ant; four-ring PAHs include Py, Flt, BaA, and Chr; five-ring PAHs include BbF, BkF, BaP, and DahA; and six-ring PAHs include Ind and BghiP. Considering the accumulation of PAHs in terms of the number of benzene rings, four-ring PAHs were dominant (32%), while two-ring PAHs were the lowest (3%). Five-ring PAHs are 25% larger than the rate of three-ring PAHs (22%) and six-ring (18%). This result is also consistent with the study by Ishwar Chandra Yadav et al. (2017) in soils in Kathmandu (Nepal) [16] with four-ring PAHs > five-ring PAHs > 3-ring PAHs > 6-ring PAHs > 2-ring PAHs.

Based on molecular weight, 16 PAHs can be divided into three groups. Low-molecular-weight (LMW) groups of PAHs with 2–3 rings include Nap, Ace, Acy, Phe, Flu, and Ant. Medium-molecular-weight groups (MMW) are groups of with four-ring PAHs, including BaA, Chr, Pyr, and Flt. High-molecular-weight groups (HMW) are groups of five- to six-ring PAHs: BbF, BkF, BaP, DahA, BghiP, and Ind. These subgroups are different in water solubility, lipid modification, and absorption of PAHs. Studies have shown that PAHs in the MMW and HMW groups are less soluble in water, less variable, and more easily absorbed lipids than PAHs in the LMW group. In addition, the toxicity and environmental stability of PAHs in the MMW and HMW groups were also higher than the LMW group.

In this study, the HMW group had the highest percentage of all samples, accounted for 36.63–56.76%. Meanwhile, the MMW group rate ranged from 17.3 to 39.77%, and the LMW group was the lowest, ranging from 17.79 to 31.52%.

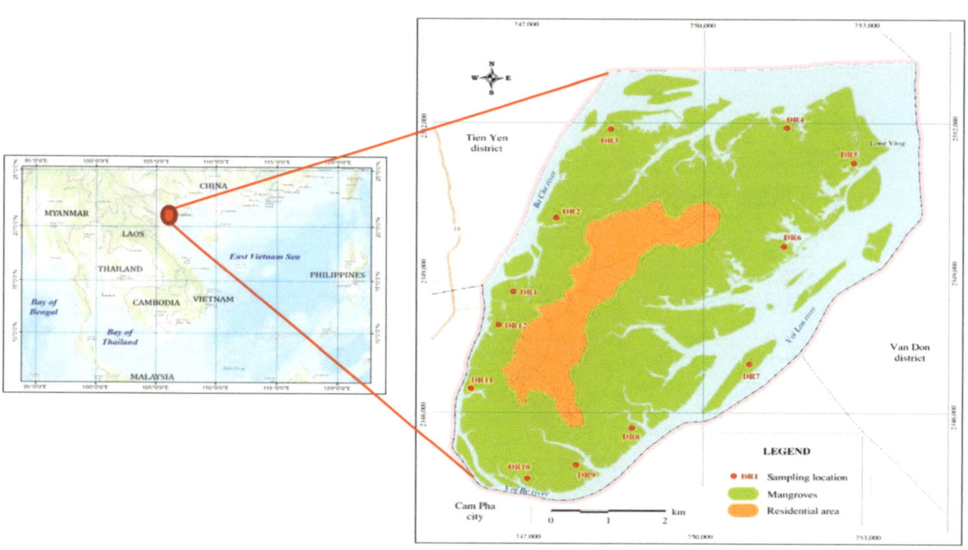

Figure 3.
Mangroves area in Dong Rui, Northern Vietnam.

2.2 PAHs emission characteristics

Determining PAH sources is difficult due to their spread and sustainability in the environment. At present, the studies are based on the characteristics of the PAHs isomer ratios such as Flt/(Flt + Pyr), Ant/(Ant + Phe), BaA/(BaA + Chyr), and Ind/(Ind + BghiP) in the environment to predict the source of PAHs (**Table 2**).

Dong Rui mangrove is surrounded by three rivers: Voi Lon, Voi Be, and Ba Che and estuaries. It is affected of coal mining and coal burning in Cam Pha and Cua Ong areas, Mong Duong I and II thermal power plants, and paper factory. During the coal mining and coal burning process, PAHs have been emitted and spread to Dong Rui mangroves due to wind and tides. Specific PAHs sources may include:

- Activities: smoking, heating, and cooking with sawdust, charcoal, honeycomb, wood, waste incineration, etc.

- Traffic: road traffic activities in island communes and national highway 18 passing through the island commune; water transportation.

- Industrial production: paper mills 2 km away from mangroves, Mong Duong thermal power plant about 7 km from mangroves, and coal mining in Cam Pha, Cua Ong area

- Other activities: burning of wood, charcoal making, burning of forest, burning of straw

The relationship between PAHs composition and source of emissions has been considered from the analysis of the proportions of PAHs in the sample. Each source of waste has the potential to produce some PAHs better than other sources. Therefore, the PAH rates determined from the sample analysis will be indicators that help determine the source of PAHs.

The Flt/(Flt + Pyr) ratio at most sampling locations is greater than 0.5. Therefore, the main source of emissions to the Dong Rui mangroves is the burning of raw materials such as coal, wood, grass, etc. At points close to the traffic

Ratios PAHs	Value	Emission source
Flt/(Flt + Pyr)	<0.4	Gasoline, oil spill
	0.4–0.5	Traffic
	>0.5	Grass, wood, coal
Ant/(Ant + Phe)	<0.1	Gasoline, oil spill
	>0.1	Fire
BaA/(BaA + Chyr)	<0.2	Gasoline, oil spill
	0.2–0.35	Gasoline, oil spill, or fire
	>0.35	Fire
Ind/(Ind + BghiP)	<0.2	Gasoline, oil spill
	0.2–0.5	Traffic
	>0.5	Grass, wood, coal

Table 2.
The relationship between the ratio of some PAHs and their emission source.

line, Flt/(Flt + Pyr) is in the range of 0.4–0.5. Thus, the main source of emissions in this area is transport.

At all sampling sites, BaA/(BaA + Chyr) ratios were greater than 0.2, and at most sampling sites, BaA/(BaA + Chyr) ratios were greater than 0.35. Therefore, it is possible that the source of the emissions is mainly due to combustion. Similarly, the Ant/(Ant+ Phe) rate at the sampling locations at the time of sampling is greater than 0.1. Thus, the source of emissions is mainly due to burning rather than oil spills. The Ind/(Ind + BghiP) ratio at most sampling points is greater than 0.5. At these locations, the source of the waste is mainly from the burning of raw materials such as coal, wood, and grass. There are some samples near the roads; Ind/(Ind + BghiP) is in the range of 0.2–0.5. As such, these points are mainly affected by the fire of gasoline from vehicles. This is in line with the actual situation in Dong Rui.

2.3 Risk assessment of PAHs

The presence of PAHs in the soil of Dong Rui mangroves has shown signs of risk to the ecological environment. To assess the risk of PAHs exposure to humans who live in mangroves area, this study used the cancer risk index (CR). This index looks at the risk of cancer through three pathways: digestive, respiratory, and the skin. Calculation formula CR digestive (cancer risk due to contaminated gastrointestinal tract), CR skin (cancer risk due to exposure to contaminated skin), and CR respiratory (cancer risk due to breathing pollutants) based on formulas 1, 2, and 3. The formulas for calculating the cancer risk index include

$$CR_{digestive} = \frac{CS \times \left(CSF_{digestive} \times \sqrt[3]{\left(\frac{BW}{70}\right)}\right) \times IR_{soil} \times EF \times ED}{BW \times AT \times 10^6} \tag{1}$$

$$CR_{skin} = \frac{CS \times \left(CSF_{skin} \times \sqrt[3]{\left(\frac{BW}{70}\right)}\right) \times SA \times FE \times AF \times ABS \times EF \times ED}{BW \times AT \times 10^6} \tag{2}$$

$$CR_{respiratory} = \frac{CS \times \left(CSF_{respiratory} \times \sqrt[3]{\left(\frac{BW}{70}\right)}\right) \times IR_{air} \times EF \times ED}{BW \times AT \times PEF} \tag{3}$$

where

CS: the concentration of PAH in the soil (μg/kg)
CSF: cancer slope index (1/(mg/kg.day))
BW: average weight of the study population (kg)
EF: frequency of exposure (day/year)
ED: length of exposure time (year)
IR air: speed of breath (m^3/ day)
IR soil: absorption rate through the gastrointestinal tract (mg/day)
SA: coefficient of contact with skin surface (cm^2/ day)
AF: adhesion of the skin when exposed to soil (mg/cm^2)
ABS: absorption coefficient across the skin
FE: skin-to-skin contact ratio
AT: average exposure time (day)
PEF: dust emission factor (m^3/kg)
CSF: BaP toxic cancer index, with CSF_{BaP} digestive = 7.3; CSF_{BaP} skin = 25; CSF_{BaP} respiratory = 3.85, that is determined by the carcinogenic potential of BaP [17]
CS: ratio between TEQ_{16PAHs} and TEQ_{BaP} [18].

$$CS = \frac{TEQ_{16PAH}}{TEQ_{BaP}} \tag{4}$$

with TEQ = TEF × the concentration of each PAH in the soil sample.

Here, TEF is equivalent toxicity.

Under the guidance of the US Environmental Protection Agency, CR ranges are categorized into five categories: very low risk, low risk, average risk, high risk, and very high risk. The majority of risk assessments used present potentially higher-risk scenarios than the actual ones, according to **Table 3**. The positive side of this approach is that the risks are not underestimated, and population health in the area is more protected.

This research split people who live in Dong Rui mangrove into two groups: group 1 (<10 years old) and group 2 (11–70 years old). This split is based on exposure time, no air intake, average balance, and also the object. All people who live in Dong Rui mangrove are allowed to be referenced. Apply the calculating 1, 2, 3 to calculate CR index (**Table 4**).

In the three components of CR index, the ratio $CR_{digestive}/CR_{Total}$ was 0.63% for group 1 and 0.55% for group 2. At the same time, the ratio $CR_{exposure}/CR_{Total}$ for group 1 was 0.37%; group 2 was 0.45%. The ratio $CR_{respiratory}/CR_{Total}$ was almost negligible in two groups. Thus, the risk of gastrointestinal cancer is highest in the exposure pathways for both groups, followed by the risk of exposure and, ultimately, the risk of breathing.

Comparing the risk of cancer between the two groups showed that the risk of cancer caused by group 2 is 1.6 times higher than that of group 1. In the risk of cancer due to exposure, group 2 is 2.3 times higher than that of group 1. The risk of cancer caused by breathing is the same for both groups. The overall risk for group 1 was 1.9 times higher than that of group 2. Thus, with PAHs in the soil of Dong Rui mangrove, group 2 had a higher risk for cancer than group 1. This could be explained by the longer exposure time of group 2 compared to group 1.

Risk level	Cancer risk index
Very low risk	$CR \leq 10^{-6}$
Low risk	$10^{-6} < CR \leq 10^{-4}$
Medium risk	$10^{-4} < CR \leq 10^{-3}$
High risk	$10^{-3} \leq CR < 10^{-1}$
Very high risk	$CR \geq 10^{-1}$

Table 3.
Classification of cancer risk.

Index	Group 1	Group 2
$CR_{digestive}$	3.81343E-06	6.22609E-06
CR_{skin}	2.2306E-06	5.18962E-06
$CR_{respiratory}$	7.3941E-11	7.3941E-11
CR_{Total}	6.04411E-06	1.14158E-05

Table 4.
Cancer risk index in groups.

3. Residue of PCBs in soil of some areas in Vietnam

3.1 General contamination status of PCBs in soil in Vietnam

Monitoring surveys of PCBs residue in soil have been conducted during the early 1992s. In the Northern Vietnam, PCBs was found in environmental soil of Hung Yen province, Bac Ninh province (Bac Ninh city, Tu Son district, Yen Phong district, Tien Du district) and Hanoi city (Hanoi downtown, Soc Son district, Gia Lam district, Dong Anh district, Thanh Tri district, Tu Liem district) [19, 20]. PCBs penetrated in the urban and rural areas. High PCBs concentrations were found in soil of Hanoi in 1995 (1070.96 ng/g dw) [20].

In the central Vietnam, PCBs was found in environmental soil of Quang Tri province and Hue city. PCBs penetrated in urban soil at significant levels (from 0.9 to 312.5 ng/g, [20]). In the southern Vietnam, PCBs were also found in Mekong River delta (Long An province, Tay Ninh province) Ho Chi Minh city. PCB distributed in wide spaces such as landfill soil (Dong Thanh landfill of Ho Chi Minh city, 17.22 ng/g), paddy field soil, and urban soil [21]. Highest PCBs concentrations were found in urban soil of Ho Chi Minh city (530.5 ng/g) [20].

According to the POP national plan of the Vietnamese government, the use of PCB oils in all equipment will have to be terminated in 2020. PCBs will have to be destroyed in 2028. Therefore, an adequate management and disposal of PCB sources would help to prevent a further PCB release to the environment.

3.2 Case study of PCBs residues in Hanoi

3.2.1 Study area and soil sampling

Our studies of PCBs residue in Hanoi, capital of Vietnam, are implemented in 2006. Hanoi city, located in the Red River Delta in the North Vietnam, is the center of culture, politics, economy, and trade of the whole country. Hanoi comprises several urban suburban districts. Due to the important role of Hanoi in safety of public health and environmental quality, an assessment of the content and distribution of PCBs in soil is therefore essential.

Soil sampling followed Vietnamese standards (TCVN). These standards are composed of:

- TCVN 4046–85: Method of soil sampling in agricultural areas
- TCVN 5297–1995: Soil quality—sampling—general requirements
- TCVN 5960–1995: Soil quality—sampling—guidance on the collection, handling and storage of soil for the assessment of aerobic microbial processes in the laboratory
- TCVN 4047–85: Method for the preparation of soil sample for analysis
- TCVN 6857–2001: Soil quality—simplified soil description

The sampling campaign for Hanoi was carried out in February 2006 (60 soil samples), during the dry season. Soil samples were collected from agricultural and industrial areas and towns of all five suburban districts (Soc Son, Dong Anh, Gia Lam, Tu Liem, Thanh Tri), as well as the center of Hanoi, for comparison. The sampling sites were chosen at random, with an attempt to get them evenly distributed over Hanoi city. The samples were taken with solvent-rinsed stainless steel scoops from the upper 5 cm of the soil and then transferred to pre-cleaned polyethylene bags. The total concentration of PCBs (ΣPCBs) and six selected PCB congeners (PCB28, 52, 101, 138, 153, 180) were analyzed following the method described by Thao et al. (2009) [20].

3.2.2 Contamination status of PCBs in soil in Hanoi

The PCB concentrations in the collected soil samples from Hanoi are all shown in **Table 5**. The ΣPCBs concentrations in industrial and urban areas ranged from not detected (N.D) to 190.42 ng g^{-1} dw (mean 41.89 ng g^{-1} dw).

Due to the historical use of PCBs in Vietnam, its main source of contamination in industrial and urban areas could originate from the dielectric oil used in old hanging transformers and capacitors which were widely used in Hanoi. From these installations, PCBs could have penetrated into the environment by mechanical damage, electrical accidents, and fire. During the retro-filling of dielectric oil containing PCBs, there is a risk of PCBs escaping into the environment [19].

With regard to the soil samples from agriculture areas, ΣPCBs concentrations ranged from N.D to 24.37 ng g^{-1} (mean 15.14 ng g^{-1} dw). These sites are not far from densely populated towns of five surrounding suburban districts. Therefore, ΣPCBs were probably deposited into the agriculture sites by atmospheric transport from urban areas. In general, the PCBs concentrations were highest in industrial soil samples, followed by those in urban soils and in agricultural soil. This also applies for the usage of PCBs in Vietnam [19].

Locations	Σ6PCBs[a]	ΣPCBs[b]
A. Agricultural areas		
Soc Son 1[c]	N.D–3.27 (2.13)	N.D–21.82 (14.22)
Dong Anh 1	N.D–4.14 (3.09)	N.D–24.37 (18.19)
Gia Lam 1	N.D–3.32 (2.15)	N.D–18.39 (11.94)
Hanoi center 1	N.D–2.27 (0.76)	N.D–11.38 (3.79)
Tu Liem 1	2.63–3.14 (2.84)	16.14–19.65 (17.84)
Thanh Tri 1	3.09–3.89 (3.37)	17.18–21.65 (18.69)
B. Industrial and urban areas		
Soc Son 2[d]	2.52–4.33 (3.72)	16.24–27.94 (23.98)
Dong Anh 2	3.42–4.95 (4.26)	N.D–37.54 (24.36)
Gia Lam 2	N.D–15.49 (8.97)	N.D–79.44 (45.99)
Hanoi center 2	3.53–39.98 (13.12)	16.82–190.42 (62.45)
Tu Liem 2	4.35–11.84 (8.09)	23.56–63.26 (43.27)
Thanh Tri 2	3.12–5.89 (4.92)	18.92–34.62 (29.76)

[a] *Σ6PCBs: sum of six selected PCB congeners.*
[b] *ΣPCB: sum of all PCB isomers and congeners.*
[c] *Soc Son 1: agricultural areas of Soc Son.*
[d] *Soc Son 2: industrial and urban areas of Soc Son.*

Table 5.
Concentrations of PCBs (ng g^{-1} dw) in the surface soil from Hanoi.

3.2.3 Temporal trends of ΣPCB in soil in Hanoi

With regard to PCBs concentrations in soil samples from Hanoi reported in the period from 1992 to 2006, the increasing temporal trend of PCB levels could be shown. It was reported that the mean ΣPCB concentration in soil samples from Hanoi in 1992 (6 soil samples), in 2000 (8 soil samples), and in 2006 (60 soil samples) range from 9.1 to 29 ng g^{-1} (mean 12.6 $\pm$ 8.9 ng g^{-1}), from 0.6 to 120 ng g^{-1} (mean 21.2 $\pm$ 25.2 ng g^{-1}), and from <0.02 to 190.24 ng g^{-1} (mean 28.08 $\pm$ 28.57 ng g^{-1}), respectively [20, 21]. There are some possible sources of PCBs from 1992 to 2006. PCBs have escaped from dielectric oil containing PCB in transformers and capacitors. It has been reported that the total amount of possible PCB-containing transformers and capacitors across Vietnam might reach 9638 units and 1784 units, respectively [22]. PCBs could have volatilized from a capacitor. The studies of Ehime University concluded that PCBs volatilize and spread easily when capacitors containing PCB that are used over their product life are destroyed. PCBs that escaped into ambient air can pollute food through biological accumulation and also pollute the environmental soil. This should not be disregarded. Besides the possible PCB sources in Vietnam, it should be noted that the inaccurate POPs management can lead to their release to a wide extent in the environment.

4. Conclusion

This work investigated the contamination status of selected persistent organic pollutants in soil of mangrove forest and urban areas in Vietnam. Wide occurrence and remarkable residue levels of S-POPs have been found in the soil of study areas. Composition analyses show that S-POPs penetrated in the soil for a long time. The main sources of S-POPs are from mix sources which have origin form anthropogenic sources. Risk assessment of S-POPs found from low- to medium-risk levels. Due to the propensity of S-POPs to accumulate in various compartments of environment, further evaluation of ecotoxicological should be undertaken as a high priority.

Acknowledgements

The authors would like to thank Thuyloi University, Trade Union University, and Institute of Physics, Vietnam Academy of Science and Technology for their support.

Conflict of interest

The authors have no conflict of interest.

Author details

Toan Vu Duc[1]*, Chi Do Thi Lan[2] and Mai Ngo Tra[3]

1 Thuyloi University, Hanoi, Vietnam

2 Trade Union University, Hanoi, Vietnam

3 Institute of Physics, Viet Nam Academy of Science and Technology, Hanoi, Vietnam

*Address all correspondence to: vuductoan2001@yahoo.com

References

[1] Werner AF, Hoogheem TJ, Staples CA. Assessment of priority pollutant concentrations in the United States using STORET database. Environmental Toxicology and Chemistry. 1985;**4**: 131-142

[2] Minister of supply and services Canada. Polycyclic Aromatic Hydrocarbons Canadian Environmental Protection Act. Canada; 1994. Catalogue No. En 40–215/42E

[3] The Centers for Disease Control and Prevention. Polycyclic Aromatic Hydrocarbons (Benzo[a]pyrene) Fact Sheet. Agency for Toxic Substances and Disease Registry: Atlanta; 2013

[4] Abdel-Shafy HI, Mansour MSM. A review on polycyclic aromatic hydrocarbons: Source, environmental impact, effect on human health and remediation. Egyptian Journal of Petroleum. 2016;**25**:107-123

[5] Sarkar SK, Bhattacharya A, Chatterjee M, Bhattacharya BD, Jover E, Albaigés J, et al. Quantification and source identification of polycyclic aromatic hydrocarbons in core sediments from Sundarban Mangrove Wetland, India. Archives of Environmental Contamination and Toxicology. 2010;**59**(1):49-61

[6] Environmental Protection Agency Washington. Polycyclic Aromatic Hydrocarbons (PAHs). United States Office of Solid Waste January: Washington; 2008, Report DC 20460

[7] Richards S, Lin Z-Q, Dixon RP, Johnson KA, Hussar E. Human health risk assessment of 16 priority polycyclic aromatic hydrocarbons in soils of Chattanooga, Tennessee, USA. Water, Air, & Soil Pollution. 2012;**223**(9): 5535-5548

[8] WHO. Selected Non-Heterocyclic Polycyclic Aromatic Hydrocarbons. WHO: Geneva; 1998, Report QD 341.H9

[9] Yasuda K. Stack sampling technique for PAHs. In: Workshop on air Pollution Monitoring and Analysis with Emphasis on PAHs; Bangkok, Thailand; 1995. pp. 87–90

[10] Wang L, Peter PF, Yu H, Yan J. Photomutagenicity of 16 polycyclic aromatic hydrocarbons from the US EPA priority pollutant list. Mutation Research. 2004;**557**(1):99-108

[11] Agency for Toxic Substances and Disease Registry. In: ATSDR, editor. Toxicological Profile for Polycyclic Aromatic Hydrocarbons. Atlanta, USA: Public Health Service; 1995

[12] Xu X, Lu X, Wang L. Composition, source and potential risk of polycyclic aromatic hydrocarbons (PAHs) in vegetable soil from the suburbs of Xianyang City, Northwest China: A case study. Environmental Earth Sciences. 2016;**75**(1):56-75

[13] Echevarria G, Sterckeman T, Dan-Badjo AT. Assessment of polycyclic aromatic hydrocarbons contamination in urban soils from Niamey, Niger. Journal of Biodiversity and Environmental Sciences. 2015;**6**(1): 275-281

[14] Tam NF. Contamination of polycyclic aromatic hydrocarbons in surface sediments of mangrove swamps. Environmental Pollution. 2001;**114**(2): 255-263

[15] Yu KSH. Natural attenuation, biostimulation and bioaugmentation on biodegradation of polycyclic aromatic hydrocarbons (PAHs) in mangrove sediments. Marine Pollution Bulletin. 2005;**51**:1071-1077

[16] Devib NL, Lia J, Zhang G, Yadava IC. Polycyclic aromatic hydrocarbons in house dust and surface soil in major urban regions of Nepal: Implication on source apportionment and toxicological effect. Science of the Total Environment. 2017;**76**(2):223-235

[17] Bai Z, Zhang L, Wang X, Zhang L, Hu Y, et al. Health risk assessment for traffic policemen exposed to polycyclic aromatic hydrocarbons (PAHs) in Tianjin, China. Science of the Total Environment. 2007;**382**(2):240-250

[18] Chen H, Li B, Yang Q. Polycyclic aromatic hydrocarbons (PAHs) in indoor dusts of Guizhou, Southwest of China: Status, sources and potential human health risk. PLoS. 2015;**1**:1-17

[19] Toan VD, Thao VD, Walder J, Schmutz H-R, Ha CT. Level and distribution of polychlorinated biphenyls (PCBs) in surface soils from Hanoi, Vietnam. Bulletin of Environmental Contamination and Toxicology. 2007;**78**(351):360

[20] Thao VD, Toan VD, Kawano M. Temporal variation of persistent organochlorine residues in soils from Vietnam. In Proceeding of Interdisciplinary Studies on Environmental Chemistry; Environmental Research in Asia: Ehime, Japan; 2009. p. 73–82. ISBN 978-4-88704-148-6

[21] Nguyen NV. Occurrence of Persistent Toxic Substances in Soils, Sediments, Fishes and Human Breast Milk in Southern Vietnam [PhD thesis], École Polytechnique Fédérale De Lausanne: Lausanne; 2009

[22] Vietnam National Environment Agency (NEA). 2006. Vietnam National Plan for Treatment of Persistent Organic Pollutant (in Vietnamese). Available from: http://www.nea.gov.vn/thongtinmt/noidung/vnn_14_08_06.htm [Access on: 1 December 2016]

Chapter 6

Formaldehyde Advantages and Disadvantages: Usage Areas and Harmful Effects on Human Beings

Nuriye Tuna Subasi

Abstract

Formaldehyde, a simple but important member of aldehydes, is highly reactive due to its strong electrophilic properties. It is a colorless, pungent, low molecular weight poisonous gas that can rapidly pass into gaseous phase at room temperature, can burn, and can dissolve very well in water. Formaldehyde, which is found in the natural structure of the organism, is used in many places from industrial areas to household materials and from the production of coatings in dentistry to the determination of cadavers in laboratories. In addition to having such a wide range of uses, it has harmful effects on human health as it can react spontaneously with various cellular elements. In this review, which is based on various sources, detailed information about the definition, properties, usage areas, and harmful effects of formaldehyde will be given.

Keywords: formaldehyde, properties of formaldehyde, benefits, harmful effects on human beings, source of formaldehyde

1. Introduction

Formaldehyde – a simple but important member of aldehydes – is a colorless, pungent, highly flammable, irritating, and poisonous low molecular weight gas in its pure form, meanwhile it dissolves very well in water, alcohols, and other polar solvents. Due to its strong electrophilic properties, it is highly reactive, readily undergoes polymerization, and can form explosive mixtures in air. It decomposes at temperatures above 150°C to methanol and carbon monoxide. In addition, it is easily photooxidized to carbon dioxide in sunlight.

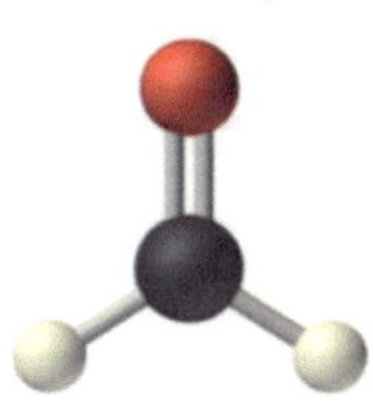

Formaldehyde

CH_2O

Pure formaldehyde is produced as a liquid through catalytic oxidation of methanol. This process is carried out in a closed facility and results in a formaldehyde

Formaldehyde (CH_2O)	
IUPAC name	**Methanal**
Chemical name	Formaldehyde, methylene oxide, oxymethylene, methyl aldehyde, oxomethane, formic aldehyde
Chemical formula	CH2O (HCHO)
Molecular weight	30.026 g/mol
Color	Clear, colorless liquid
Density	0.8153 g/cm3 (−20°C)
Melting point	93–96°C (at 37% concentration)
Boiling point	−15°C (at 37% concentration)

Table 1.
Physical and chemical properties of formaldehyde.

solution in the water together with methanol in various concentrations. This product may be further refined or converted to the paraformaldehyde (polymerized form of formaldehyde) which is in the form of a white powder or flake. Formaldehyde gas is slowly given by paraformaldehyde. Pure formaldehyde is not available commercially, so it is usually transported or stored as a 37% (by weight) aqueous solution, which is known as formalin [1, 2]. The technical (specific) properties of formaldehyde, which must be taken into account during use of it and also appropriate equipment should be used with it, are given in **Table 1**.

The most common methods for formaldehyde detection are based on spectrophotometry. Besides spectrophotometric ways other methods such as high-performance liquid chromatography, gas chromatography, colorimetry, infrared detection, fluorimetry, polarography, and gas detector tubes are also used. Organic and inorganic chemicals, such as sulfur dioxide, other aldehydes, and amines, can interfere with these detection methods. The most sensitive of these methods is flow injection, which has a detection limit of 9 ppt (0.011 $\mu g/m^3$) and is high-performance liquid chromatography, which offers a detection limit of 0.0017 ppm (0.002 mg/m^3) [3, 4].

Formaldehyde is found in small quantities in every human cell because it is taken from outside the organism or it is derived from the metabolism of serine, glycine, choline, and methionine [5, 6]. Formaldehyde is excreted from the body through urine and stool, by metabolizing formic acid catalyzed formaldehyde dehydrogenase (FDH) enzyme in the liver and erythrocytes, or excreted through respiration by converting to carbon dioxide [7–9]. Formaldehyde tends to combine strongly with protein, nucleic acids, and unsaturated fatty acids in a nonenzymatic way. This combination causes cytotoxicity, inflammatory reaction, necrosis, allergy, and mutagenic effect to be seen by producing denaturation in proteins. In addition, formaldehyde shows antimicrobial activity and function detection in tissues that have lost their vitality [7, 10, 11].

2. Formaldehyde, usage areas, and harmful effects

2.1 Usage areas

Formaldehyde is a chemical that is widely used due to its chemical properties and is also found in the natural structure of the organism. It is particularly important in the chemical industry because formaldehyde is an inexpensive starting material for a number of chemical reactions. It is used in the industrial field in the construction of plywood, chipboard, insulation materials, paint and plastic materials, textile industry, carpets, furniture, wall coverings, and household cleaning products [7, 12].

Formaldehyde is used in the storage of biological samples and mummification as it hardens proteins and prevents them from decomposition. Also, it is used as disinfectant because it kills insects and many microorganisms [13]. Formaldehyde, which has an important place in the field of medicine, is used in the anatomy laboratory for the determination of the cadaver and its long-term storage without decomposition and used in histology and pathology laboratories during the fixation stage of tissues. It is benefited from formaldehyde for the structure of coatings in dentistry, in the clinic for the treatment of persistent cystitis, and as a preservative in some drugs. In addition, the solution used in hemodialysis unit contains formalin [1, 14–16].

The use of formaldehyde in medical and other fields is 1.5% of the total production compared with its use in the manufacture of synthetic resins and chemical compounds. However, its use in these areas has great significance for human beings, because it can reach many people by means of various consumer goods. These products containing formaldehyde in medicinal and other technical areas are listed in **Table 2** [7].

Area	Use
Agriculture	Preservation of grain, seed dressing, soil disinfection, rot protection of feed, nitrogen fertilizer in soils, and protection of dietary protein in ruminants (animal nutrition)
Cleaning agent industry	Preservative in soaps, detergents, and cleaning agents against microbial contamination
Cosmetics industry	Preservative in soaps, deodorants, shampoos, etc. against microbial contamination; additive in nail hardeners, products for oral hygiene, makeup, hand cream, and shaving cream; and plant and equipment sanitation
Food industry	Preservation of dried foods, disinfection of containers, and preservation of fish and certain oils and fats, modifying starch for cold swelling
Leather industry	Additive to tanning agents
Medicine	Disinfection, sterilization, and preservation of preparations
Metal industry	Anticorrosive agent; vehicle in vapor depositing and electroplating processes
Petroleum industry	Biocide in oil well-drilling fluids and auxiliary agent in refining
Photographic industry	Developing accelerator and hardener for gelatin layers
Rubber industry	Biocide for latex, adhesive additive, and anti-oxidizer additive also for synthetic rubber
Sugar industry	Infection inhibitor in producing juices
Textile industry	Formaldehyde-releasing agents[a] provide crease resistance, dimensional stability, and flame retardance and binders in textile printing
Wood industry	Preservative

[a]Some preservatives are formaldehyde releasers. Formaldehyde release upon decomposition depends mainly on the temperature and pH. Industrial and household cleaning agents, soaps, shampoos, paints/lacquers, and cutting fluids have formed the most common product categories for formaldehyde releasers. The three most common recorded formaldehyde release agents are bromonitropropanediol, bromonitrodioxane, and 2-chloroallylhexaminium chloride [17].

Table 2.
Use of products containing formaldehyde in medicinal and other technical areas.

2.2 Impact area and harmful effects

Formaldehyde contains significant harm to human health as well as widespread use. Formaldehyde has a sharp odor that can be detectable at low concentrations, and its vapor and solutions are known as skin and eye irritants in human beings. The common effects of formaldehyde exposure are various symptoms caused by irritation of the mucosa in the eyes and upper respiratory tract.

Formaldehyde is classified by the International Cancer Research Institute as a Group 2A carcinogenic agent in 1995. As a result of the studies, formaldehyde is reported to contribute to the development of cancer of the nose and upper respiratory tract and skin cancer [18, 19].

OSHA has identified 52 professions that are risky in terms of formaldehyde exposure. The most frequently studied groups were the ones who were at risk for the effect of formaldehyde, which are listed below:

- Workers working at the production stage of formaldehyde-containing compounds
- Industry workers working in formaldehyde-containing products and adhesives (furniture and goods produced from the chipboard, MDF, plywood, varnish, lacquer, fire retardants, etc.)
- Workers in traffic or garages
- Anatomy, pathology, and histology laboratory staff (medicine and veterinary)
- Those who sterilize dialysis equipment and other medical supplies— dentists and nurses,
- Foundry employees
- Workers in paper, paper products, and recycling [20–22].

Research on persons working in industrial areas where formaldehyde production is performed or used showed that there is an increase in the number of people dying from brain cancer, blood cancer, and colon cancer compared to the normal population [2, 13]. Furthermore, the use of formaldehyde-containing products in homes and workplaces in daily life (wall paint, furniture, lacquer coatings, deodorants, cleaning products, etc.) and exposure to environmental factors (such as fuel oil and wood burning, exhaust gas, and cigarette smoke) further increase the impact of formaldehyde. It has been shown that formaldehyde, which is emphasized as carcinogenic by experimental studies, has harmful effects on many systems such as the respiratory system, nervous system, and digestive system [1, 7, 23]. Furthermore, it is stated that formaldehyde, which has adverse effects on the reproductive system, causes fertility problems by damaging to germinal cells, disrupts the morphological structure of testicle, and decreases sperm count and serum testosterone levels [24–26].

Formaldehyde is a genotoxic, mutagenic, teratogenic, embryotoxic, and carcinogenic chemical that includes gene mutations, chromosomal errors, single-chain fractures, sister chromatid exchange, and cell changes [2, 27, 28]. Respiratory system toxicity of formaldehyde occurs even in low concentrations (0.5 ppm). It causes clinical symptoms such as burning sensation in the nose and throat, difficulty of breathing, coughing, and wheezing in acute effects. At higher concentrations, pulmonary edema, inflammation, and pneumonia are developing [2, 11, 12, 29]. It is stated that among workers exposed to formaldehyde, the mortality rate of lung cancer is 30% higher [30, 31].

Formaldehyde has been reported to have toxic effects on the central nervous system, skin, eyes, testes, and menstrual functions as well as the respiratory system [24, 32, 33]. After oral ingestion, formaldehyde produces a local corrosive effect in the upper gastrointestinal system. Necrosis, perforation, and bleeding develop after following symptoms such as nausea, severe diarrhea, and abdominal pain. Then, circulatory failure and severe metabolic acidosis occur and result in death within a few days [1]. In addition, in some studies, it has been stated that formaldehyde inhibits the activity of some enzymes and increases some enzyme activity [13, 34].

Formaldehyde tends to perform toxic effects by combining strongly with DNA, RNA, protein, and unsaturated fatty acids in a nonenzymatic way [10]. The neurotoxicity effects of formaldehyde are shown up in the form of headache, dizziness, depression, insomnia, and loss of appetite, while in long-term exposure, permanent neurotoxicity such as mood disorders, behavioral disorders, and epilepsy occur [32, 35, 36].

2.3 Formaldehyde sources in the environment

Formaldehyde enters to the environment from natural sources (including forest fires) and comes directly from human resources. Formaldehyde occurs naturally in large quantities in the troposphere during the oxidation of hydrocarbons. These hydrocarbons react with OH radicals and ozone forming formaldehyde and/or other aldehydes as intermediates in a series of reactions resulting in the formation of carbon monoxide and carbon dioxide, hydrogen, and water [37, 38]. In addition, terpenes and isoprene spread around by foliage and react with the OH radicals to form formaldehyde as an intermediate product. Because of their short lifetimes, this potentially important formaldehyde source is only important around the vegetation [39].

Human sources of formaldehyde include direct sources such as industrial uses in the field, fuel combustion, and off-gassing from building materials and consumer products. Formaldehyde, although is not present in gasoline, is an incomplete combustion product and consequently is released from internal combustion engines. The formaldehyde amount produced depends mainly on the composition of the fuel, the type of engine, the emission control applied, the operating temperature, and the age and condition of the vehicle being repaired. Therefore, emission rates are variable.

The major man-made sources affecting human beings are in the indoor environment. Primary sources (covering a range of fuels from wood to plastics) include cigarette smoke, chipboard and plywood, wood-burning stoves, fireplaces, furnaces, power plants, agricultural burns, furniture and fabrics, waste incinerators, gas from by heating systems, and cooking [40–47].

Furniture made from wood materials are widely used in indoor and outdoor living spaces. Depending on the developments in the glue sector, the rate of using synthetic materials in the furniture industry is increasing. This situation brings with it air pollution. Urea-formaldehyde (UF) glue, which is the most widely used adhesive for wood paneling and furniture production around the world, is one of the most common contaminants in indoor environments. For this reason, formaldehyde can be found in our daily indoor areas, in homes and in offices. Formaldehyde release value can be increased by increasing the ambient temperature and humidity. The formaldehyde level should normally be below 0.03 ppm in indoor environments. The level at which symptoms occurred was determined as 0.10–1.1 ppm range [18, 48].

Therefore, the indoor formaldehyde levels are clearly different from the concentrations in the outdoor air. Temperature, humidity, ventilation rate, age of the building, product usage, the presence of combustion sources, and the smoking habits of occupants affect indoor formaldehyde concentrations.

3. Conclusion

As a result, since formaldehyde has a harmful and even toxic effect on many tissues and organs in the body, it is necessary to keep the formaldehyde concentration below the 0.3 ppm level, which is the permitted limit in formaldehyde-working environments.

In macroscopic anatomy laboratories where formaldehyde is used more frequently, some precautions should be taken to prevent the harmful effects of formaldehyde. For this purpose, a sufficient concentration of 10% should not be exceeded for the determination of a suitable tissue. Materials waiting for detection should be closed in a way that does not contain air. The area in which the macroscopic examination is performed must be equipped to remove the formaldehyde vapor immediately from the environment. Laboratory personnel with chronic conjunctivitis and upper and lower respiratory diseases are removed from this environment until they are completely passed. The contact times of formaldehyde should be reduced as much as possible by providing appropriate conversions between laboratory personnel.

In addition, employees should be trained on environmental risk factors, toxic chemicals and protection from risk factors, and the use of gloves and masks, and it is also necessary to identify and map important emission areas and operations and to arrange/adjust the existing equipment [28, 49, 50]. Measures to be taken to against emission sources include increased ventilation, treatment of cadavers, and tissues with ammonium chloride in anatomy laboratories [51], covering machines, the use of local exhaust systems [52], and improvement of general ventilation [53]. Taking these measures in environments exposed to formaldehyde is necessary to reduce the exposure and minimize the health effects that may occur.

In spite of all these harmful effects, formaldehyde is still in use all over the world because of its cheap and good detection solution.

Author details

Nuriye Tuna Subasi
Department of Food Engineering, Ahi Evran University, Kırşehir, Turkey

*Address all correspondence to: tunasubasi@gmail.com

References

[1] Smith AE. Formaldehyde. Occupational Medicine. 1992;**42**:83-88

[2] Shaham J, Bomstein Y, Meltzer A, Kaufman Z, Palma E, Ribak J. DNA-protein crosslinks, a biomark.er of exposure to formaldehyde in vitro and in vivo studies. Carcinogenesis. 1996;**17**:121-125

[3] Fan Q, Dasgupta PK. Continuous automated determination of atmospheric formaldehyde at the parts per trillion level. Analytical Chemistry. 1994;**66**(4):551-556

[4] IARC Monographs on the Evaluation of Carcinogenic Risks to Humans. Wood Dust and Formaldehyde. Vol. 62. Lyon: International Agency for Research on Cancer; 1995. pp. 217-375

[5] Unsaldi E, Ciftci MK. Formaldehyde and its using areas, risk group, harmful effects and protective precautions against it. YYU Journal of Veterinary Faculty. 2010;**21**(1):71-75

[6] International Program on Chemical Safety (IPCS). Formaldehyde. In: Environmental Health Criteria. Vol. 89. Geneva: World Health Organisation; 1989. pp. 11-176

[7] Usanmaz SE, Akarsu ES, Vural N. Neurotoxic effects of acute and subacute formaldehyde exposures in mice. Environmental Toxicology and Pharmacology. 2002; **11**:93-100

[8] Eells JT, Mc Martin KE, Black K, Vırayotha V, Tısdell RH, Tephly TR. Formaldehyde poisoning. Rapid metabolism to formic acid. Journal of the American Medical Association. 1981;**246**:1237-1238

[9] Koivusalo M, Koivula T, Uotila L. Oxidation of formaldehyde by nicotinamid dependent dehydrogenases. Progress in Clinical and Biological Research. 1982;**114**:155-168

[10] Bolt HM. Experimental toxicology of formaldehyde. Journal of Cancer Research and Clinical Oncology. 1987;**113**:305-309

[11] Heck H, Casanova M. Pharmacodynamics of formaldehyde. Applications of a model for the arrest of DNA replication by DNA-protein cross- links. Toxicology and Applied Pharmacology. 1999;**160**:86-100

[12] Blair A, Stewart PA, Hoover RN. Mortality from lung cancer among workers employed in formaldehyde industries. American Journal of Industrial Medicine. 1990;**17**:683-699

[13] Schlink K, Janßen K, Nitzsche S, Gebhard S, Hengstler JG, Klein S, et al. Activity of O6-methylguanine DNA methyltransferase in mononuclear blood cells of formaldehyde-exposed medical students. Archives of Toxicology. 1999;**73**:15-21

[14] Khanzadeh FA, Vaquerano MU, Khanzadeh MA, Bisesi MS. Formaldehyde exposure, acute pulmoner response and exposure control options in a gross anatomy laboratory. American Journal of Industrial Medicine. 1994;**26**:61-68

[15] Cohen BI, Pagnillo MK, Musikant BL, Deutsch AS. Formaldehyde evaluation from endodontic materials. Oral Health. 1998;**88**:37-39

[16] Sarnak MJ, Long J, King AJ. Intravesicular formaldehyde instillation and renal complications. Clinical Nephrology. 1999;**51**:122-125

[17] Flyvholm MA, Andersen P. Identification of formaldehyde releasers and occurrence of formaldehyde and formaldehyde releasers in registered

chemical products. American Journal of Industrial Medicine. 1993;**24**:533-552

[18] Soysal A, Demiral Y. Indoor air pollution. TAF Preventive Medicine Bulletin. 2007;**6**(3):221-226

[19] Muzi G, Dell'omo M, Murgia N, Abritti G. Chemical pollution of indoor air and its effect on health. Giornale Italiano di Medicina del Lavoro ed Ergonomia. 2004;**26**(4):364-369

[20] Rosenstock L, Cullen MR, Brodkin CA, Redlich CA. Textbook of Clinical Occupational and Environmental Medicine. 2nd ed. China: Elsevier Saunders; 2005

[21] Pecka I, Wiglusz R, Madeja-Gryzb A, DziewanowskaPudliszak A. Formaldehyde emissions from wooden products and office furniture. Roczniki Państwowego Zakładu Higieny. 2001;**52**(1):49-54

[22] Tanaka K, Nishiyama K, Yaginuma H, Sasaki A, Maeda T, Kaneko SY, et al. Formaldehyde exposure levels and exposure control measures during an anatomy dissecting course. Kaibogaku Zasshi. 2003;**78**(2):43-51

[23] Zararsiz I, Kus I, Akpolat N, Songur A, Ogeturk M, Sarsilmaz M. Protective effects of O-3 essential fatty acids against formaldehyde-induced neuronal damage in prefrontal cortex of rats. Cell Biochemistry and Function. 2006a;**24**:237-244

[24] Chowdhury AR, Gautam AK, Patel KG, Trivedi HS. Steroidogenic inhibition in testicular tissue of formaldehyde exposed rats. Indian Journal of Physiology and Pharmacology. 1992;**36**:162-168

[25] Thrasher JD, Kilburn KH. Embryo toxicity and teratogenicity of formaldehyde. Archives of Environmental Health. 2001;**56**: 300-311

[26] Özen OA, Akpolat N, Songur A. Effect of formaldehyde inhalation on Hsp70 in seminiferous tubules of rat testes: An immunohistochemical study. Toxicology and Industrial Health. 2005;**21**:249-254

[27] Casanova M, Heck HAD, Everitt JI, Harrington WW, Popp JA. Formaldehyde concentrations in the blood of rhesus monkeys after inhalation exposure. Food and Chemical Toxicology. 1988;**26**:715-716

[28] McLaughlin JK. Formaldehyde and cancer. International Archives of Occupational and Environmental Health. 1994;**66**:295-301

[29] Kriebel D, Myers D, Cheng M, Woskie S, Cocanour B. Short term effect of formaldehyde on peak expiratory flow and irritant symptoms. Archives of Environmental Health. 2001;**56**:11-18

[30] Halperin WE, Goodman M, Stayner L, Elliot LJ, Keenlyside RA, Landrigan PJ. Nasal cancer in a worker exposed to formaldehyde. Journal of the American Medical Association. 1983;**249**:510-512

[31] Hayes RB, Raatgever JW, de Bruyn A, Gerin M. Cancer of the nasal cavity and paranasal sinuses and formaldehyde exposure. Indian Journal of Cancer. 1986;**37**:487-492

[32] Kilburn KH, Warshaw R, Thornton JC. Formaldehyde impairs memory, equilibrium, and dexterity in histology technicians: Effects which persist for days after exposure. Archives of Environmental Health. 1987;**42**:117-120

[33] Hayasaka Y, Hayasaka S, Nagaki Y. Ocular changes after intravitreal injection of methanol, formaldehyde, or formate in rabbits. Pharmacology & Toxicology. 2001;**89**(2):74-78

[34] Cassee FR, Feron VJ. Biochemical and histopathological changes in nasal epithelium of rats after 3-day intermittent exposure to formaldehyde and ozone alone or in combination. Toxicology Letters. 1994;**72**:257-268

[35] Stroup NE, Blair A, Erikson GE. Brain cancer and other causes of deaths in anatomists. Journal of the National Cancer Institute. 1986;**77**:1217-1224

[36] Kilburn KH. Neurobehavioral impairment and seizures from formaldehyde. Archives of Environmental Health. 1994;**49**:37-44

[37] Zimmermann PR, Chatfield RB, Fishman J, Crutzen PJ, Hanst PL. Estimates on the production of CO and H2 from the oxidation of hydrocarbon emissions from vegetation. Geophysical Research Letters. 1978;**5**:679-682

[38] Calvert JG. The Homogeneous Chemistry of Formaldehyde: Generation and Destruction within the Atmosphere. Washington, DC: Federal Aviation Agency; 1980. pp. 153-190

[39] Lowe DC, Schmidt U, Ehhalt DH. The Tropospheric Distribution of Formaldehyde. Jülich: Kernforschungsanlage; 1981. (Chemie Institut 3: No. 1756)

[40] Jermini C, Weber A, Grandjean E. Quantitative determination of various gas-phase components of the side-stream smoke of cigarettes in the room air as a contribution to the problem of passive smoking. International Archives of Occupational and Environmental Health. 1976;**36**:169-181

[41] Kitchens JF, Casner RE, Edwards GS, Harward WE, Macri BJ Investigation of Selected Potential Environmental Contaminants: Formaldehyde. Washington, DC: US Environmental Protection Agency; 1976. p. 204. (EPA 560/2-76-009)

[42] Klus H, Kuhn H. Distribution of different components of tobacco smoke between main-current and side-current smoke. Beiträge zur Tabakforschung International. 1982;**11**:229-265

[43] Ramdahl T, Alfheim I, Rustad S, Olsen T. Chemical and biological characterization of emissions from small residential stove burning wood and charcoal. Chemosphere. 1982;**11**(4):601-611

[44] Schriever E, Marutzky R, Merkel D. Examination of emissions from small wood-fired combustion furnaces. Staub - Reinhaltung der Luft. 1983;**43**:62-65

[45] Lipari F, Dasch JM, Scruggs WF. Aldehyde emissions from wood-burning fireplaces. Environmental Science & Technology. 1984;**18**:326-330

[46] Walker BL, Cooper CD. Air pollution emission factors for medical waste incinerators. Journal of the Air & Waste Management Association. 1992;**42**:784-791

[47] Baker DC. Projected emissions of hazardous air pollutants from a Shell coal gasification process-combined-cycle power plant. Fuel. 1994;**73**(7):1082-1086

[48] Marutzky R. Release of Formaldehyde by Wood Products. Forest Product Society. Report No: 94RS100R; 1994

[49] Rosen G, Andersson IM, Juringe L. Reduction of exposure to solvents and formaldehyde in surface-coating operations in the woodworking industry. The Annals of Occupational Hygiene. 1990;**34**(3):293-303

[50] Priha E, Pennanen S, Rantio T, Uitti J, Liesivuori J. Exposure to and acute effects of medium-density fiber board dust. Journal of Occupational and Environmental Hygiene. 2004;**1**(11):738-744

[51] Kawamata S, Kodera H. Reduction of formaldehyde concentrations in the air and cadaveric tissues by ammonium carbonate. Anatomical Science International. 2004;**79**(3):152-157

[52] Linnainmaa M, Kiviranta H, Laitinen J, Laitinen S. Control of workers' exposure to airborne endotoxins and formaldehyde during the use of metalworking fluids. AIHA Journal. 2003;**64**(4):496-500

[53] Hiipakka DW, Dyrdahl KS, Garcia Cardenas M. Successful reduction of mortician's exposure to formaldehyde during embalming procedures. AIHAJ-American Industrial Hygiene Association. 2001;**62**(6):689-696

Section 3

Relationship of Heavy Metals - Nanomaterials

Chapter 7

Biomedical Applications of Nanomaterials: Nanotubes and Metal-Organic Frameworks (MOFs)

Miguel Martell-Mendoza, Cuauhtémoc Pérez-González, Hiram I. Beltrán, Roberto Serrano-Vega and Carlos Alberto Méndez-Cuesta

Abstract

Nanomedicine plays an important role in the diagnosis, treatment, monitoring and control of biological systems in the area of nanotechnology and has been referred by the National Institute of Health (NIH) as an emergent way of medicine. Nanoparticles are new delivery vehicles with the ability to release drugs to a specific cell type or tissue, which may also improve the pharmacological activity of those drugs by controlling their release, as well as prolonging their short half-lives in blood. The aim of this review is to gather several options of MOFs and nanotubes synthesised with different nanoparticles and processes, some including compound loading and release studies, with particular focus on 13 anti-cancer compounds e.g. doxorubicin, curcumin, methotrexate, etc.; 3 anti-inflammatory compounds, namely ibuprofen, salicylic acid and chlorogenic acid; and with 5 miscellaneous bioactive compounds, including rifampicin, griseofulvin, enoxacin, etc. Finally, other biomedical applications for these composites are shown, like being enzyme immobilisation agents, for water treatment e.g. in swimming pools, and other becoming support to carry & secure integrity of drugs.

Keywords: nano MOFs, nanotubes, drug delivery, biomedical applications, composite materials

1. Introduction

Any material could be described as a (semi) solid entity, substance or device that things could be made from, with the purpose to resolve a present or future need. There are a lot of daily examples that we are able define as materials, for instance, cloth, wood and electronic devices, such as computers, cell phones and smart TVs. Materials could be divided into natural and synthetic groups and, at the same time, they are commonly classified depending on their composition or physicochemical properties. Nowadays, the search for synthetic materials has been fast growing, because of their electrical, thermal, mechanical, structural and in many cases, their emergent properties, that make them suitable for many fields of science.

IntechOpen

In recent years, the development and modification of materials at the nanoscale for biomedical purposes has been extensively reported in the literature. One of the most significant of these has been the encapsulation or capture of drugs with the purpose of increasing dosage, providing protection against body's metabolism and directing the drug to the therapeutic target or a specific site. Despite these benefits, the principal limitations include the host-guest compatibility, very closely related with toxicity, the degradation and the half-life of the nanomaterial. For this reason, these side studies should be included when a new material is developed for biomedical purposes.

Metal Organic Frameworks (MOFs) are a class of microporous 1D, 2D or 3D crystalline materials, constructed from a metal ion held together by organic polyfunctional ligands, that confer special characteristics to this arrangement. Some of these features are their high/tunable surface area, homogenous porosity, their great stability and crystallinity, among other. Due to these characteristics, MOFs are widely applied in the storage and separation of gases, as sensors, and in matrices to capture/deliver a large amount of several kinds of molecules and in particular drugs even showing specificity towards therapeutic targets and thus improving the effect of the drugs and their bioavailability.

Besides, nanotubes have the potential to revolutionise biomedical research, due to their important electrical, chemical, thermal, mechanical and structural properties which have made them an area of great research interest. With this in mind, they are capable to display metallic, semiconducting and superconducting electron transport properties. Although carbon nanotubes (CNTs) are the most common, they also could be constructed from peptides and organometallic moieties or materials. The CNTs could be used in numerous applications, including nanofluidic systems, biopharmaceutical applications such as drug delivery, implantable biomedical devices, diagnostic tools and devices in radiation oncology, biosensors, probes and quantum dots, such as nanosensors and nanorobots and also for tissue engineering applications [1].

Hence, the gathering criteria of all these research examples in this chapter is focused on evidencing some of the most relevant examples from the last 5 years (2014–2018) in terms of nanomaterials, with capability to act as (i) drug delivery systems and for (ii) general biomedical applications, addressing aspects such as the composition of these materials, type of loaded/tested/delivered drugs interacting with both, (nano) MOFs or nanotube materials and their perspectives on the synthesis and modification of these new composites for such applicability.

2. Drug delivery

2.1 Anti-cancer

In this first contribution, the MIL-100(Fe) was prepared using a hydrothermal microwave-assisted method. Synthetic procedure required a mixture of $FeCl_3$ hexahydrate and 1,3,5-benzenetricarboxylic acid settled in deionised water, which was heated at 130°C during a period of 6 min. The characterisation of the crystalline substance was performed by X-ray powder diffraction (XRPD), meanwhile particle size and morphology were determined by Dynamic Light Scattering (DLS) and Transmission Electron Microscopy (TEM). Additionally, surface morphology was characterised using Field-Emission Scanning Electron Microscopy (FESEM) and the pore size was determined by nitrogen sorption experiments. The measured Langmuir surface was of 1350 ± 100 $m^2\ g^{-1}$. The pore size of this material measured a free diameter of *ca.* 25 and 29 Å, which is accessible through the pentagonal and hexagonal microporous windows present in this material (5.5 and 8.6 Å). The incorporation of doxorubicin (DOXO) in MIL-100(Fe) was determined by UV-Vis, circular dichroism (CD) and fluorescence spectroscopies, and the determined concentration of DOXO present in this material was 9 wt% (**Figure 1**) [2].

In this other piece of work, Gemcitabine-5′-monophosphate (Gem-MP) was appropriately loaded into MIL-100(Fe) MOF material, reaching a top concentration of 30.7 ± 0.8 wt%; this was confirmed by High Performance Liquid Chromatography (HPLC) and radioactivity counting methods (**Figure 2**). The Gem-MP@MIL-100(Fe) release studies were performed in PBS media and 100% of release of this drug molecule was reached at 4 h. The Half Maximal Inhibitory Concentration (IC_{50}) of both empty and loaded materials were tested in pancreatic cancer cell lines (PANC-1) using the MTT method. This experiment has shown that the unloaded material had no effect on the viability of cells. However, when Gem-MP and Gem-MP@MIL-100(Fe) were tested, the IC_{50} were 17.5 μM and 45 nM, respectively. This finding clearly confirmed that the activity of Gem-MP is improved *ca.* 389 times when it is loaded into MIL-100(Fe) material [3].

Moreover, a phytochemical-ligand-containing metal-organic framework of the formula {[Zn_2(fer)$_2$]}n, (Zn-fer MOF) was prepared, where the organic ligand named H_2fer = ferulic acid, and its structural elucidation revealed the presence of large nanocage-based pores suitable for ionic or molecular guest incorporation. With the latter in mind, Zn-fer MOF was employed as interaction matrix for the adsorption and *in vitro* carriage of 5-fluorouracil (5-FU), obtaining 5-FU@Zn-fer material. The ability of 5-FU@Zn-fer to deliver 5-FU, biodegradation and cytotoxicity assays were also determined. Additionally, the grand canonical ensemble Monte Carlo (GCMC) simulation was performed to *in silico* investigate the loading of 5-FU to Zn-fer at the molecular level. With these results, authors determined that 5-FU could be adsorbed into this BioMOF with a high loading. GCMC simulations validated the experimental trend, showing that 5-FU could be incorporated into desolvated Zn-fer MOF reaching loadings as high as 0.388 g g^{-1}. The analysis of radial distribution function (RDF) and configuration snapshot analysis, showed that the most important interaction between 5-FU and Zn-fer MOF are hydrogen bonding and dipolar interactions (**Figure 3**). Furthermore, the delivery of 5-FU occurred within 100 h and at that time, 99% of the loaded drug was already released. For further sights, this may lead to the desired modulated release of anti-cancer agents over a long-time and probably reducing side-effects for patients. Finally, according

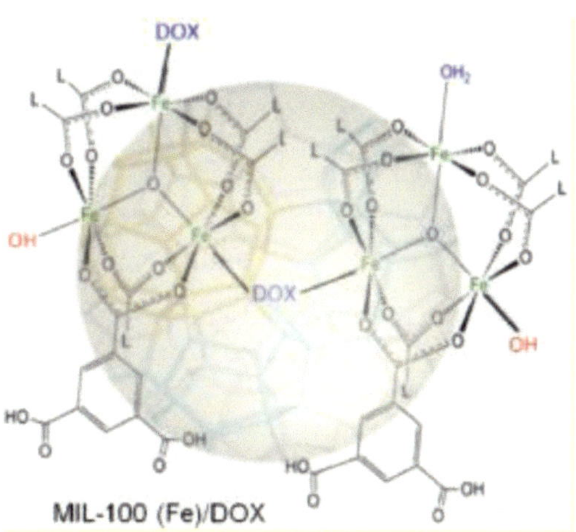

Figure 1.
MIL-100 (Fe)/DOX [2].

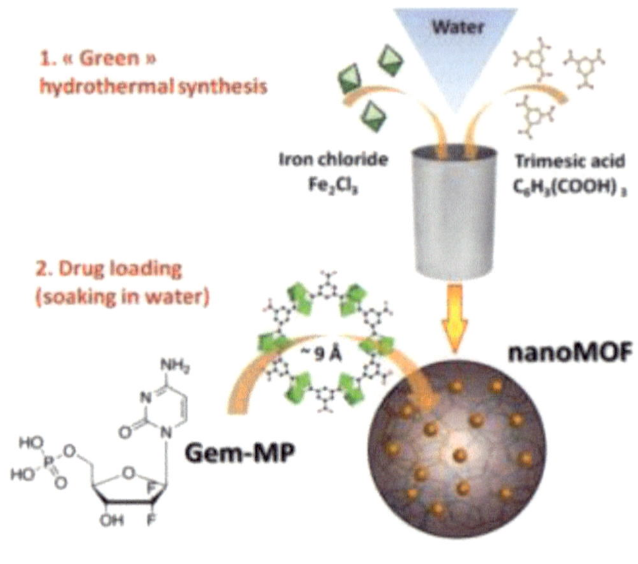

Figure 2.
Representation of Gem-MP encapsulation into MIL-100(Fe) [3].

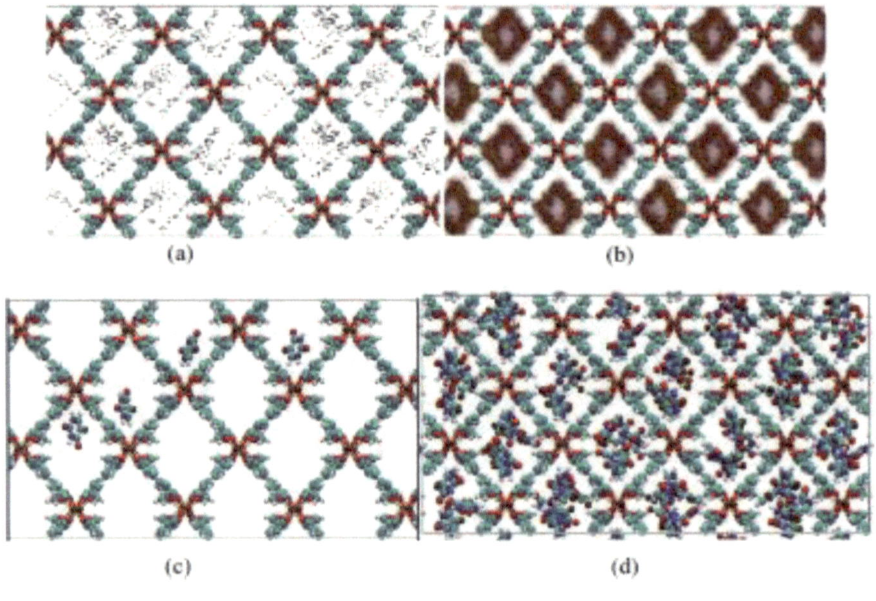

Figure 3.
The density of 5-FU under 10-5 mPa, 1 mPa for (a) and (b) (top pictures) and the snapshot of 5-FU in Znfer-MOF for (c) and (d) (down pictures) [4].

to our criteria, this investigation has provided impetus to design and develop similar structured biocompatible MOFs which are able to offer relatively superior drug carrying and drug release properties [4].

Some other investigation aims for the incorporation of target molecules based on a multistep post-functionalization procedure. In the cited research, the authors report a novel approach combining MOF synthesis and molecule encapsulation in a one-pot process. Researchers have therein demonstrated that large molecules are appropriate to be entrapment in the composite zeolitic imidazolate framework (ZIF). The distribution was homogeneous into the ZIF, and in this way their loadings could be improvement. The ZIF-8 crystals were carried with DOXO to obtain DOXO@ZIF-8 composites, like efficient drug delivery vehicles for cancer therapy using pH-dependent release (**Figure 4**). The DOXO@ZIF-8 showed higher efficiency than DOXO against breast cancer cell lines, due to well-known composite enhancements. This one-pot process opens new possibilities to construct multifunctional delivery systems for a wide range of applications [5].

The incorporation of drugs in biodegradable polymeric particles is one of many processes that controllably and significantly increase their release and action. The synthesis and physicochemical characterisation of ZnBDC-MOF (MOF-5) + DOXO giving place to DOXO@ZnBDC hybrid, and the effectiveness of this composite in the sustained release of the DOXO drug has been described. In a first procedure, the MOF-5 was obtained by mixing sodium terephthalate (Na_2BDC), $Zn(NO_3)_2{\cdot}6H_2O$ and H_2O; the suspension was then transferred to a CEM (Microwave reactor) S-Class System with vessel temperature set at 120°C. The loading of DOXO into MOF-5 was performed by stirring 0.034 g of the dehydrated MOF-5 powder in 4 mL of aqueous solution containing 0.1 g of DOXO during 1 day interaction period. An experimental and theoretical study is presented of the interaction between the MOF-5 material and DOXO molecule (**Figure 5**). The synthesis was carried on, and the resulting material was characterised by elemental analysis and XRPD. The experimental incorporation was accomplished and analysed by Fourier Transform Infrared Spectroscopy (FTIR) and UV-Vis spectroscopies, as well as by XRPD. An analysis of the adsorption of the DOXO@ZnBDC system confirmed the successful incorporation of the drug, revealing 0.0163 g of DOXO included into the composite, or an equivalent to 96% of the drug. The stability and drug release profile of DOXO@ZnBDC confirmed that the system released DOXO in a sustained or bimodal manner, like other systems, releasing 51.4% of the DOXO molecule in 48 h. The behaviour described in the article demonstrates that the DOXO@ZnBDC system has the potential against cytotoxic cancer cell lines NCI-H292 (human pulmonary mucoepidermoid carcinoma), HT-29 (human colorectal adenocarcinoma) and MCF-7 (human breast adenocarcinoma). The cytotoxic effect, an intensity scale for the cytotoxic potential of the system under study, was as stated in the following tendency related to cell growth inhibition [CGI], zero activity, ranging from 1 to 20%; little activity, 20–50%; moderate activity, 50–70%; and significant activity, 70–100%. *In vitro* cytotoxicity of unloaded MOF-5 was HT29 CGI = 72.6%, MCF-7 CGI = 47.4%, NCI-H-292 CGI = 77.0%; for free DOXO, HT29 CGI = 57.0%, MCF-7 CGI = 55.2%, NCI-H-292 CGI = 76.3%; and for DOXO@ZnBDC was HT29 CGI = 70.7%; MCF-7 CGI = 20.1%; NCI-H-292 CGI = 26.4% at different

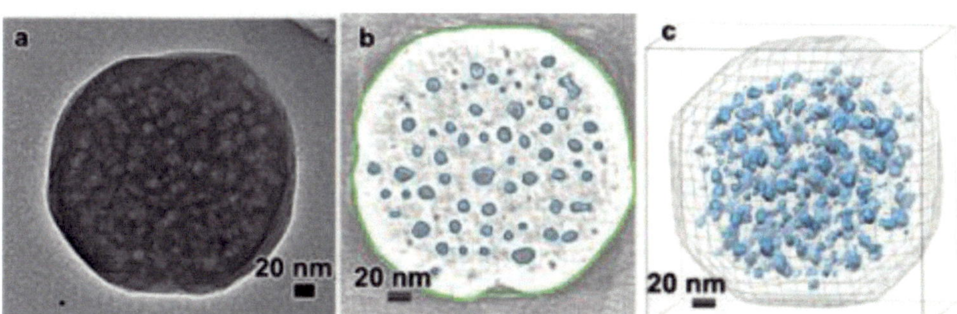

Figure 4.
Distribution of mesopores in DOX@ZIF-8 particles illustrated by electron tomography. (a) TEM image of a DOX@ZIF-8 single crystal. (b) Cross-section of the electron tomogram with the mesopores marked by blue lines. (c) 3D distribution of the mesopores in the DOX@ZIF-8 particles [5].

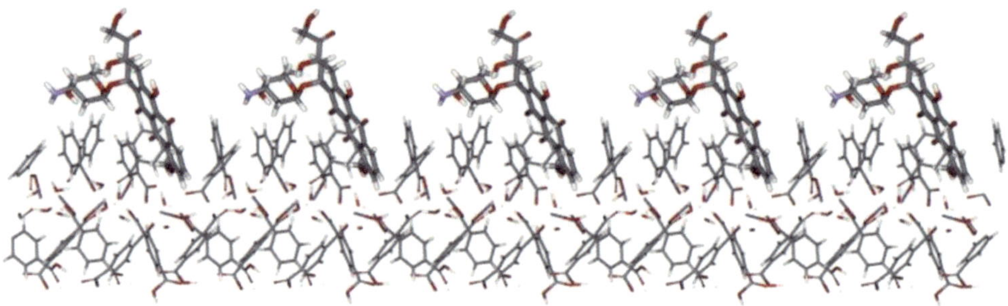

Figure 5.
Simulated adsorption of the DOXO in surface of MOF by means of PM6 calculation [6].

concentrations after 72 h. As can be seen, the MCF-7 & NCI-H-292 proved to be the most sensitive strains, because of the activity of composite material [6].

Another work of ZIF-8 crystal as a functional material was used to control the release of an autophagy inhibitor, 3-methyladenine (3-MA), and avoid the decomposition of large quantities of the drug and enhance their bioavailability (**Figure 6**). The HeLa cells treated with 3-MA@ZIF-8 NPs has shown that the autophagosome development was successfully blocked. The pH-sensitive dissociation rises the efficiency of autophagy inhibition at the same concentration of 3-MA. *In vivo* test data showed higher efficacy to repress the expression of autophagy-related markers, Beclin 1 and LC3, in 3-MA@ZIF-8 NPs more than free 3-MA. Some of the most important features underlined by the authors is that ZIF-8 resulted an efficient drug delivery vehicle in antitumor therapy, especially in inhibiting autophagy of cancer cells. The cytotoxicity of 3-MA@ZIF-8 nanoparticles was evaluated by determining cellular viability through an MTT assay. The 3-MA@ZIF-8 NPs system was found to be toxic to HeLa cells in a dose-dependent manner, after treatment at a concentration of 7.5 μg mL^{-1} (equivalent to a concentration of 3-MA of 1.5 μg mL^{-1}) for 24 h. The values were even lower after the cells had been treated with 3-MA@ZIF-8 NPs at a concentration of 10 μg mL^{-1} [7].

Following the versatility of ZIF-8 system, in other studies, DOXO was loaded into this MOF via a one pot process. The *in situ* loading process implied the water dissolution of the DOXO bioactive at 4 mg mL^{-1}, then 0.2 g (0.66 mmol) of $Zn(NO_3)_2{\cdot}6H_2O$ were dissolved in 0.8 mL of water, into which 4 mL of DOXO solution was added. After that 2 g of 2-methylimidazole were dissolved in 8 mL water and this was slowly dropped into the previous mixture. The *in situ* assembled DOXO@ZIF-8 composite was then coated with polydopamine, successively chelated with Fe^{3+} and conjugated with hyaluronic acid (HA). Finally, all these resulted in a multifunctional ZIF-8 nanocarrier of DOXO@ZIF@HA nature (**Figure 7**).

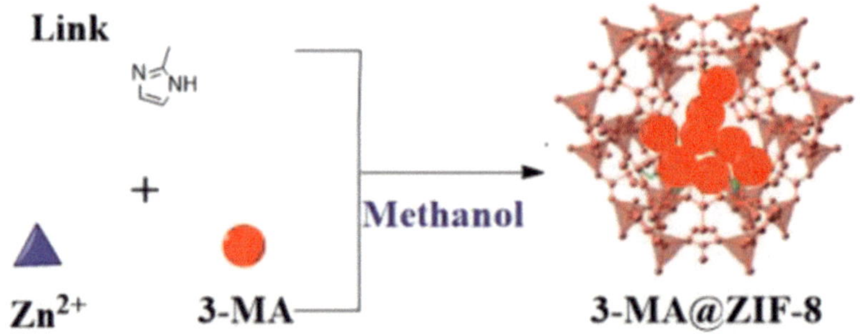

Figure 6.
Schematic representation of 3-MA@ZIF-8 [7].

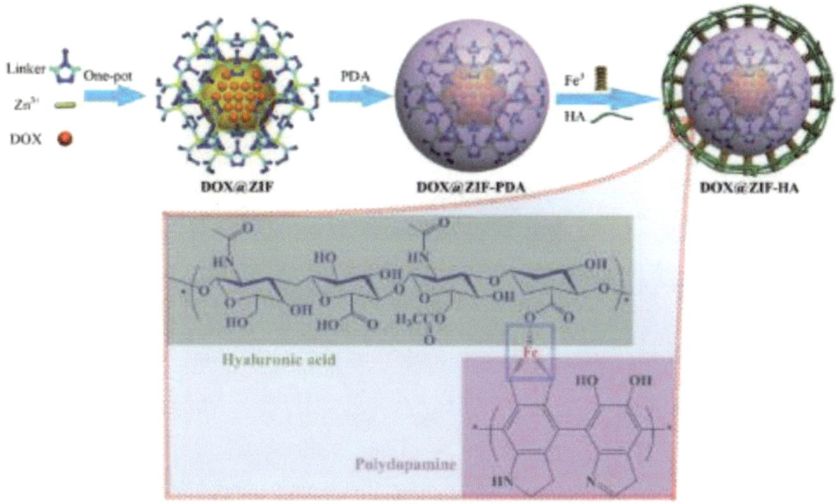

Figure 7.
Diagram for the preparation of DOX@ZIF-HA and the Fe^{3+}-mediated coordination interaction between HA and PDA [8].

The characterisation results confirmed the successful formation of the hybrid nanocarrier. The loading efficacy was determined to be 8.92 ± 0.53%. The data suggest that the release of DOXO from the nanocarrier demonstrated a sustained nature, but in this case regardless of the pH value. The cumulative amount of DOXO released at pH 5.0 and 7.4 was 70.1 and 9.8%, respectively, clearly showing a pH dependent behavior. The results of flow cytometry and confocal laser scanning microscope shown the targeting ability of DOXO@ZIF-HA towards prostate cancer PC-3 cells. In order to make notice the effect of composite assembly, the therapeutic efficacy of DOXO@ZIF-HA was clearly improved when compared with free DOXO. The cells were treated with different formulations of free DOXO and DOXO@ZIF-HA for 24 h and untreated cells were used as a control. At a DOXO concentration of 1 mg mL^{-1}, the cell viability for free DOXO and DOXO@ZIF-HA was 65.61 and 48.59%, respectively. This is mainly since the efficient internalisation of the targeted carrier DOXO@ZIF-HA could improve the intracellular DOXO concentration. Hence, authors state that the constructed ZIF-8 based multifunctional nanocarrier could be a candidate for cancer theranostics [8].

Another method to effectively carry DOXO to the breast cancer sites is the use of halloysite nanotubes (HNTs) coated with poly(ethylene glycol) (PEG) and folate (HNTs-PEG-FA), which have been used as drug delivery systems. The HNTs were reduced to ~200 nm by ultrasonic scission and then functionalised with N-hydroxylsuccinimide-polyethylene glycol carboxylic acid (NHS-PEG-COOH) and folate (FA) moieties. The DOXO@HNTs-PEG-FA was prepared by filling with DOXO on HNTs-PEG-FA via physical adsorption (**Figure 8**). The maximum release of DOXO from DOXO@HNTs-PEG-FA was reached to 35 h at pH 5.3. The DOXO@HNTs-PEG-FA ensemble showed significant inhibition of proliferation and induction of apoptosis in MCF-7 cells with positive FA receptors but this is not true for L02 cells without FA receptors. The *in vivo* anti-breast cancer activity of DOXO@HNTs-PEG-FA was confirmed using 4T1-bearing mice. The DOXO@HNTs-PEG-FA reduced toxicity and inhibited tumour growth associated with higher levels of caspase-3 protein. These results suggest that FA-conjugated HNTs may be designed to be a novel drug delivery system for targeted therapy of breast cancer via intravenous [9].

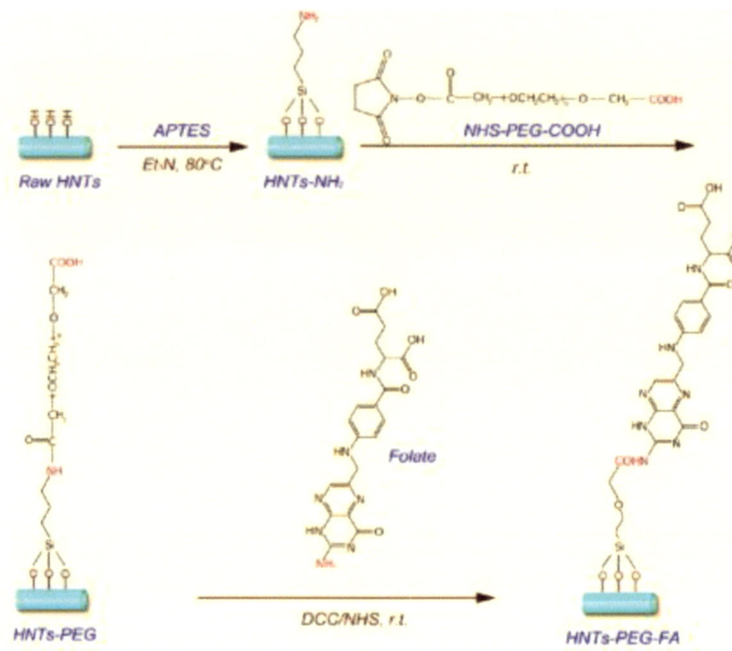

Figure 8.
Schematic representation of HNTs-PEG-FA preparation [9].

Another drug delivery strategy is when some peptides were used in the synthesis of nanotubes capable of this method of carrying. Nanotubes was synthetized using two dipeptides based on their flexibility, one of them using the Phe-Phe backbone (βPhe-Phe and βPhe-ΔPhe); containing βPhe amino acid, and the other containing βPhe like a backbone constraining ΔPhe (α,β-dehydrophenylalanine) amino acid. Both were characterised by X-ray diffraction, DLS, TEM, FTIR and CD. Small drugs like riboflavin, DOXO, chloramphenicol and chloroquine, were tested in encapsulation experiments in these new nanotubes. The results have shown comparable encapsulation in both types of nanotubes, and the loaded contents were 7, 15, 35 and 18%, respectively. Moreover, these dipeptides have not shown cytotoxicity towards HeLa (cervical uterine cancer), B6F10 (melanoma mouse) and L-929 (fibroblast mouse) cells with different concentrations of peptide nanostructure. Mitoxantrone free and encapsulated in βPhe-Phe and βPhe-Phe/βPhe-ΔPhe nanotubes was tested in equals amounts against cell lines HeLa and B6F10. The viability of HeLa cells treated with free mitoxantrone at 3 mg mL^{-1} was 77%, while when encapsulated in βPhe-Phe or βPhe-ΔPhe nanotubes, the viability reduced to 58 and 53%, respectively. However, the value of viability for B6F10 cells changed from 85 to 60% and 31%, respectively. These results suggest that administration of mitoxantrone with dipeptide nanotubes was more effective against HeLa and B6F10 cancerous cells [10].

There are reports that by combining the advantage of multi-walled carbon nanotubes (MWCNTs) and interpolymer supramolecular complexes, a new carrier system consisting of poly (acrylic acid)/PEG/carbon nanotubes (PAA/PEG/CNT) has been assembled. The oxidised MWCNTs were obtained with nitric acid treatment, yielding HOOC-MWCNTs, and then submitted to an activation reaction with $SOCl_2$ to get MWCNT-COCl. The PEGylation of acyl chloride groups on the oxidised MWCNTs was completed by refluxing with PEG4000 and subsequently complexing with the second polymer (PAA). Then, methotrexate (MTX) and cyclophosphamide (CPP) were loaded on PAA/PEG/CNT, and nanoparticles were characterised by FTIR, SEM, TGA and NMR. The efficiency of loaded drugs was determinate, an *in vitro* drug release study was carried out with UV spectroscopy in buffer human body (pH = 7.4) and buffer at pH of cancer cells (pH = 4). The *in vitro* release of drugs from nanoparticles showed an initial burst release followed by sustained release, this fact was due to the presence of the drug on the surface of the nanoparticles. The rate of release at this stage was very high and after 1 h, the drug concentration was constant [11].

Another kind of composite is based in the synthesis of the bio-compatible polymer PEG-400 and MWCNTs. The MWCNTs were PEG-400-broken-assisted into small tubes by vortex mechanical mixing with tungsten-carbide balls for about 15 h. Length separation of MWCNTs was then carried out using differential centrifugation also PEG-400-assisted with various concentrations of the polyether. Novel cocoon nanoparticles of sizes ranging about 100–200 nm were observed in one of the centrifuged fractions. The cocoon pellets were re-dispersed in water using ultrasonication for 2 min and characterised using Field Emission SEM, TEM and FTIR. Energy Dispersive Spectroscopy (EDS) and diffraction patterns were also obtained using TEM. Curcumin (CUR) was added as the bioactive, anticancer drug, to these cocoons, and it was observed that it was distributed in these motifs while it was not attached to the CNT-PEG solution without cocoon structures (**Figure 9**). The cocoon and CUR@cocoon samples exhibited much lower haemolysis than CUR alone, with a value of 0.04, 0.03 and 0.09%, respectively. Also, it was observed that all cocoon and CUR@cocoon samples were non-toxic at the concentrations tested. The cell viability of CUR@cocoon samples were less than 95% at 50 μg, indicating cytotoxicity on L-929 cells at higher concentrations. The CUR@cocoon assemblies were dispersible in saline solution and could be internalised by brain cancer cells (C6 glioma), while free CUR dispersed in saline solution could not enter C6 glioma cells, this clearly evidenced differential diffusion and selectivity in this trial [12].

In this work was prepared HNT@CUR-Au/CS NPs by an *in situ* preparation. First, gold, HNTs and CUR were mixed to obtain HNT@CUR-Au and subsequently coating with bio-adhesive chitosan (CS). The HNT@CUR-Au/CS has been characterised by FTIR, XRPD, XPS and STEM methods (**Figure 10**). The loading efficiency of drug into the nanostructures was 12% at most. The release of the drug was more efficient under pH = 5.5 than pH = 7.4. The anticancer potential of HNT@CUR-Au/CS against MCF-7 cells shown more efficient anticancer activity in

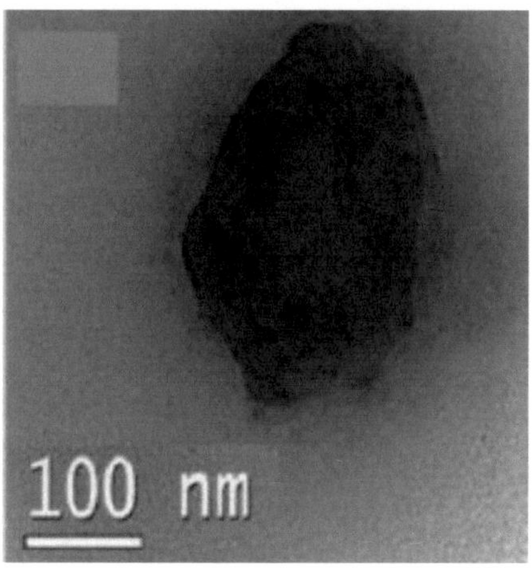

Figure 9.
High resolution TEM of curcumin added to nano-cocoons [12].

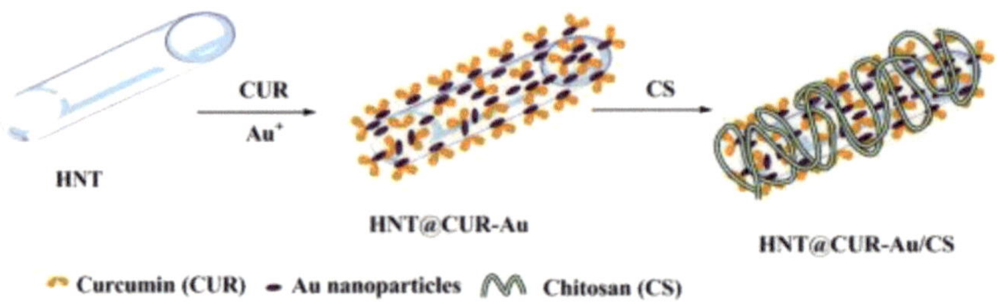

Figure 10.
Schematic representation of formation of HNT@CUR-Au/CS [13].

the intracellular environment than in extracellular conditions, in agreement with their own previous differential pH physicochemical CUR-release tests. Moreover, the development of this composite consisting of Au NPs and pH-responsive CUR release could make it suitable for cancer cell-targeted drug delivery platforms, also with the possibility to develop NIR-imaging [13].

In an another research group, a new design of hydroxypropyl-β-cyclodextrin (HP-β-CD) modified carboxylated single-walled carbon nanotube (CD-SWCNTs) assembly was employed to improve the biocompatibility and reduce the toxicity of the self-carbon nanotubes for the release of the anticancer drug formononetin (FMN). According to the analysis of results developed by the authors related to findings in FTIR, HP-β-CD was successfully grafted into carboxylated single-walled carbon nanotubes (SWCNTs-COOH). The samples were characterised by XRPD, differential scanning calorimetry (DSC), DLS and SEM. The loading of FMN in CD-SWCNTs to develop FMN@CD-SWCNTs system was determined by HPLC. The entrapment efficiency and loading capacity were determinate to be 88.66 ± 3.13% and 8.43 ± 1.11%, respectively. The HP-β-CD system possesses a hydrophobic inner cavity and a hydrophilic exterior, which could bind/inner entrap hydrophobic drug molecules to form stable host-guest supramolecular assemblies. The SWCNTs have a high aspect ratio and surface area, and they could interact with FMN via π-π stacking interactions, which resulted in a high entrapment efficiency (**Figure 11**). The cumulative release of FMN from FMN@CD-SWCNTs nanocarrier achieved 4.11 ± 0.62% within 48 h at a pH = 5.3, compared with 16.75 ± 0.88% when exposed to pH = 7.4. This kind of drug release kinetics demonstrated a slow and sustained release, but in this particular case resulted more efficient at physiologic

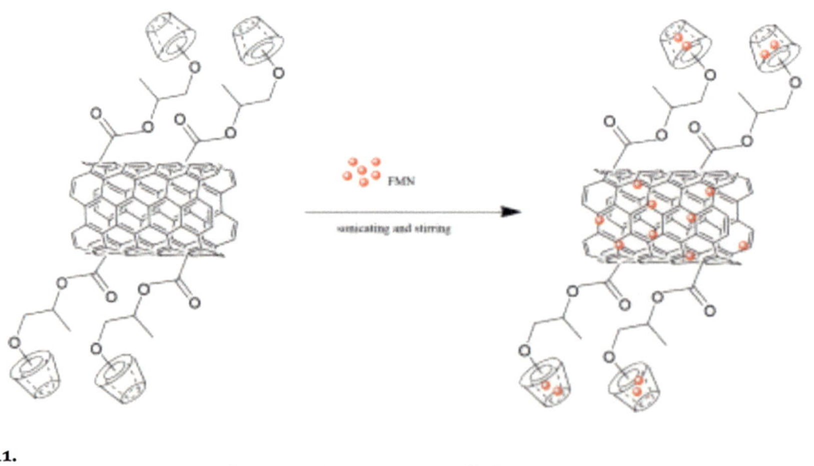

Figure 11.
Scheme of the possible interaction of FMN with CD-SWCNTs [14].

pH, in comparison with other related systems. The *in vitro* cytotoxic activity of FMN@CD-SWCNTs nanocarriers against MCF-7 and HeLa cells was tested by using the WST-1 assay. The antitumour activity of FMN@CD-SWCNTs had an IC_{50} = 17.989 ± 1.255 and 21.775 ± 1.338 μmol L^{-1} for MCF-7 and HeLa cells, respectively. This latter was higher than that of lone FMN with an IC_{50} = 55.986 ± 2.479 and 72.995 ± 0.551 μmol L^{-1} for MCF-7 and HeLa cells, respectively. These results confirm that FMN@CD-SWCNTs complexes exhibit a higher cytotoxic activity than free drug [14].

In this review, f-SWCNTs were used as the starting material to react with the anticancer drug betulinic acid (BA) to produce f-SWCNTs-BA conjugate via π-π stacking interactions. The BA@f-SWCNTs composite was assembled by dispersed f-SWCNT in a solution with BA in methanol and sonicated for 30 min. The BA@f-SWCNTs conjugate was characterised by XRPD, TGA, FE-SEM and FTIR spectroscopy to elucidate and quantify the concentration of the drug in BA@f-SWCNTs and the structure of the conjugate (**Figure 12**). The results indicated that the drug loading capacity was around 20 wt%. The release of the drug from BA@f-SWCNTs was tested in a human body media at pH 7.4 and 4.8 value; this study has shown that the release rate of BA is higher in pH 7.4 than pH 4.8, again another example of controlled release but an higher pH values, and for this reason drug delivery resulted to behave pH-dependent. The maximum percentage release of BA reached 89.2% (24 h) and 78.7% (10 h) when exposed to pH 7.4 and 4.8, respectively. The cytotoxicity assays for BA, f-SWCNT and conjugated BA@f-SWCNTs were performed in a healthy fibroblast cell line (3T3) and two cancer human lines, liver cancer (HepG2) and lung cancer (A549), at various concentrations ranging from 0.78 to 50 μg mL^{-1} at 72 h and were measured by the MTT method. The experiment has shown that at several doses the f-SWCNT did not have a significant impact on the viability of any cell lines. However, at a dose of 25 μg mL^{-1} of BA@f-SWCNTs, the viability of HepG2 and A549 were reduced by more than 50%, in comparison with lone BA that shown low cytotoxicity at the same concentration [15].

Also, there are reports describing the preparation of a biocompatible and pH sensitive biodegradable hydroxyapatite material using mesoporous nanoplates (Hap PNPs) employing a hydrothermal technique with carboxymethylcellulose calcium salt. This material was characterised using FESEM; the length of spindle structures was 20 nm and the diameter was 10 nm on average, the specific area was 180 $m^2\ g^{-1}$ and a crystallite size of 17 nm was calculated using the Debye-Scherer equation. This material was tested as a nanocarrier, and the model loaded drugs were MTX and andrographolide. The UV-vis analysis confirmed that the HAp PNPs have a drug loading efficiency of 50–55.5% at pH = 7.0, which is greater than the conventional HAp nanostructure loading capacity, showing a sustained release at a pH = 4.4. The andrographolide anticancer drug was readily loaded onto prepared HAp PNPs and released in a pH-controlled manner, where for an acidic pH = 4.4

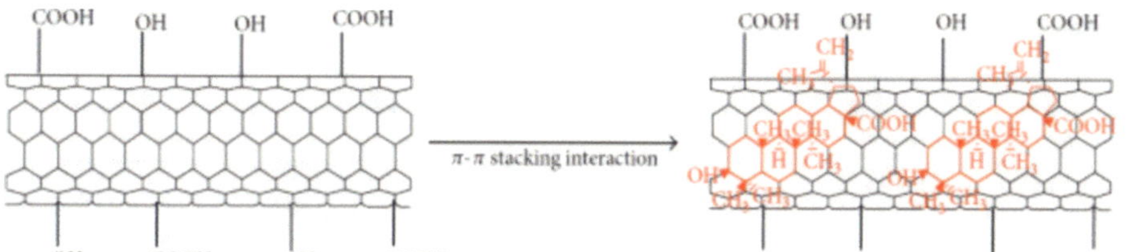

Figure 12.
Scheme for the functionalization of BA molecule onto the f-SWCNTs nanocarrier via π-π stacking interaction [15].

the liberation is higher as compared with a pH of 7.0 or 9.0. The MTT assay was used for the determination of the cytotoxicity in A431 cell lines at different doses of HAp PNPs (0–1000 μg mL^{-1}) and andrographolide loaded (25, 50, 75, 100, 125 and 150 μM) on HAp PNPs (fixed concentration of 100 μg mL^{-1}) at different pHs of 9.0, 7.0 and 4.4 for 24 h. The results have shown that the prepared HAp PNPs exhibited biocompatibility at higher doses of 1000 μg mL^{-1}. Also, they demonstrated that the cytotoxic effect increased by increasing the dose of andrographolide loaded HAp PNPs at pH = 9.0 with an IC_{50} = 125 μM [16].

In the next work nanotubes of SiO_2 were prepared with a uniform diameter of 2.5 nm and shell thickness of 1–5 nm and the exterior surface was silane functionalised and had a negative charge; hence could be selectively loaded with compounds positively charges. The synthesis was carried out using (3-chloropropyl) trimethoxysilane (CPTMS) and tetraethylorthosilicate (TEOS). The characterisation was performed with TEM, X-ray spectroscopy elemental mapping and the particle size was determined by dynamic analysis. The concentration of organic material was quantified using FTIR. This material had a transmittance of aprox. 84% at 550 nm. The load of organic material was 63.6% and determinate by TGA. Positively charged DOXO was loaded in the material; 80% of material was released over 2 weeks, due to size of the elongated nanochannel that suppressed the diffusion [17].

2.2 Anti-inflammatory

Other method to prepare porous MOF materials is the union of an organic linker with other secondary building unit (SBU). For example $[M_2(COO)_4]$ (M = Cu, Zn, Mn, Ni, etc.), $[M_3O(COO)_6]$ (M = Fe, Ni, etc.), $[Zn_4O(COO)_6]$ and $[M_6O_4(OH)_4(COO)_{12}]$ (M = Zr, Hf) MOF systems. Calcium ion possess acid properties, large atom radii and large coordination number, for these reasons is not frequently found it in MOFs structures in comparation with other transition metal-based MOFs. However, the assembly of calcium ions with a big triangle aromatic carboxylic acid ligand has been reported and resulted in a unique porous Ca-MOF structure with nano-sized $\{Ca_{11}\}$ carboxylate SBU and a 2D square channel with a size of 10.8 Å × 10.7 Å. The crystal structure was solved by single crystal X-ray diffraction methods. To determine the thermal stability of the material TGA method was used, where it was found that a continuous slow weight loss was observed until 550°C, the authors state that this should correspond to the release of the coordinated water, at the beginning, and DMF molecules, later on at the thermogram. Drug molecular storage experiments revealed that the porous structure could be dosed with guaiacol molecules at a ratio of 0.19 g g^{-1}; the molecular size of guaiacol was 4.9 × 4.1 Å, which is smaller than the channel size of Ca-MOF. On the other hand, the same probes were made with ibuprofen. The TGA measurement for ibuprofen was performed as well; however, there was no obvious signal pointing to the residual of ibuprofen in the framework of Ca-MOF, since all the guest molecules in the sample were gone when the temperature was lower than 100°C. The drug release experiments were performed by guaiacol samples immersed in PBS solution (pH = 7) and the UV-Vis spectroscopy of the guaiacol release solution was monitored *in situ* for 24 h. The results showed that the guaiacol molecules were released slowly from Ca-MOF, and after 15 h the absorbance reached the maximum value, demonstrating a slow molecule release process and its potential application in medical use. Further work should explore the anionic property of the Ca-MOF, so the drug candidate would be extended from the neutral one to a cationic one, which may achieve the required drug release controlled by strong electro interaction [18].

Halloysite (Hal), a clay mineral of the kaolin group, is of great interest due to a variety of its potential applications. Many Hal nanotubes were functionalised with a polyamidoamine (PAMAM) dendrimer to obtain polyamidoamine dendrimer-functionalised halloysite nanotubes (Hal_PAMAM). These were obtained with single tube lengths between 200 and 1000 nm, the external diameter = 25–50 nm, internal diameter = 9–20 nm, these materials were characterised by FTIR, XRPD, TGA, SEM and TEM. The Hal_PAMAM was tested as a carrier of three different drugs, chlorogenic acid (CHLG), ibuprofen (IBU) and salicylic acid (SAL). The higher adsorption capacity was 123.16 mg g^{-1} for CHLG; 182.72 mg g^{-1} for IBU; 39.52 mg g^{-1} for SAL as compared to raw halloysite and 3-aminopropyltrimethoxysilane (APTS) functionalised-halloysite nanotubes. As a result of surface functionalisation of halloysite with the dendrimer, the release rate of CHLG and SAL decreased, while the release profile of IBU was like that of APTS functionalised nanotubes. The accumulative CHLG release decreased from 90% for Hal to about 55% for Hal_PAMAM, while the IBU release rates slowed down and for SAL the release rate decreased with respect to the other materials. The *in vivo* toxicity studies showed that the Hal_PAMAM had no effect on the living organisms used in the bioassays against *Acutodesmus acuminatus* and *Daphnia magna* [19].

Clay nanotubes are a nanomaterial carrier for sustained drug delivery that provide an extended 10–20 h release profile. These 50 nm diameter aluminosilicate tubes, with inner-alumina and outer-silica surface layers, could be loaded with 10–30 wt% of drug molecules, DNA and enzymes (**Figure 13**). Clay nanotubes were evaluated for the delivery of different drug types, such as the anti-cancer drug Paclitaxel (release pattern initiation after 6 h, slow release over 24 h), and anti-inflammatory drugs such as SAL (burst 89% release within; then slow rate release over 100 min) and IBU (initial burst within 10 min; slow rate release over 7 h) [20].

Novel nanohybrids have been used for the local release of drugs, particularly layered double hydroxides (LDHs), widely known as hydrotalcite-like compounds. These anionic clays are synthetic positively charged thin layer structures with exchangeable interlayer of anions. Many of these materials were synthesised with different molar ratios of Zn/Al-NO_3 and Zn/Al-CO_3 LDHs and were prepared by three different ion-exchange techniques. Three molar ratios were used: 0.3:1 to 0.5:1 and 1:1. The resulting materials were intercalated with dexamethasone (DEXA) and deposited into nanotubes of anodised titanium (ATS-NL-1D), and the resulting nanotubes were characterised using FTIR and XRPD. The incorporation of DEXA anions in LDHs increased and this fact was confirmed by a diffraction lines $d_{(003)}$ to lower Θ with a maximum spacing from 8.9 to 15.09 Å, 16.70 and 21.215 Å for the nanohybrids, with a loading capacity of 12% (**Figure 14**). The test of cell viability revealed that the material was not toxic, the value of release of material was 80% of DEXA in 800 min, and the viability was 81.8% when this material was used for bone implants [21].

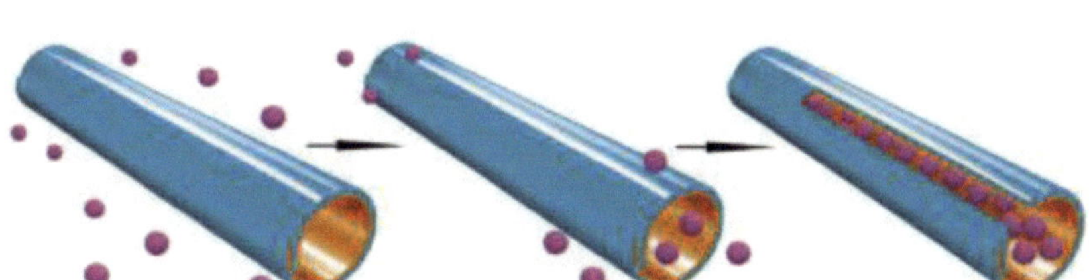

Figure 13.
Scheme of drug molecules loading into clay nanotubes [20].

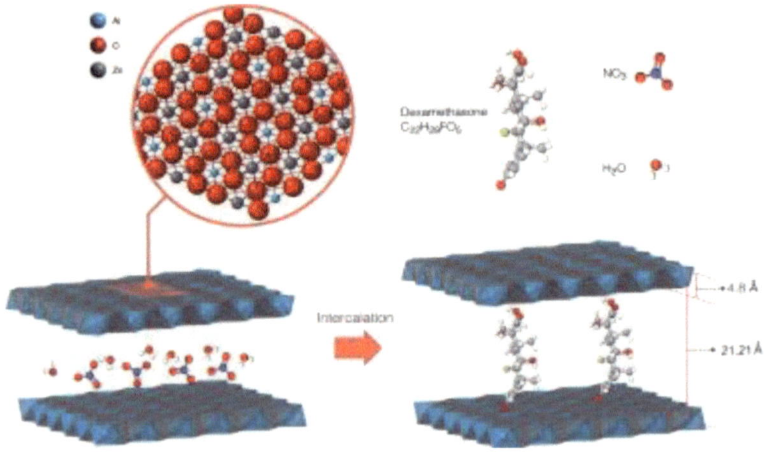

Figure 14.
Schematic illustration of the nitrate layered double hydroxide before and after intercalation of DEXA [21].

2.3 Miscellaneous

Despite the increasing interest in MOFs for biomedical applications, the development of suitable formulations for different administration ways is still a major challenge. A simple, fast and bio-friendly press-moulding method has been proposed for the obtention of cutaneous patches using composites of MIL-100(Fe). The physicochemical properties of the patches implying structure, hydration, bio adhesivity, swelling properties, as well as their encapsulation and release capabilities, both in *ex vitro* and *ex vivo* models were evaluated using different active ingredients like challenging cosmetic liporeductor, caffeine and IBU. High concentrations of caffeine were taken up for these patches with sustained releases under experimental cutaneous physiological conditions due the swelling of these devices. These patches afforded progressive and adequate permeation of their loaded molecules across the skin, reaching the adipose tissue. These characteristics make MOF-based patches as promising candidates for cosmetic applications (**Figure 15**) [22].

The Cu-BTC (BTC =1,3,5-benzenetricarboxylate) is a MOF considered the ideal porous framework in comparison with activated carbon due to its exceptional thermal and mechanical stability. The ultrasound assisted synthesis of Cu-BTC nanoparticles has been studied *vs* bulk Cu-BTC and activated carbon. To test the absorption capacity of the Cu-BTC for Rifampicin (Rif), a sample of Cu-BTC was put in an aqueous solution of Rif and the absorption was measured in real time with UV-vis technique. The samples were characterised with XRPD, SEM, FTIR and UV-vis spectroscopy. The adsorbed quantity of Rif over nano Cu-BTC (Rif@Cu-BTCNANO) was much higher (42.15 mg g^{-1}) than those over a bulk Cu-BTC (Rif@Cu-BTC) (25.62 mg g^{-1}) and activated carbon (18.85 mg g^{-1}) (**Figure 16**). In compound Rif@Cu-BTCNANO and all the nano-MOFs the channel length is decreased so that the amount of adsorption is increased a little. The delivery of Rif in ethanol increases with time, indicating that the Rif release is governed by the host-guest interaction. At 7 days of treatment, Rif release from Rif@Cu-BTCNANO, Rif@Cu-BTC and activated carbon was 78.47, 64.91 and 37.78%, respectively [23].

The direct incorporation of carboxylated carbon nanotubes (f-CNTs) into hydrophobic drug particles has been reported for the first time. The antifungal griseofulvin (GF) and the antibiotic sulfamethoxazole (SMZ) via anti-solvent precipitation, it consists that GF and SMZ were dissolved in acetone, and then added to a dispersion of f-CNTs in water, with the mixture turning cloudy when the crystals

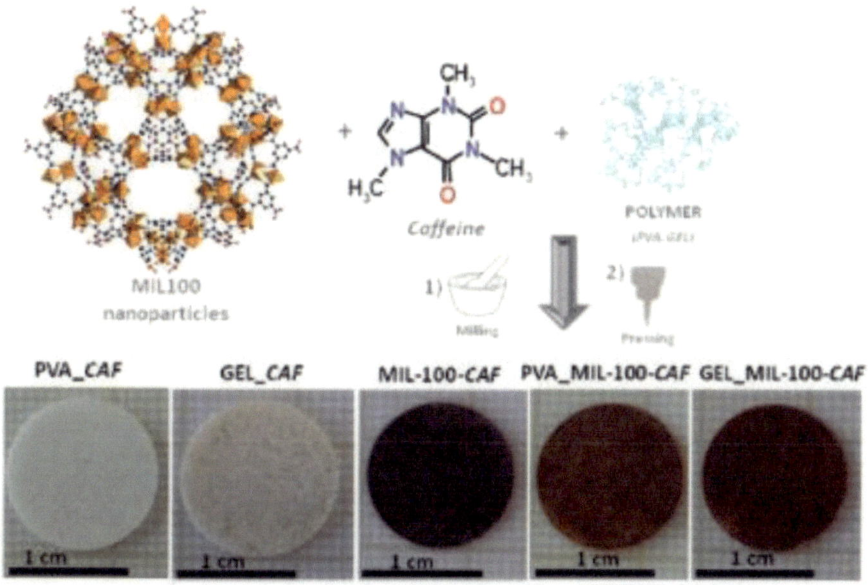

Figure 15.
Schematic view of the composite patch preparation together with images of the different obtained patches [22].

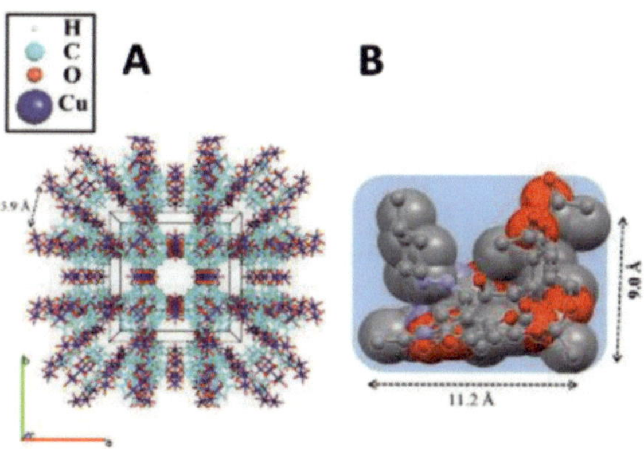

Figure 16.
(A) The pore of Cu-BTC. (B) Size of the Rif in comparison with pore size [23].

were formed. When f-CNTs were dispersed in water they acted as a nucleating site for the crystals and this fact allowed the rapid incorporation of the drug particles and increased the solubility. The time necessary to reach 80% dissolution (t_{80}) of the drugs decreased from 67 to 10 min with the incorporation of 5.1% of f-CNTs in the case of SMZ. For GF, the decrease was from 66 to 18 minutes with the addition 4% of f-CNTs (**Figure 17**) [24].

Also, there are nanotubes of carbon with cisplatin bonded that were synthesised and tested against promastigotes and amastigotes of *Leishmania major*. The cisplatin was bonded to single walled (CP-SWCNT) and multiwalled (CP-MWCNT) carbon nanotubes, and both materials were evaluated using TEM and FTIR. The value of size was between 100 and 1000 nm in the longitudinal direction, and the diameter was <10 nm and <30 nm for CP-SWCNT and CP-MWCNT, respectively (**Figure 18**). The IC_{50} obtained with CP-SWCNT was 0.39 μM and for CP-MWCNT was 0.24 μM against promastigote, while against amastigote the IC_{50} was 0.17 and 0.11 μM, respectively [25].

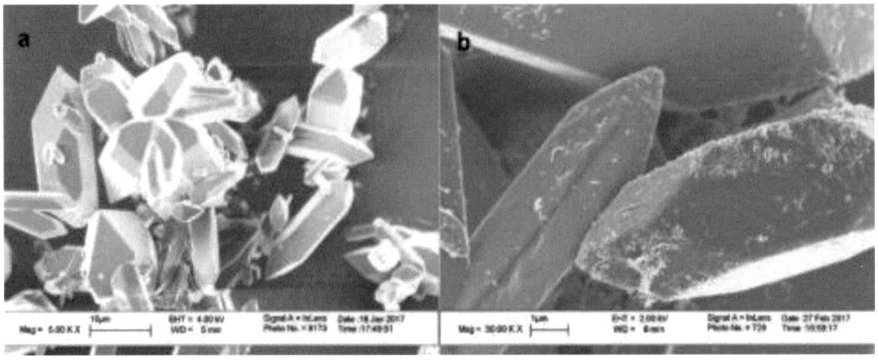

Figure 17.
SEM images of (a) GF and (b) GF-CNTs [24].

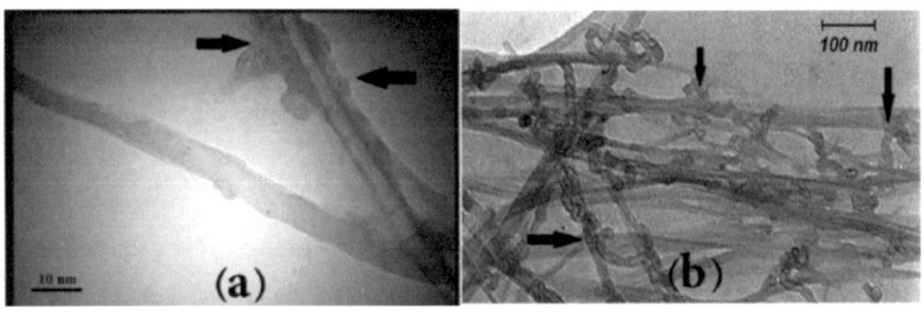

Figure 18.
TEM images of (a) CP-SWCNT and (b) CP-MWCNT [25].

Peripheral nerve injury (PNI) often results in a loss of sensory, motor, and autonomic functions in the affected region. Current treatments depend largely upon surgical intervention, most popularly the use of autografts and allografts. For that reason, the use of HNTs to form a stronger chitosan-HNT composite structure has been investigated. HNTs with biodegradable chitosan were synthesised, with interconnected, longitudinally-aligned pores with an average size of 59.3 ± 14.2 μm. This material was used for sustained delivery of 4-aminopyridine (4-AP), to improve the rate of nerve regeneration. TGA profiles indicated a 7.69 wt% overall drug loading, compared with unmodified HNTs where average load is 5–10 wt%. On the first 7 days 30 ± 2% of encapsulated drug was release (**Figure 19**). *In vivo* studies carried out in Wistar rats with a primary focus on sciatic nerve studies showed an increase in strength and mobility over a period of 4 weeks after the implantation of 4-AP. Histological evaluation demonstrated biocompatibility and regeneration of the nerve. These studies demonstrated that the development of HNTs has a high potential to improve peripheral nerve regeneration and repair [26].

Titania nanotubes (Ti-NTs) have been proven to be good drug carriers and could release drugs efficiently around implants. Enoxacin (EN), an antibiotic with the possibility to be used for anti-osteoclastogenesis, was loaded into the Ti-NTs to obtain the complex Ti-NT + EN, and then was coated with type I collagen and HA to obtain Ti-NT + EN + Col/HA, both materials were characterised by X-ray photoelectron spectroscopy (XPS) (**Figure 20**). The results indicated that the loading efficiency of EN was 75% after the initial rinse. EN release was measured by HPLC and on the 10th day the total amount of EN released by Ti-NT + EN and Ti-NT + EN + Col/HyA was 41.03 and 37.61 μg, respectively. Ti-NT + EN and Ti-NT + EN + Col/HyA were tested in the model of ovariectomised rats to evaluate the effect of osteogenesis and osteoclastogenesis. The results indicated that Ti-NT + EN + Col/HyA could promote osseointegration in ovariectomised rats better than Ti-NT + EN [27].

DOI: http://dx.doi.org/10.5772/intechopen.89626

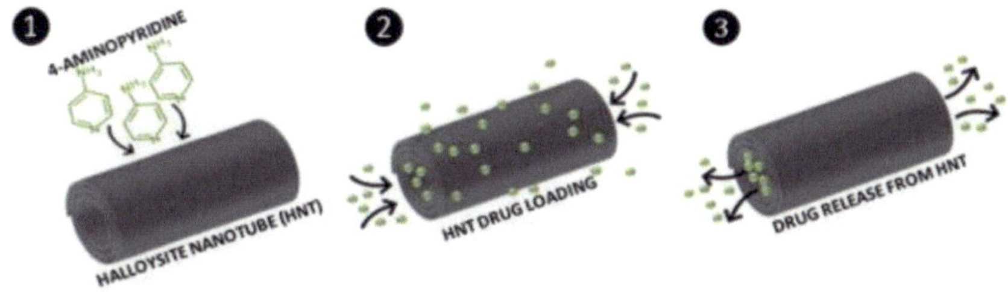

Figure 19.
Schematic of 4-AP drug loading into HNT, followed by sustained release of drug from lumne [26].

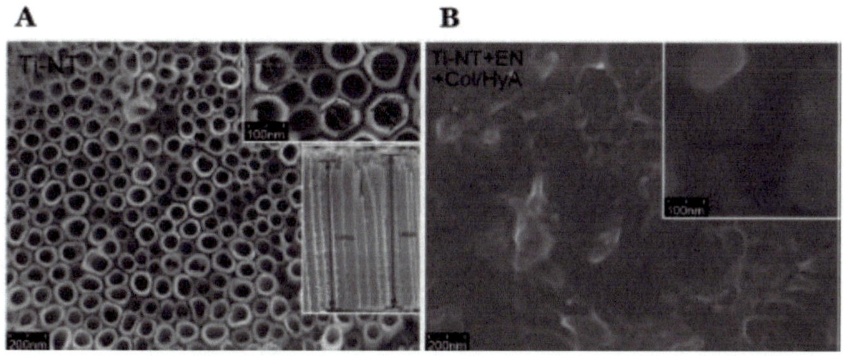

Figure 20.
SEM images of the surface morphology of (A) Ti-NT and (B) Ti-NT + EN + Col/HyA [27].

3. Biomedical applications

The HNTs have been widely used for controlled drug delivery, immobilisation of enzymes and for the capture of circulating tumour cells. These nanotubes were functionalised by two different organosilane reagents, Trimethoxy (propyl) silane (TMPS) and Triethoxy (octyl) silane (EOS), to improve their properties. Functionalisation was carried out by mixing HNTs and the organosilane reagent in acetone, and was heated at 50°C for 48 h. Both HNTs and their modifications were characterised by SEM, XRD, TGA and FTIR (**Figure 21**). The biocompatibility and cytotoxicity of these nanomaterials were determined using C6 rat glioblastoma cells. The results suggested that before being functionalised the nanotubes showed a high biocompatibility and low cytotoxicity. In contrast with their organosilane derivatives, increased cell mortality was observed after incubating under the same conditions [28].

Trichloroisocyanuric acid (TCCA) tablets are used for water treatment in swimming pools. This has been a widely used and safe way of releasing hypochlorous acid with wide biological capabilities, for instance, disinfectant, algaecide and bactericide application. The cited paper studied the incorporation of insect repellents (geranic acid, citronellic acid, geraniol and IR3535) in TCCA tablets with a simultaneous perfume/essence function. Although the mixture of TCCA with the repellents is not possible due to the incompatibility between both components, the researchers proposed a strategy of incorporation in silica and MOFs MIL-53(Al) and MIL-88A(Al) (**Figure 22**). The formulation of TCCA with the incorporated repellents resolved the incompatibility and produced a new tablet that could be used in water treatment, insect repellency and perfume [29].

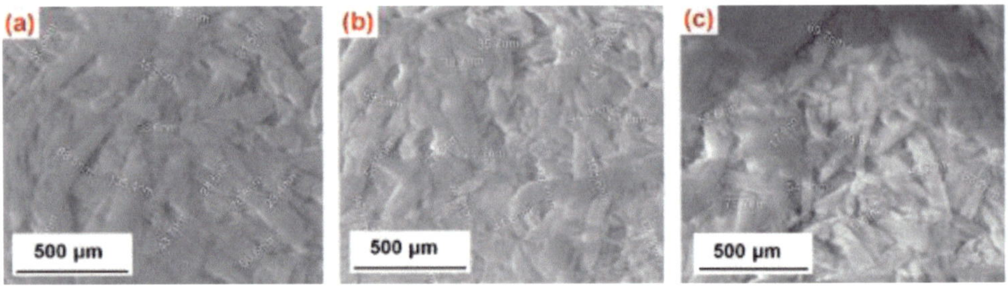

Figure 21.
SEM images of (a) HNTs, (b) HNTs-TMPS and (c) HNTs-EOS [28].

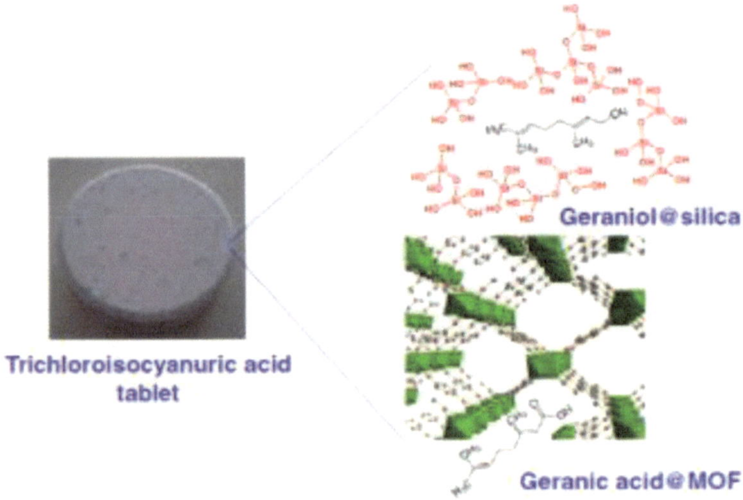

Figure 22.
Trichloroisocyanuric acid tablet [29].

In this contribution, the authors defined that a well-controlled three-step green synthetic method allowed the synthesis of composite materials based on the highly stable chromium (III) terephthalate MIL-101(Cr) MOF with Au NPs and polyoxometalates (POMs) inside its mesopores, developing (Au)POM@MOF ensembles. The strategy included, as a first step, the inclusion of POM into the MIL-101(Cr) cages by direct synthesis method of MIL-101(Cr) in the presence of $H_3PMo_{12}O_{40}$ (POM). Then, POM was reduced using H_2 and finally a soft reduction of $HAuCl_4$ was performed to obtain Au NPs and oxidised POM into the MIL-101(Cr) structure [(Au)H_2redPOM@101] (**Figure 23**). The final atomic ratio of 1.8 for Au/POM was reached. Characterisation studies revealed that the chemical and structural stabilities of both MIL-101(Cr) and the POM were preserved during the whole process. Although the crystalline structure of the MOF was pre-served, the Au NPs were successfully incorporated within the MOF and are strongly associated with the framework, as confirmed by their exceptional stability under physiological conditions (cell culture medium). These results clearly underline the potential applications of these composites to the *in situ* formation of other interesting metal NPs within the pores of MOFs. In addition to the potential physicochemical properties of these highly porous composite systems, the authors state their promising performance as optical contrast agents. The (Au)H_2red-POM@101 composites exhibited excellent biostability and were rapidly internalised in macrophage cells, as observed by fluorescence confocal microscopy. In this line, a suitable biological interaction was evidenced, as confirmed

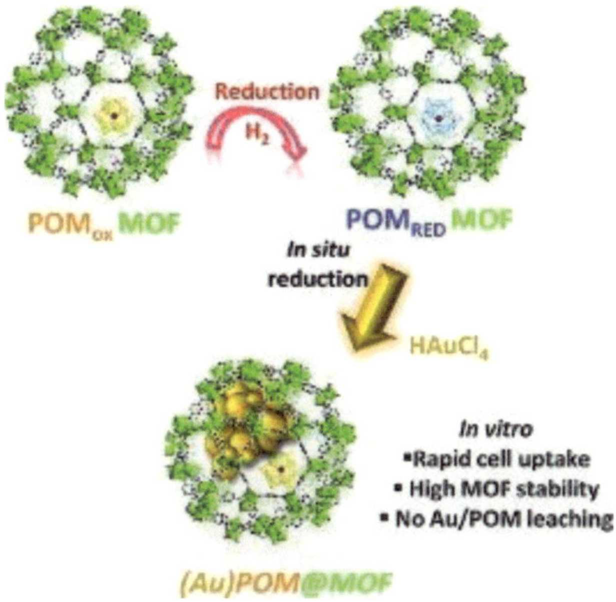

Figure 23.
Schematic representation of (Au)POM@MOF [30].

by the rapid cell internalisation of these (Au)POM@MOF composites. In addition, the previously proven important capacity to encapsulate and progressively release drugs from MOFs, together with the potential antitumoral and antiviral activity of POMs, make them interesting candidates in theranostics field [30].

In biotechnology, protein and especially enzyme immobilisation provides technical and economic advantages since the molecules could be used multiple times for the same reaction, demonstrating enhanced stability under extreme conditions of temperature, pH, salts and denaturing solvents. Therefore, they have longer half-lives since they degrade less and recover better and they are suitable for continuous processes. Conjugated protein-carbon nanotubes possess unique physicochemical properties that make them attractive to a wide range of applications. Thus, the effects of covalent conjugation of lysozymes with the activity and stability of SWCNTs were analysed. The carbodiimide method was used to coupling the lysozyme with SWCNTs (**Figure 24**). After the enzyme was analysed using fluorescence methods, plots of protein unfolding using different concentrations from 0 and 6 M of guanidine hydrochloride (Gn-HCl) were generated. Free lysozyme showed a notable increase in the fluorescence value at 287 nm, besides to a red

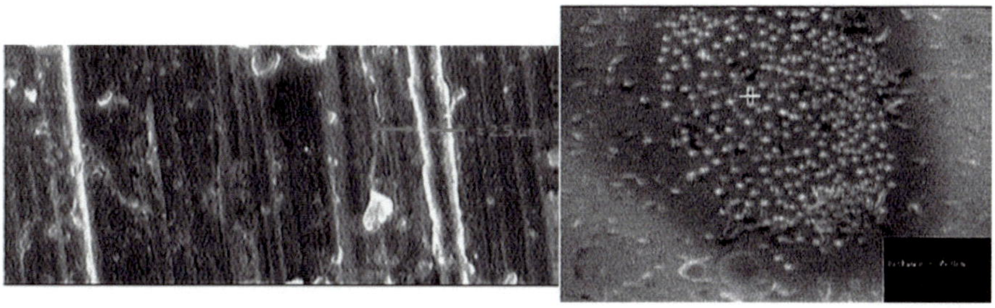

Figure 24.
SEM of conjugated lysozyme-SWCNTs (a) diameter of a bundle of lysozyme-SWCNTs = 2.5 μm, (b) average diameter of each conjugated lysozyme-SWCNTs = 95 nm [31].

shift from 343 to 352 nm. The emission spectrum of conjugated lysozyme showed a substantial increase in the fluorescence at 287 nm and an important decrease in the value at 348 nm. These results support the important role of tryptophan and phenylalanine residues in the fluorescence of conjugated and free lysozymes. Kinetic parameters were observed in KM from 4.8 to 5.6 mM and Vmax from 193 to 197 nmol min^{-1}. The conjugated lysozyme showed a notable increase in pH stability from 3.0 to 10.0 at 70°C. The inactivation kinetic showed a behaviour of first-order for free and conjugated lysozymes when they were incubated for 10 min at 70°C obtaining a value of K = 0.139 min^{-1}, in the presence of KCl and KSCN. The results of this study confirmed the excellent potential of the SWCNTs as a support for enzyme immobilisation [31].

4. Conclusions

In recent years the development of these composite materials has been grown due to their emergent biomedical applications. This 5 years survey evidenced that these materials have been employed with the intend to treat cancer, as anti-inflammatory agents, behaving as controlled-drug delivery systems or enzyme enhancers-immobilisers, and other potential applications such as theranostics, also were found intends to develop combined therapeutics like photodynamic-chemotherapy, among other applications. Some of the most featured findings in this research gathering revealed that even 2–3 orders of magnitude of efficacy have been determined for the loaded drug@material composites in comparison to the free drug state. Some other important features are that imidazolate materials resulted to be efficient drug delivery vehicles in antitumor therapy, especially in inhibiting autophagy of cancer cells. In general, it has been settled that acidic media is more feasible to release molecular contents of composites, but nevertheless this is also depending on chemical nature of composite itself, e.g. the physicochemical properties of drug as well as material confiner. Moreover, the broad applicability of these materials is just emerging, and we are going to presence very important developments in these lines in the near future.

Conflict of interest

The authors declare no conflict of interest.

DOI: http://dx.doi.org/10.5772/intechopen.89626

Author details

Miguel Martell-Mendoza[1], Cuauhtémoc Pérez-González[1], Hiram I. Beltrán[2], Roberto Serrano-Vega[1] and Carlos Alberto Méndez-Cuesta[1*]

1 Universidad Autónoma Metropolitana-Xochimilco, Mexico City, Mexico

2 Universidad Autónoma Metropolitana-Azcapotzalco, Mexico City, Mexico

*Address all correspondence to: cmendezc@correo.xoc.uam.mx

References

[1] Alshehri R, Muhammad A, Hasan A, Arnaout A, Ahmed F, Memic A. Carbon nanotubes in biomedical applications: Factors, mechanisms, and remedies of toxicity. Journal of Medicinal Chemistry. 2016;**59**:8149-8167. DOI: 10.1021/acs.jmedchem.5b01770

[2] Anand R, Borghi F, Manoli F, Manet I, Agostoni V, Reschiglian P, et al. Host-guest interactions in Fe(III)-trimesate MOF nanoparticles loaded with doxorubicin. The Journal of Physical Chemistry. B. 2014;**118**:8532-8539. DOI: 10.1021/jp503809w

[3] Rodriguez V, Maksimenko A, Anand R, Monti S, Agostoni V, Couvreur P, et al. Efficient "green" encapsulation of a highly hydrophilic anticancer drug in metal-organic framework nanoparticles. Journal of Drug Targeting. 2015;**23**:759-767. DOI: 10.3109/1061186X.2015.1073294

[4] Fumei L, Baohong L, Chunfeng W, Yongping Z, Jianqiang L, Chu-Ying G, et al. Encapsulation of pharmaceutical ingredient linker in metal–organic framework: Combined experimental and theoretical insight into the drug delivery. RSC Advances. 2016;**6**:47959-47965. DOI: 10.1039/c6ra06178h

[5] Zheng H, Zhang Y, Liu L, Wan W, Guo P, Nyström A, et al. One-pot synthesis of metal–organic frameworks with encapsulated target molecules and their applications for controlled drug delivery. Journal of the American Chemical Society. 2016;**138**:962-968. DOI: 10.1021/jacs.5b11720

[6] Vasconcelos I, Wanderley K, Rodrigues N, da Costa N, Freire R, Junior S. Host-guest interaction of ZnBDC-MOF + doxorubicin: A theoretical and experimental study. Journal of Molecular Structure. 2017;**1131**:36-42. DOI: 10.1016/j.molstruc.2016.11.034

[7] Chen X, Tong R, Shi Z, Yang B, Liu H, Ding S, et al. MOF nanoparticles with encapsulated autophagy inhibitor in controlled drug delivery system for antitumor. ACS Applied Materials & Interfaces. 2018;**10**(3):2328-2337. DOI: 10.1021/acsami.7b16522

[8] Shu F, Lv D, Song XL, Huang B, Wang C, Yu Y, et al. Fabrication of a hyaluronic acid conjugated metal organic framework for targeted drug delivery and magnetic resonance imaging. RSC Advances. 2018;**8**(12):6581-6589. DOI: 10.1039/C7RA12969F

[9] Wu Y, Yang J, Gao HY, Shen Y, Jiang L, Zhou C, et al. Folate-conjugated halloysite nanotubes, an efficient drug carrier, deliver doxorubicin for targeted therapy of breast cancer. ACS Applied Nano Materials. 2018;**1**(2):595-608. DOI: 10.1021/acsanm.7b00087

[10] Perween S, Misra A, Ramakumar S, Singh V. Self-assembled dipeptide nanotubes constituted by flexible β-phenylalanine and conformationally constrained α, β-dehydrophenylalanine residues as drug delivery system. Journal of Materials Chemistry B. 2014;**2**:3096-3106. DOI: 10.1039/c3tb21856b

[11] Azqhandi M, Farahani B, Dehghani N. Encapsulation of methotrexate and cyclophosphamide in interpolymer complexes formed between poly acrylic acid and polyethylene glycol on multi-walled carbon nanotubes as drug delivery systems. Materials Science and Engineering: C. 2017;**79**:841-847. DOI: 10.1016/j.msec.2017.05.089

[12] Hindumathi R, Jagannatham M, Haridoss P, Sharma CP. Novel nano-cocoon like structures of polyethylene glycol–multiwalled carbon nanotubes for biomedical applications. Nano-Structures & Nano-Objects.

2018;**13**:30-35. DOI: 10.1016/j.nanoso.2017.11.001

[13] Rao KM, Kumar A, Suneetha M, Han SS. pH and near-infrared active; chitosan-coated halloysite nanotubes loaded with curcumin-Au hybrid nanoparticles for cancer drug delivery. International Journal of Biological Macromolecules. 2018;**112**:119-125. DOI: 10.1016/j.ijbiomac.2018.01.163

[14] Liu X, Xu D, Liao C, Fang Y, Guo B. Development of a promising drug delivery for formononetin: Cyclodextrin-modified single-walled carbon nanotubes. Journal of Drug Delivery Science and Technology. 2018;**43**:461-468. DOI: 10.1016/j.jddst.2017.11.018

[15] Tan M, Karthivashan G, Arulselvan P, Fakurazi S, Zobir M. Sustained release and cytotoxicity evaluation of carbon nanotube-mediated drug delivery system for betulinic acid. Journal of Nanomaterials. 2014;**2014**:862148. DOI: 10.1155/2014/862148

[16] Bharath G, Rambabu K, Banat F, Anwer S, Lee S, BinSaleh N, et al. Mesoporous hydroxyapatite nanoplate arrays as pH-sensitive drug carrier for cancer therapy. Materials Research Express. 2019;**6**:085409. DOI: 10.1088/2053-1591/ab2348

[17] Deng C, Zhang Q, Fu C, Zhou F, Yang W, Yi D, et al. Template-free synthesis of chemically asymmetric silica nanotubes for selective cargo loading and sustained drug release. Chemistry of Materials. 2019;**31**:4291-4298. DOI: 10.1021/acs.chemmater.9b01530

[18] Wei L, Lu J, Li Q, Zhou Y, Tang L, Li F. A porous Ca-MOF with nano-sized $\{Ca_{11}\}$ as building unit: Structure, drug loading and release properties. Inorganic Chemistry Communications. 2017;**78**:43-47. DOI: 10.1016/j.inoche.2017.02.010

[19] Kurczewska J, Cegłowski M, Messyasz B, Schroeder G. Dendrimer-functionalized halloysite nanotubes for effective drug delivery. Applied Clay Science. 2018;**153**:134-143. DOI: 10.1016/j.clay.2017.12.019

[20] Santos AC, Ferreira C, Veiga F, Ribeiro AJ, Panchal A, Lvov Y, et al. Halloysite clay nanotubes for life sciences applications: From drug encapsulation to bioscaffold. Advances in Colloid and Interface Science. 2018;**257**:58-70. DOI: 10.1016/j.cis.2018.05.007

[21] Kamyar A, Khakbiz M, Zamanian A, Yasaei M, Yarmand B. Synthesis of a novel dexamethasone intercalated layered double hydroxide nanohybrids and their deposition on anodized titanium nanotubes for drug delivery purposes. Journal of Solid State Chemistry. 2019;**271**:144-153. DOI: 10.1016/j.jssc.2018.12.043

[22] García A, Hidalgo T, Lana H, Cunha D, Blanco M, Álvarez C, et al. Biocompatible polymer–metal–organic framework composite patches for cutaneous administration of cosmetic molecules. Journal of Materials Chemistry B. 2016;**4**:7031-7040. DOI: 10.1039/c6tb01652a

[23] Abbasi AR, Rizvandi M. Influence of the ultrasound-assisted synthesis of Cu-BTC metal-organic frameworks nanoparticles on uptake and release properties of rifampicin. Ultrasonics Sonochemistry. 2018;**40**:465-471. DOI: 10.1016/j.ultsonch.2017.07.041

[24] Chen K, Mitra S. Incorporation of functionalized carbon nanotubes into hydrophobic drug crystals for enhancing aqueous dissolution. Colloids and Surfaces B. 2019;**173**:386-391. DOI: 10.1016/j.colsurfb.2018.09.080

[25] Akhtaria J, Faridniab R, Kalanic H, Bastanid R, Fakhard M, Rezvane H, et al. Potent in vitro antileishmanial

activity of a nanoformulation of cisplatin with carbon nanotubes against *Leishmania major*. Journal of Global Antimicrobial Resistance. 2019;**16**:11-16. DOI: 10.1016/j.jgar.2018.09.004

[26] Manoukianab O, Arulb M, Rudraiahbc S, Kalajzicd I, KumbarS. Aligned microchannel polymer-nanotube composites for peripheral nerve regeneration: Small molecule drug delivery. Journal of Controlled Release. 2019;**296**:54-67. DOI: 10.1016/j.jconrel.2019.01.013

[27] Li H, Nie B, Zhang S, Long T, Yue B. Immobilization of type I collagen/hyaluronic acid multilayer coating on enoxacin loaded titania nanotubes for improved osteogenesis and osseointegration in ovariectomized rats. Colloids and Surfaces B. 2019;**175**:409-420. DOI: 10.1016/j.colsurfb.2018.12.033

[28] Sánchez A, Peña L, Vidaltamayo R, Cué R, Mendoza A, Zomosa V, et al. Synthesization, characterization, and in vitro evaluation of cytotoxicity of biomaterial son halloysite nanotubes. Materials. 2014;**7**:7770-7780. DOI: 10.3390/ma7127770

[29] Paseta L, Simón-Gaudó E, Gracia F, Coronas J. Encapsulation of essential oils in porous silica and MOFs for trichloroisocyanuric acid tablets used for water treatment in swimming pools. Chemical Engineering Journal. 2016;**292**:28-34. DOI: 10.1016/j.cej.2016.02.001

[30] Roch-Marchal C, Hidalgo T, Banh H, Fischer R, Horcajada P. A promising catalytic and theranostic agent obtained through the in-situ synthesis of Au nanoparticles with a reduced polyoxometalate incorporated within mesoporous MIL-101. European Journal of Inorganic Chemistry. 2016;**2016**:4387-4394. DOI: 10.1002/ejic.201600359

[31] Borzooeian Z, Taslim M, Borzooeian G, Ghasemi O, Aminlari M. Activity and stability analysis of covalent conjugated lysozyme-single walled carbon nanotubes: Potential biomedical and industrial applications. RSC Advances. 2017;**7**:48692-48701. DOI: 10.1039/c7ra07189b

Section 4

Nanoscience and Nanoengineering

Chapter 8

Biochemical Toxicology: Heavy Metals and Nanomaterials

Sibi Raj and Dhruv Kumar

Abstract

The synthesis and application of nanoparticles have been actively studied in the modern era as it holds promises for effective and targeted strategies to deliver drugs inside the human body. Nanoparticles (NPs) play a big role in cancer diagnosis and have various advantages over other conventional chemotherapeutic drug delivery systems. But, the application of emerging engineered NPs to heavy toxic metals such as zinc, cobalt, and iron has resulted in a major source of toxicity. The toxicity of nanomaterials is majorly determined by their physical and chemical properties such as size, charge, and surface area. Also, the mechanism of nanotoxicity is majorly via the production of reactive oxygen species that create oxidative stress, thereby activating inflammatory cytokines and the mechanism of DNA damage that ultimately results in the cell death. So, mechanistic study needs to be done on nanomaterials to elucidate the mechanism involved in nanotoxicity and to generate less toxic and efficient nanomaterials.

Keywords: nanoparticle, heavy metals, nanotoxicity, ROS, inflammation

1. Introduction

Nanotechnology is one of the rapidly emerging fields in the twenty-first century with extensive increase of nanoparticle application for the treatment of a wide variety of chronic diseases such as cancer. P. Ehrlich's visionary concept of "magic bullet" based on the use of targeted medicines to effectively attack cancer cells has provided a promising field for cancer therapy [1]. Targeted delivery to solid cancers provides more bioavailability and effective approach for cancer treatment. The characteristics of nanocarriers such as their nanoscale, high surface-to-volume ratio, favorable drug release profiles, and targeting modifications allow them to target tumor tissue in an effective manner and release drugs in a stable and controlled manner [2]. NPs can accumulate in the leaky vasculatures of tumor tissue in an enhanced permeability and retention effect (EPR). The potential of nanomedicine can be explored in the field of early detection of cancer as well as in combination therapies for treating tumor earlier and effectively. NPs effectively solve the physiological barriers such as renal, hepatic, and immune related for effective drug delivery of conventional chemotherapeutic drugs [3]. NPs may be modified to utilize passive and active targeting mechanism to reach the tumor tissue. The nanodelivery-based carriers range from natural polymeric materials to nonbiodegradable gold NP, and magnetic mesoporous silica-based, metal-based NP. The surface of the NP can be suitably modified with ligands or drugs to offer multimodular treatment options [4]. The nanoparticle shape also plays an important role

IntechOpen

in specific and effective nanodrug delivery. Nano-based drug delivery system has enhanced pharmacokinetic parameters, such as clearance value, volume distribution, and bioavailability to cancer cells through EPR. Unfortunately, these novel drug delivery systems still face barriers when delivered into the body, which can reduce the targeting efficiency as well as have increased toxic side effects. NPs have shown distinct toxicity patterns as compared with their larger counterparts [5]. As the size of NPs gets reduced for effective targeting, the number of surface molecules and surface area increase exponentially, which leads to complex bio-physiochemical interactions at the bio-nano interfaces when exposed to physiological environments. The potential paradigms of nanotoxicity can be understood possibly by understanding these bio-nano interactions. Since nanomaterials and therapeutic drug in combination work against cancer, the unfavorable toxicity of nanomaterials causes side effects and dysfunctions. Since the nanomedicines and therapeutic drugs share the same fate in the body, understanding the interconnections between nanotoxicity and drug delivery can widen our knowledge to improve the possibilities for cancer therapy. The effect of NPs can be divided into two categories, that is, primary and secondary depending upon the exposure time period [6]. The direct contact of NPs with cells results in primary effect, which involves toxicity, oxidative stress, DNA damage, and inflammation. Due to their nano-based size, the nanoparticles can translocate into the blood through tissue barriers where they can circulate and eventually accumulate in other organs, thereby, generating a secondary response of the NP. The secondary toxic effect of NPs might occur at the site of nanoparticle accumulation in organs such as the liver, spleen, or kidneys, and can stimulate systemic inflammation or can alter their systemic function [7]. The toxicity of NPs has been studied in different biological systems involving the cell lines as well as different organisms, which involve humans, rodents, zebra fish, catfish, algae, and macrophages. Carbon and metallic NPs are the most widely studied and used engineered nanomaterials. Nanometals, such as nanogold (nano-Au), nanosilver (nano-Ag), nanocopper, nanoaluminum, nanonickel, nanocobalt, and other NPs, have also been extensively studied. Toxic effect of metal oxide NPs such as nano-TiO_2, nano-ZnO, nano-CuO, nano-CuZn, nano-Fe_3O_4, and nano-Fe_2O_3, with nano-TiO_2 and nano-ZnO in particular, has been reported [8]. As expected, different nanomaterials exhibit different toxic potency. For example, Zhu et al. compared the toxicity of three nanometal oxides, nano-CuO, nano-CdO, and nano-TiO_2. Nano-CuO was determined to be the most potent in cytotoxicity and DNA damage, leading to 8-hydroxy-2′-deoxyguanosine (8-OHdG) formation, while nano-TiO_2 was the least, without inducing a significant level of 8-OHdG [9]. The production of carbon nanotubes (CNTs) and graphene oxide is becoming commercially important. Under some experimental conditions, investigators have found that CNTs and graphene oxide are toxic. So, understanding the matter of safety and toxicity of nanomaterials has become an issue of interest to the public. Therefore, understanding the interactions of nanomaterials with biological systems is a particularly important scientific issue.

2. Physical and chemical properties of NPs in nanotoxicity

Toxic effect of NPs can proceed through a variety of mechanisms. Toxicity from a nanoparticle depends on its physical and chemical properties as well as the testing systems such as different cell types. The fundamental physical and chemical properties, which include molecular shape, size, oxidation status, surface area, bonded surface species, surface coating, solubility, and degree of aggregation and agglomeration of nanomaterials, majorly lead to the generation of reactive oxygen species and toxicity [10]. These intrinsic properties of nanomaterials can stimulate and generate toxic effects inside the biological system. Also, interaction with environmental factors such as light also determines how nanomaterials interact with the biological factors and lead to the mechanism of toxicity.

2.1 Size and shape

Their nanosize and large surface area are the unique physiochemical properties of nanomaterials that determine their toxicity. Due to their very small size, they have the ability to penetrate into cell membrane and other biological barriers into living organisms and can inhibit cellular functions [11]. The increased nanoparticle size decreases its ability for cellular uptake. Majorly due to their nanosize, nanomaterials can even target the lungs and give rise to several toxic effects. Yoshida et al. had reported that particle size plays a major role in intracellular disruption of amorphous silica and its induced reactive oxygen species (ROS) formation, leading to DNA damage in human skin HaCaT cells [12]. Moreover, as the size of nanoparticle decreases, the toxic effects increase. Alpha-MnO_2 nanowire, which is a wire-shaped nanomaterial, induces cytotoxicity, DNA oxidative damage, and apoptosis in HeLa cells [13]. In support of this statement, it was shown that long nanowires in cultured fibroblasts inhibited cell division, DNA damage, and increased ROS. Similarly, WISH cells when exposed to TiO_2 induced cytotoxicity alterations in morphology, production of ROS, and DNA damage. Sohaebuddin et al. determined the effects of the chemical composition of nano-TiO_2, nano-SiO_2, and multiwall CNTs on their toxicity in 3T3 fibroblasts, RAW 264.7 macrophages, and telomerase-immortalized bronchiolar epithelial cells [14]. The results indicated that the composition, molecular size, and target cell type are all critical determinants of intracellular responses, degree of cytotoxicity, and potential mechanisms of toxicity. Moreover, these nanomaterials induced cell-specific responses, resulting in variable toxicity and subsequent cell damage. A study by Yin et al. showed that the smaller the particle size, the greater the cellular damage induced. He studied the photocytotoxicity of four different sized (<25, 31, <100, and 325 nm) nano-TiO_2 and two different crystal forms antase and rutile in human skin keratinocytes. Upon exposure to UVA radiation, all nano-TiO_2 particles induced cytotoxicity and cell membrane damage in a light- and dose-dependent manner. Similarly, in a study with different sizes of silica-titania hollow particle with uniform diameters of 25, 50, 75, 100, and 125 nm, the 50-nm silica-titania hollow NP showed the largest toxicity effect in macrophages [15].

The shape of the nanoparticle is one of the major determinants of nanomaterial-induced cytotoxicity. This was supported by the study done by Ray and his coworkers where they determined that a set of gold NPs with different shapes had similar cytotoxicity [16]. The shape of the nanoparticle is considered as a major determinant in the process of engineering and application. The characteristic shapes of NP are mainly spherical, ellipsoidal, sheet-like, cubic, and rod-like. Spherical NPs have shown to be more prone to endocytosis than nanotubes and nanofibers. Similarly, a study with different shapes (needle-like, plate-like, rod-like, and spherical) of hydroxyapatite NPs on cultured BEAS-2B cells showed that plant-like and needle-like NPs showed higher cell death than spherical and rod-like NPs [17]. This might be due to the fact that needle-like NPs have the capacity of damaging cells upon direct contact to the cell surface. An interesting study with graphene oxide nanosheets showed that the toxicity of these NPs was determined by their shape allowing them to physically damage the cell membrane. However, the toxicity of these NPs was reduced with increasing concentration of the fetal calf serum in the cell culture media. This phenomenon was explained on the basis that graphene oxide NPs had the capacity to adsorb the protein molecules, which covered the nanoparticle surface which changed the shape of the nanoparticle and partly prevented cell damage.

2.2 Surface charge

The surface charge of NPs plays an important role in determining the nanotoxicity as it largely determines the interactions of the NP with biological systems. Positively charged NPs have been reported to have high toxicity due to their easy penetration into cells rather than the negatively charged nanoparticles [18]. This is due to the electrostatic attraction between the negatively charged cell membrane and positively charged NP. A comparative study of the toxic effects of negatively and positively charged polystyrene NPs on HeLa and HIH/3T3 cells has shown that the positively charged NPs were relatively more toxic. This is due to the ability of positively charged cells to easily penetrate through the cell membrane; also, they strongly bind to the negatively charged DNA, causing its damage, and prolong the G0/G1 phase of the cells. Negatively charged NPs have not been reported to have any effect on cell cycle. Similar observations have been reported with gold NPs where positively charged NPs were highly adsorbed and showed toxic effects rather than the negatively charged gold nanoparticle. Positively charged NPs have increased capacity of opsonization, which involves the process of adsorption of proteins facilitating phagocytosis, including antibodies and complement components from blood and biological fluids [19]. The adsorbed protein to the surface of nanoparticle which is normally referred to as protein crown may affect the surface properties of the NP. The protein crown contains serum proteins such as albumin, fibrinogens, and immunoglobulin G and several other functional molecules. *In vitro* experiments with quantum dots coated with a hydrophilic polymer enhance the fibril formation of human β_2 microglobulin, which is arranged into multilayered structures on the surface of nanoparticle resulting in local increase in the protein concentration on the nanoparticle surface, precipitation, and formation of oligomers [20]. The charge of the nanoparticle can be modified from negative to positive via various modifications of the surface. So, Xu et al. had developed a method of changing the charge in polymer NP with the help of a pH-sensitive polymer that helps the negatively charged particles in a neutral medium acquire a positive charge in an acidic medium of pH 5–6 [21]. The cytotoxic effect estimated from surface-modified cerium oxide NP in H9C2, HEK293, A549, and MCF-7 cells showed that different polymers enable the nanoparticle charge modification, thereby showing different biological and toxic effects. Specifically, positive and neutral charged NPs are absorbed by all cell types at the same rate, whereas negatively charged NPs have the tendency to accumulate inside the biological tissues. So, modifying the charge of NPs allows to control their localization and toxicity, which can help in improving effective systems for targeted chemotherapeutic drug delivery to the tumor site.

3. Nanoparticle shell

Improving the optical, magnetic, and electrical properties of nanomaterials application of a shell onto the surface of NP is quite important as it also improves the biocompatibility and solubility of NPs in water and other biological fluids by decreasing their capacity to aggregate and increasing their stability. Therefore, the shell reduces the toxic effect of NPs and provides them the capacity to selectively interact with different types of cells and biological molecules [22]. In addition, the shell influences the pharmacokinetics of NP, which considerably changes the pattern of nanoparticle distribution and accumulation inside the body. Most of the nanoparticle toxicity has been reported due to the formation of free radicals inside the cells [23]. However, the shell has the capability to: reduce or eliminate these negative side effects as well as stabilize the NP, increase the resistance of NPs toward environmental factors, and enable them to acquire the capacity to selectively interact with the biological molecules. In regard to this point, Cho et al. demonstrated that polymer NPs could be modified with lectins and were able to selectively bind to the tumor cells presenting sialic acid on their surface, which made the nanoparticle suitable for specifically labeling cancer cells [24]. The surface of the NP can be modified using both organic and inorganic compounds such as polyethylene glycol, polyglycolic acid, lipids, proteins, low-molecular weight compounds and silicon. These modifiers make complex nanoparticle surface and change the nanoparticle properties for their specific transport and accumulation. The toxicity of quantum dots is significantly reduced using shells as the core of quantum dots is mostly hydrophobic and mainly consists of toxic heavy metals such as cadmium, tellurium, and mercury [25]. The shell enhances the stability of the core of quantum dots, thereby preventing its desalinization and oxidative or photolytic degradation. This ultimately prevents the leakage of heavy metal ions from the quantum core, thereby preventing nanotoxicity [26].

4. Mechanism of nanotoxicity

Nanotechnology has been an emerging field to determine the set standards or to formulate a set of designed rules for designing safe nanomaterials. The ability of nanomaterials to accumulate in different organs has resulted in some severe side effects and has hindered their use in the field of nanomedicine. So, understanding the mechanism that underlies the toxicity of nanomaterials may provide clues for overcoming the toxic effects of NPs. A major mechanism of nanotoxicity is by the generation of reactive oxygen species (ROS), which results in the subsequent formation of oxidative stress in tissues [27]. The induction of oxidative stress simultaneously activates the pro-inflammatory mediators via the principle cascades such as the nuclear factor-κB (NF-κb), mitogen-activated protein kinase (MAPK), and phosphoinositide 3-kinase (PI3K) pathways [28]. The most widely used nanomaterials are mostly the carbon nanotubes and metallic nanomaterials. Radomski et al. reported that engineered carbon NPs and nanotubes induced the aggregation of platelets in vitro, and enhanced vascular thrombosis in rat carotid artery [29]. Similarly, the single-walled carbon nanotubes showed enhanced cell apoptosis and decreased cell adhesion by upregulating genes involved in cell death or downregulating genes involved in cell proliferation and survival in cellular models of human kidney and bronchi. With the application of skin lotion and creams that majorly contain nano-TiO_2 and nano-ZnO, the skin is in continuous exposure to the toxic nanometals that can accumulate in the brain and can cause auxiliary toxicity resulting in the disruption of normal metabolism of neurotransmitters and ultimately leading to the cause of brain damage. While comparing the toxicity of three nanometal oxides, nano-CuO, nano-CdO, and nano-TiO_2, nano-CuO was determined to be the most potent in regard to cytotoxicity and DNA damage, leading to 8-hydroxy-20-deoxyguanosine (8-OHdG) formation, while nano-TiO_2 was the least potent, without inducing a significant level of 8-OHdG [9] (**Figure 1**).

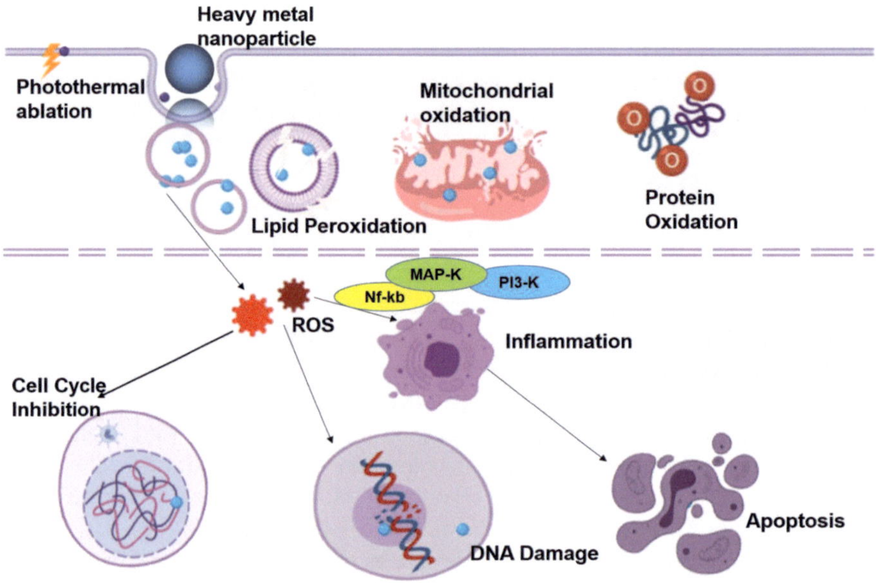

Figure 1.
Mechanism of nanotoxicity. The major mechanism of nanotoxicity is by the generation of reactive oxygen species (ROS), which results in the subsequent formation of oxidative stress in tissues. The induction of oxidative stress simultaneously activates the pro-inflammatory mediators via the principle cascades such as the nuclear factor-κB (NF-κB), mitogen-activated protein kinase (MAPK), and phosphoinositide 3-kinase (PI3K) pathways. The other major effects are protein oxidation and DNA damage, which leads to apoptosis or cell cycle inhibition.

4.1 Nanotoxicity via ROS production

The ROS generation and the subsequent production of oxidative stress are major causes of nanotoxicity, which involves DNA damage, unregulated cell signaling, changes in cell motility, cytotoxicity, apoptosis, and cancer initiation and progression. The amount and effect of ROS generation are completely dependent on the chemical nature of the nanomaterials [30]. Engineered nanomaterials have relatively small size, high specific volume-to-area ratio, and high surface reactivity, which results in higher production of ROS, simultaneously resulting in cytotoxicity and genotoxicity [31]. A variety of nanomaterials has been reported to induce nanotoxicity, that is, mediated by ROS in many biological systems such as human erythrocytes and fibroblasts. Quantum dots have been reported to have toxic effects produced by ROS-mediated oxidative stress and cell death. Akhtar et al. reported that silica NPs induced cellular stress and cytotoxicity in a dose-dependent manner, which is mediated by the induction of ROS and lipid peroxidation in cell membranes [32]. Nano-CuO induced cytotoxicity in mouse embryonic fibroblasts (BALB 3T3) by releasing lactate dehydrogenase, causing oxidative stress in a dose-dependent manner mediated by the induction of ROS and lipid peroxidation. Nano-ZnO has been reported to induce cytotoxicity that is mostly mediated by the induction of ROS, causing oxidative injury simultaneously releasing inflammatory mediators resulting in cell death in phagocytic RAW 264.7 cells, and transformation in human bronchial epithelial BEAS-2B cells [17]. Nano-Ag has been reported to induce apoptosis in NIH3T3 cells, which is mainly mediated via ROS and C-Jun terminal kinase-dependent mechanism involving the mitochondrial pathway. Also, nano-Ag–induced mutation and oxidative stress in mouse lymphoma cells. Shvedova et al. reported that keratinocytes incubated with high doses of single-walled CNTs resulted in ROS production, thereby leading to cellular and mitochondrial dysfunction. Comparison of cytotoxicity of the four nanometal oxides nano-ZnO, nano-TiO_2, nano-Co_3O_4, and nano-CuO in catfish hepatocytes and human HepG2 cells induced toxicity in the order of TiO_2 < Co_3O_4 < ZnO < CuO and the major cause was the ROS generation leading to cell and mitochondrial damage [15, 33].

4.2 DNA damage

DNA is one of the major targets of ROS. Toxicity of NPs is often specified for ROS production that ultimately damages the genetic material, thereby causing cell death. NPs are responsible for a wide variety of DNA damage such as chromosomal fragmentation, DNA strand breakages, and the induction of mutation in genes [34]. Gold NPs 20 nm in size at concentration of 1 nM have been reported to exhibit DNA damage in the form of 8-hydroxydeoxyguanosine (8OHdG), adduct formation in the embryonic lung fibroblasts, having a very low expression for DNA repair and cell cycle check point genes [35]. Several reports have also confirmed that metal oxide NPs induce DNA fragmentation and formation of oxidation-induced DNA adducts. The main functional molecule that comes into play in response to DNA damage is p53. Metal oxide NPs including TiO_2, ZnO, Fe_3O_4, Al_2O_3, and CrO_3 of particle sizes ranging from 30 to 45 nm have been reported to induce apoptosis [36]. Cadmium telluride quantum dots were found to significantly increase p53 levels and upregulate the p53-downstream effectors Bax, Puma, and Noxa in human breast carcinoma cells [37].

4.3 Inflammation

Oxidative stress induction is relatively linked to inflammation through the release of pro-inflammatory mediators through the cascade such as the NF-κB (nuclear factor-κB), mitogen-activated protein kinase (MAPK), and phosphoinositide 3-kinase (PI3K) pathways [38]. Inflammation is majorly a type of defense mechanism of the body that involves several immune regulatory molecules followed by the infiltration of phagocytic cells. The induction of inflammation in several cell types such as the alveolar and bronchial epithelial cells, epidermal keratinocytes, and cultured monocyte-macrophage cells has been reported with single and multi-walled carbon nanotubes and fullerene derivatives. A recent study has been able to provide a mechanistic explanation for immune and inflammatory responses initiated upon exposure to carbon NPs [39]. This observation reported that the immune system receptors like toll-like receptors recognize carbon nanotubes and C60 fullerenes as pathogens and thereby trigger the inflammatory responses by secreting inflammatory protein mediators such as interleukins and chemokines. Similarly, exposure of liposomes and other lipid-based NPs trigger the activation of the complementary cascade leading to hypersensitivity reactions and anaphylaxis [40]. However, the exact mechanism through which these complement proteins mediate nanotoxicity has not been elucidated. In the absence of a stimulus, NF-κB is degraded in the cytoplasm by the Inhibitor of κB (IκB) family of inhibitors. The reactive oxygen species play a major role in the induction of the NF-κB, resulting in the inflammatory responses. Both *in vitro* and *in vivo* studies showed that nanoparticle-induced lung injury and pulmonary fibrosis lead to the ROS-mediated activation of NF-κB and production of pro-inflammatory mediators such as TNF-α, IL-8, IL-2, and IL-6 [41]. Metal oxide NPs such as zinc, cadmium, silica, and iron have also been reported to show toxic effects via the induction of inflammatory-related cytokine release induced by NF-κB. The single-walled and multiple-walled carbon nanotubes were also shown to promote inflammatory responses in mice by generating the TNF-α and monocyte chemoattractant protein-1 (MCP-1) [42].

The MAP-kinase pathway regulates critical cellular processes such as cell proliferation, differentiation, mitosis, cell survival, and apoptosis. Treatment of human bronchial epithelial cell lines with titanium dioxide NPs showed interleukin (IL)-8 production via p38 MAPK and/or ERK pathway and mediated toxicity in the cell lines [43]. The model organism *C. elegans* used for in vivo toxicity assay studies of silver NPs with a size range of 20–30 nm showed that the toxicity mediated was due to the production of ROS, which consequently increased the expression of PMK-1 p38 MAPK and hypoxia-inducible factor (HIF-1) [44]. The toxicity of silica NPs, which hinders their application as drug delivery systems, has been attributed to the activation of JNK, p53, and NF-κB pathways and an elevated expression of pro-inflammatory factors IL-6, IL-8, and MCP-1 [45]. Also, single-walled nanocarbon of size range 0.8–2 nm was reported to have potential adverse cytotoxic effects in mesothelial cells via the activation of signaling molecules, including PARP, AP-1, NF-κB, p38, and Akt, in a dose-dependent manner [46].

5. Organ-/tissue-specific nanotoxicity

Nanoparticles can easily penetrate the tissue system and damage body organs because of their smaller size and high specificity to the tissue system. It has been observed that nanoparticles can move fast in the blood stream and easily cross the blood-brain barrier, this may induce toxicity, which can be harmful for the human organ system (e.g., pulmonary system, reticuloendothelial systems, cardiovascular systems, central nervous system, skin, and embryonic cells) (**Figure 2**).

5.1 Toxicity in pulmonary system

The small-sized NPs have the ability to penetrate easily through the lungs and can cause lung injuries and generate ROS [47]. The pulmonary toxicity studies in rats with ultrafine and fine NPs such as carbon black, nickel, and TiO_2 particles have shown enhanced pulmonary inflammation by the ultrafine NPs [48]. It is being reported that the toxic effects of NPs on lungs show characteristics such as development of exaggerated lung responses, high rate of pulmonary inflammation, failed clearance, cellular proliferation, fibroproliferative effects, and inflammatory-derived mutagenesis, ultimately leading to chronic effects like tumor development in lungs. Factors that mainly influence nanotoxicity in lungs are the particulate characteristics of NPs, such as particle size, number, surface area, surface dose, surface modifications, degree of aggregation, and method of particle synthesis [49, 50].

5.2 Toxicity in reticuloendothelial systems

The reticuloendothelial system in the liver is the main source of biological system where all the NPs get absorbed from the gastrointestinal tract into the cardiovascular systems, as all blood exiting from the gastrointestinal tract transport from the hepatic portal vein that directly diffuses to the liver. Carbon black and polystyrene NPs being less toxic NPs stimulate macrophages by the generation of ROS and activation of calcium signaling to release pro-inflammatory cytokines such as tumor necrosis factor-alpha [51]. Pro-inflammatory cytokines are also associated with pathology of liver disease where the generation of ROS molecule inhibits the hepatocyte function and bile formation.

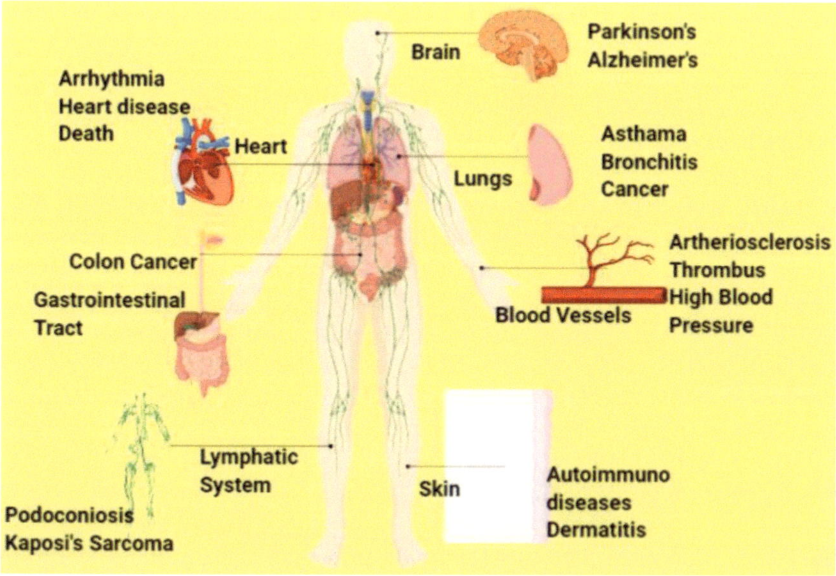

Figure 2.
Tissue- and organ-specific nanotoxicity. The toxic accumulation of nanoparticles can affect any of the tissue types in the body. The small-sized nanoparticles have the ability to penetrate easily through the lungs and can cause lung injuries and have an ability to generate ROS that lead to toxic effects in lungs. The reticuloendothelial system in the liver is the main source of biological system where all the nanoparticles get absorbed from the gastrointestinal tract into the cardiovascular systems, as all blood exiting from the gastrointestinal tract transport from the hepatic portal vein that directly diffuses to the liver. Increased exposure to nanoparticles majorly happens through the process of inhalation, which results in altered heart rate. The inhalation of nanoparticles acquires the ability to reach the brain system mainly through the route of olfactory epithelium by the mechanism of transsynaptic transport or through their uptake via the blood-brain barrier. Nanoparticles acquire the ability to penetrate inside the skin and cause toxic effects such as dermatitis and auto immune disorders.

5.3 Toxicity in cardiovascular systems

The positively charged NPs such as gold and polystyrene have been reported to cause hemolysis and clotting of blood, while the negatively charged NPs are reported to be nontoxic in nature. Increased exposure to diesel-exposed particles (DEP) in hypertensive rats through the process of inhalation resulted in altered heart rate in rats as interpreted through the pacemaker that determines the activity of the heart [52]. Exposure to single-walled NPs also showed altered cardiovascular effects [53]. The injection of ultrafine carbon black NPs into the blood of normal rats caused platelet accumulation in the hepatic microvasculature of the rats and also caused prothrombotic changes on the endothelial surface of the hepatic microvessels [54].

5.4 Toxicity in central nervous system

NPs on inhalation of acquire the ability to reach the brain system mainly through the route of olfactory epithelium by the mechanism of transsynaptic transport or through their uptake via the blood-brain barrier [55]. Enhanced permeability of NPs through the blood-brain barrier has been reported to have increased the number of pathologies including hypertension and allergic encephalomyelitis. The surface charge of the nanoparticle has also been shown to have toxic effects on the brain leading to brain toxicity altering the blood-brain integrity [56]. NPs have also been associated with the production of reactive oxidative species and oxidative stress, which are also associated with brain diseases such as Parkinson's and Alzheimer's [57].

5.5 Toxicity in skin

The widely used cosmetic products for application in the skin contains mostly 3% NPs of size range approximately 50–500 nm [58]. These NPs behold the scattering properties that enhance the entering of UV photons from the optical source into the skin layer although the dermatological effects of NPs able to penetrate the skin are still under investigation. In vitro study with multi-walled carbon nanotubes reported that the carbon NPs have the ability to localize within and initiate an irritation response in human keratinocytes, which are the primary route of occupational exposure [59].

5.6 Toxicity in embryonic cells

Fluorescence correlation spectroscopy played a major role in identifying the toxicity of nanomaterials in embryonic cells. The observation through this microscopy revealed that the accumulation of NPs especially NPs with carboxylate group on their surface takes place more in smaller blood vessels rather than larger blood vessels [60]. These findings are majorly important for finding the aggregation state that can likely influence nanoparticle accumulation in angiogenic tissue. The fluorescence correlation spectroscopy helps to measure the loss of NPs from the blood streams of live embryo [61]. This kinetic loss of NPs can be correlated to surface characteristics of NPs such as surface charge and size. Also, it has been reported that in a mature organism, the renal clearance of nanoparticles occurs only for NPs with size less than 5 nm in lateral dimension. NPs are being reported to act as effective targeted delivery agents in angiogenic tissues of adults as well as embryonic tissues. Larson et al. reported that quantum dots could be used to image vasculature (using two-photon excitation) in the dermis of mice [61]. Semiconductor quantum dots are NPs with intense, stable fluorescence and are a very good source to detect ten to hundreds of cancer biomarkers in blood assays, on cancer tissue biopsies, or as contrast agents for medical imaging. Smith and coworkers have developed some functionalized quantum dots for tumor targeting in mice; however, no study has been made to measure directly the concentration of the quantum dots in the blood or whether or not they were aggregated; hence, the toxicity level of these quantum dots has not been checked [62].

6. Conclusion

The use of nanomaterials in biomedical sciences and health sciences has increased in recent years due to their size and surface characteristics appropriate for targeted and site-specific delivery of drugs to the affected areas. In cancer research, nanomedicine holds the massive potential for cancer therapy. The surface and tiny size and shape of NPs have been used as unique properties of NPs to play a key role for an efficient treatment and specific targeting. Nano-based therapeutic and diagnostic strategies pose as highly promising tools for easy and cost-effective diagnosis of cancer. But, the public interest's in accurate, relevant, and predictive nanotoxicological assessments also has been growing. Due to the complication of ROS formation and disruption to the normal biological events, the use of nanomaterials has created complicated situation. The usage of nanomaterials has been highly reported

DOI: http://dx.doi.org/10.5772/intechopen.90928

to cause toxic events such as DNA damage, oxidative stress damage, and inflammatory responses. Major organs such as heart, brain, skin, etc. have been reported to have toxic responses related to nanoparticle applications. So, the development of a set of rules is needed for developing safe engineered nanomaterials, which can be determined by *in vitro* toxicity studies.

Author details

Sibi Raj and Dhruv Kumar*
Amity Institute of Molecular Medicine and Stem Cell Research (AIMMSCR), Amity University, Noida, Uttar Pradesh, India

*Address all correspondence to: dhruvbhu@gmail.com; dkumar13@amity.edu

References

[1] Tan SY, Grimes S. Paul Ehrlich (1854-1915): Man with the magic bullet. Singapore Medical Journal. 2010

[2] Truong NP, Whittaker MR, Mak CW, Davis TP. The importance of nanoparticle shape in cancer drug delivery. Expert Opinion on Drug Delivery. 2015

[3] Singh AP, Biswas A, Shukla A, Maiti P. Targeted therapy in chronic diseases using nanomaterial-based drug delivery vehicles. Signal Transduction and Targeted Therapy. 2019

[4] Heinz H et al. Nanoparticle decoration with surfactants: Molecular interactions, assembly, and applications. Surface Science Reports. 2017

[5] Hofmann-Amtenbrink M, Grainger DW, Hofmann H. NP in medicine: Current challenges facing inorganic nanoparticle toxicity assessments and standardizations. Nanomedicine: Nanotechnology, Biology, and Medicine. 2015

[6] Song Y et al. Nanomaterials in humans: Identification, characteristics, and potential damage. Toxicologic Pathology. 2011

[7] Nurkiewicz TR et al. Systemic microvascular dysfunction and inflammation after pulmonary particulate matter exposure. Environmental Health Perspectives. 2006

[8] Liu LZ et al. Tungsten carbide-cobalt NP induce reactive oxygen species, AKT, ERK, AP-1, NF-κB, VEGF, and angiogenesis. Biological Trace Element Research. 2015

[9] Zhu X, Hondroulis E, Liu W, Li CZ. Biosensing approaches for rapid geno-toxicity and cytotoxicity assays upon nanomaterial exposure. Small. 2013

[10] Bantz C et al. The surface properties of NP determine the agglomeration state and the size of the particles under physiological conditions. Beilstein Journal of Nanotechnology. 2014

[11] Singh R, Lillard JW. Nanoparticle-based targeted drug delivery. Experimental and Molecular Pathology. 2009

[12] Yoshida T, Yoshikawa T, Nabeshi H, Tsutsumi Y. Relation analysis between intracellular distribution of nanomateriarls, ROS generation and DNA damage. Yakugaku Zasshi. 2012

[13] Li Y et al. Mechanism for α-MnO_2 nanowire-induced cytotoxicity in HeLa cells. Journal of Nanoscience and Nanotechnology. 2010

[14] Sohaebuddin SK, Thevenot PT, Baker D, Eaton JW, Tang L. Nanomaterial cytotoxicity is composition, size, and cell type dependent. Particle and Fibre Toxicology. 2010

[15] Yin JJ et al. Phototoxicity of nano titanium dioxides in HaCaT keratinocytes-generation of reactive oxygen species and cell damage. Toxicology and Applied Pharmacology. 2012

[16] Wang S, Lu W, Tovmachenko O, Rai US, Yu H, Ray PC. Challenge in understanding size and shape dependent toxicity of gold nanomaterials in human skin keratinocytes. Chemical Physics Letters. 2008

[17] Xia T et al. Comparison of the mechanism of toxicity of zinc oxide and cerium oxide NP based on dissolution and oxidative stress properties. ACS Nano. 2008

[18] Liu Y et al. Intracellular dynamics of cationic and anionic polystyrene NP

without direct interaction with mitotic spindle and chromosomes. Biomaterials. 2011

[19] Hühn D et al. Polymer-coated NP interacting with proteins and cells: Focusing on the sign of the net charge. ACS Nano. 2013

[20] Linse S et al. Nucleation of protein fibrillation by NP. Proceedings of the National Academy of Sciences of the United States of America. 2007

[21] Xu P, Van Kirk EA, Zhan Y, Murdoch WJ, Radosz M, Shen Y. Targeted charge-reversal NP for nuclear drug delivery. Angewandte Chemie, International Edition. 2007

[22] Arami H, Khandhar A, Liggitt D, Krishnan KM. In vivo delivery, pharmacokinetics, biodistribution and toxicity of iron oxide NP. Chemical Society Reviews. 2015

[23] Nguyen KC, Rippstein P, Tayabali AF, Willmore WG. Mitochondrial toxicity of cadmium telluride quantum dot NP in mammalian hepatocytes. Toxicological Sciences. 2015

[24] Cho J, Kushiro K, Teramura Y, Takai M. Lectin-tagged fluorescent polymeric NP for targeting of sialic acid on living cells. Biomacromolecules. 2014

[25] Derfus AM, Chan WCW, Bhatia SN. Probing the cytotoxicity of semiconductor quantum dots. Nano Letters. 2004

[26] Huang J et al. Casein-coated iron oxide NP for high MRI contrast enhancement and efficient cell targeting. ACS Applied Materials and Interfaces. 2013

[27] Beckman KB, Ames BN. The free radical theory of aging matures. Physiological Reviews. 1998

[28] Azad MB, Chen Y, Gibson SB. Regulation of autophagy by reactive oxygen species (ROS): Implications for cancer progression and treatment. Antioxidants and Redox Signaling. 2009

[29] Radomski A et al. Nanoparticle-induced platelet aggregation and vascular thrombosis. British Journal of Pharmacology. 2005

[30] Valko M, Rhodes CJ, Moncol J, Izakovic M, Mazur M. Free radicals, metals and antioxidants in oxidative stress-induced cancer. Chemico-Biological Interactions. 2006

[31] Dröge W. Free radicals in the physiological control of cell function. Physiological Reviews. 2002

[32] Akhtar MJ et al. Nanotoxicity of pure silica mediated through oxidant generation rather than glutathione depletion in human lung epithelial cells. Toxicology. 2010

[33] Chiang HM et al. Nanoscale ZnO induces cytotoxicity and DNA damage in human cell lines and rat primary neuronal cells. Journal of Nanoscience and Nanotechnology. 2012

[34] Singh N et al. NanoGenotoxicology: The DNA damaging potential of engineered nanomaterials. Biomaterials. 2009

[35] Li JJ, Zou L, Hartono D, Ong CN, Bay BH, Yung LYL. Gold NP induce oxidative damage in lung fibroblasts in vitro. Advanced Materials. 2008

[36] Poli G, Leonarduzzi G, Biasi F, Chiarpotto E. Oxidative stress and cell signalling. Current Medicinal Chemistry. 2012

[37] Choi AO, Brown SE, Szyf M, Maysinger D. Quantum dot-induced epigenetic and genotoxic changes in human breast cancer cells. Journal of Molecular Medicine. 2008

[38] Huang YW, Wu CH, Aronstam RS. Toxicity of transition metal oxide NP: Recent insights from in vitro studies. Materials. 2010

[39] Yuan X, Zhang X, Sun L, Wei Y, Wei X. Cellular toxicity and immunological effects of carbon-based nanomaterials. Particle and Fibre Toxicology. 2019

[40] Szebeni J et al. Animal models of complement-mediated hypersensitivity reactions to liposomes and other lipid-based NP. Journal of Liposome Research. 2007

[41] Monteiller C et al. The pro-inflammatory effects of low-toxicity low-solubility particles, NP and fine particles, on epithelial cells in vitro: The role of surface area. Occupational and Environmental Medicine. 2007

[42] Nygaard UC, Hansen JS, Samuelsen M, Alberg T, Marioara CD, Løvik M. Single-walled and multi-walled carbon nanotubes promote allergic immune responses in mice. Toxicological Sciences. 2009

[43] Torres M, Forman HJ. Redox signaling and the MAP kinase pathways. BioFactors. 2003

[44] Lim D, Roh JY, Eom HJ, Choi JY, Hyun J, Choi J. Oxidative stress-related PMK-1 P38 MAPK activation as a mechanism for toxicity of silver NP to reproduction in the nematode *Caenorhabditis elegans*. Environmental Toxicology and Chemistry. 2012

[45] Liu X, Sun J. Endothelial cells dysfunction induced by silica NP through oxidative stress via JNK/P53 and NF-κB pathways. Biomaterials. 2010

[46] Pacurari M et al. Raw single-wall carbon nanotubes induce oxidative stress and activate MAPKs, AP-1, NF-κB, and Akt in normal and malignant human mesothelial cells. Environmental Health Perspectives. 2008

[47] Warheit DB, Webb TR, Sayes CM, Colvin VL, Reed KL. Pulmonary instillation studies with nanoscale TiO_2 rods and dots in rats: Toxicity is not dependent upon particle size and surface area. Toxicological Sciences. 2006

[48] Pettibone JM, Adamcakova-Dodd A, Thorne PS, O'Shaughnessy PT, Weydert JA, Grassian VH. Inflammatory response of mice following inhalation exposure to iron and copper NP. Nanotoxicology. 2008

[49] Nemmar A, Hoylaerts MF, Hoet PHM, Vermylen J, Nemery B. Size effect of intratracheally instilled particles on pulmonary inflammation and vascular thrombosis. Toxicology and Applied Pharmacology. 2003

[50] Oberdorster G, Ferin J, Lehnert BE. Correlation between particle size, in vivo particle persistence, and lung injury. Environmental Health Perspectives. 1994

[51] Brown DM et al. Calcium and ROS-mediated activation of transcription factors and TNF-α cytokine gene expression in macrophages exposed to ultrafine particles. The American Journal of Physiology-Lung Cellular and Molecular Physiology. 2004

[52] Hansen CS et al. Diesel exhaust particles induce endothelial dysfunction in apoE−/− mice. Toxicology and Applied Pharmacology. 2007

[53] Li Z et al. Cardiovascular effects of pulmonary exposure to single-wall carbon nanotubes. Environmental Health Perspectives. 2007

[54] Simeonova PP, Erdely A. Engineered nanoparticle respiratory exposure and potential risks for

cardiovascular toxicity: Predictive tests and biomarkers. Inhalation Toxicology. 2009

[55] Lockman PR, Koziara JM, Mumper RJ, Allen D. Nanoparticle surface charges alter blood-brain barrier integrity and permeability. Journal of Drug Targeting. 2004

[56] Jallouli Y, Paillard A, Chang J, Sevin E, Betbeder D. Influence of surface charge and inner composition of porous NP to cross blood-brain barrier in vitro. International Journal of Pharmaceutics. 2007

[57] Long TC, Saleh N, Tilton RD, Lowry GV, Veronesi B. Titanium dioxide (P25) produces reactive oxygen species in immortalized brain microglia (BV2): Implications for nanoparticle neurotoxicity. Environmental Science and Technology. 2006

[58] Baroli B, Ennas MG, Loffredo F, Isola M, Pinna R, López-Quintela MA. Penetration of metallic NP in human full-thickness skin. The Journal of Investigative Dermatology. 2007

[59] Zvyagin AV, Zhao X, Gierden A, Sanchez W, Ross JA, Roberts MS. Imaging of zinc oxide nanoparticle penetration in human skin in vitro and in vivo. Journal of Biomedical Optics. 2008

[60] Clancy AA, Gregoriou Y, Yaehne K, Cramb DT. Measuring properties of NP in embryonic blood vessels: Towards a physicochemical basis for nanotoxicity. Chemical Physics Letters. 2010

[61] Larson DR et al. Water-soluble quantum dots for multiphoton fluorescence imaging in vivo. Science. 2003

[62] Smith AM, Dave S, Nie S, True L, Gao X. Multicolor quantum dots for molecular diagnostics of cancer. Expert Review of Molecular Diagnostics. 2006

Chapter 9

Few-Layered Hexagonal Boron Nitride: Functionalization, Nanocomposites, and Physicochemical and Biological Properties

Magdalena Jedrzejczak-Silicka, Martyna Trukawka, Katarzyna Piotrowska and Ewa Mijowska

Abstract

Hexagonal boron nitride (h-BN) is an analogue of graphite called "white graphene." In the structure of h-BN, B and N atoms substitute C atoms. The boron and nitrogen atoms are linked via strong B-N covalent bonds and form interlocking hexagonal rings. h-BN is used in different areas due to its interesting physical and chemical properties, e.g., in electronics as an insulator and in ceramics, resins, plastics, and paints. Therefore, boron nitride (BN) is also a popular inorganic compound in cosmetic industry (the highest BN concentration up to 25% can be found in eye shadow formulation). It is also widely used in dental cement production (for dental and orthodontic applications). Boron nitride seems to be suitable for biomedical applications; therefore, the cytotoxicity in vitro and in vivo observations of h-BN nanoplates and novel few-layered h-BN-based nanocomposites are still needed. The short-time studies confirm their low cytotoxicity and suggest that BN can be used as a novel drug delivery system; however, medical application needs additional verification in long-term studies.

Keywords: boron nitride, few-layered hexagonal boron nitride, exfoliation, functionalization, hydroxyl groups, gold nanoparticles, h-BN nanocomposites, biocompatibility, cellular uptake

1. Introduction

Nanotechnology became a crucial technology in many science fields, not only in organic and inorganic chemistry, materials and surface sciences, semiconductor physics, microfabrication, and molecular engineering but also has significant impact on biological and medical science. The results of nanotechnology activity create a new reality. On the one hand, it gives the possibility to develop novel methods of diagnosis, drug delivery, and cancer treatment. On the other hand, methods implemented in nanomaterial production and development can affect human health and the state of the environment. The knowledge of the effect on

IntechOpen

living organisms is limited due to relatively short-time *in vitro* and especially *in vivo* experiments that highlight mechanism of nanomaterials—cell-tissue-organism interactions.

Application of nanomaterials in biology and medicine has a multidirectional character. The different nanomaterials with many unique physicochemical properties are tested to develop new nanomaterial-based approaches: fluorescent labels (e.g., quantum dots), detection of pathogens and other biological samples (e.g., nucleic acids, proteins), methods of separation and purification of single biomolecules or cells, pharmacokinetic analysis, biosensing, final drug or gene delivery, cancer treatment via hyperthermia method, tissue engineering, and contrast enhancement of medical imaging technique (e.g., magnetic resonance imaging) [1].

Hexagonal boron nitride (h-BN) is one of the most unique and promising layered nanomaterial widely used as in cosmetic production. As it was stated by Fiume and co-workers [2], although the *International Cosmetic Ingredient Dictionary and Handbook* does not specify which crystal form/forms is/are used in cosmetics, it is presumed that the hexagonal form of boron nitride is applied for that proposes. The form of h-BN presents the most appropriate functionality in cosmetic production/properties (e.g., as a slip modifier). The use of h-BN in cosmetic formulation suggests the lack of toxicity/cytotoxicity [2–4]; thus, the new approach of h-BN, or its exfoliated form, to study its modification and functionalization to obtain a potentially interesting nanomaterial in, e.g., the context of theranostic concept is expected.

2. General information about hexagonal boron nitride (h-BN)

In recent years, 2D materials have become very attractive due to their properties. The most popular among them are graphene, graphene oxide (GO), and reduced graphene oxide (rGO). The big advantage of these materials is their potential multifunctionality, so they can be applied, for example, in transistors, sensing, energy devices [5] and biomedical devices [6], or nanomedicine [7]. Even though these materials are studied widely, there is a plenty of room to explore their properties, e.g., very complexed bio-response on many levels. Another attractive layered material, which is not fully explored, is hexagonal boron nitride. Its exfoliated form is considered as a graphene analogue.

Boron nitride is a chemical compound with equal number of boron and nitrogen atoms. Just like carbon, it occurs in amorphous and crystalline forms. The major crystalline forms are hexagonal boron nitride (h-BN) compared to graphite, sphalerite boron nitride (β-BN) similar to cubic diamond, and rhombohedral (r-BN) and wurtzite boron nitride (γ-BN), which is in hexagonal diamond form [3, 8–10]. Boron nitride nanotubes (BNNT) are also known. All the forms are electrical insulators [11]. The most popular form of BN, due to its stability, is hexagonal boron nitride. In its structure the boron and nitrogen atoms are linked with each other via strong B-N covalent bonds and form interlocking hexagonal rings [12, 13]. Atoms are bound via strong covalent bonds in-plane, and each layer is held together via van der Waals forces [12] (**Figure 1**).

The multilayered form stabilizes the whole structure. Hexagonal boron nitride systems (e.g., nanotubes, flakes) are highly thermally and chemically stable, but at the same time, they are equally thermally conductive and mechanically robust. **Table 1** presents the basic properties of hexagonal boron nitride. Thus, h-BN systems are widely used for durable high-temperature crucibles, antioxidation lubricants, and protective coatings and as a substrate for semiconductors, lens coatings, etc. in industry [2, 15].

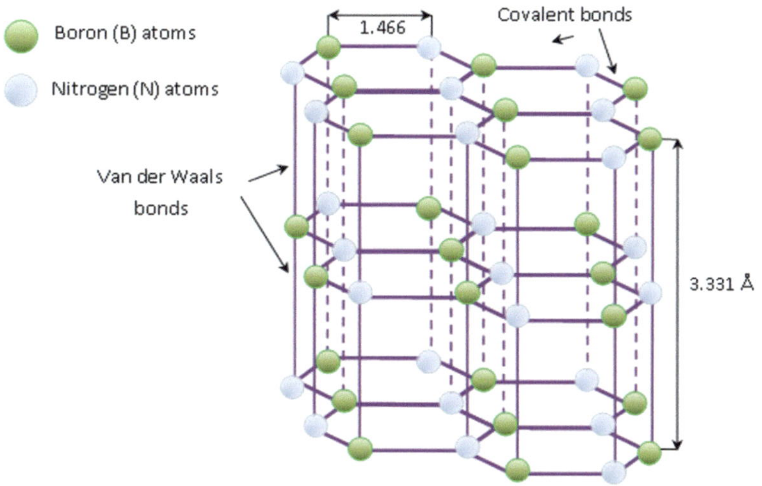

Figure 1.
Hexagonal boron nitride structure [13].

Properties of hexagonal boron nitride (h-BN)	
Appearance	White powder, photostable, odorless (hexagonal, cosmetic grade)
Bond length	1.466 Å (with interlayer spacing of 3.331 Å)
Molar mass	24.82 g mol^{-1}
Density	~2.1 g/cm^3
Structure	Crystal; hexagonal
Melting point	2.973°C; sublimes
Surface area	0.82–30 m^2/g (varies by grade)
Refractive index (n_D)	1.74
Stability	Chemical inert and stable
Hardness	1–2 on the Mohs scale
Specific heat capacity (C)	19.7 J/(K·mol)
Std enthalpy of formation ($\Delta_f H^o{}_{298}$)	−254.4 kJ/mol
Gibbs free energy ($\Delta_f G^o$)	−22 kJ/mol
Coefficient of friction	<0.3

Table 1.
Properties of hexagonal boron nitride [2, 14].

Boron nitride nanosheets (BNNSs) were found to be used in polymeric film reinforcement, for example, the elastic modulus of polymethyl methacrylate (PMMA) film was increased when BN nanosheets were incorporated into the polymer [16]. It is also a popular inorganic compound in cosmetic industry used as a slip modifier [13, 17]. The data from the US Food and Drug Administration (FDA) report showed that boron nitride was used in 643 cosmetic formulations (data from 2013). The highest BN concentration (up to 25%) can be found in eye shadow formulation, up to 16% in powders and 2% in lipstick formulation [2, 13]. The successful use of BNNTs in dental adhesive and sealants has been also reported. Moreover, h-BN nanoplatelets modified by the presence of quaternary ammonium compounds (QACs) loaded on h-BN's surface to form fillers for linear low-density polyethylene (LLDPE) were tested for inhibition of growth of both *E. coli* and *S. aureus* bacteria [18–20].

Therefore, boron nitride seems to be suitable for biomedical applications as well. Several cytotoxicity studies based on boron nitride nanotubes confirmed its low cytotoxicity and suggested that BN can be used as a novel drug delivery system. In contrast, other studies showed that BNNT was cytotoxic and affected relative cell viability even at low concentrations [14, 21–24].

For the sake of discrepancies occurring in the literature, a deeper understanding of the toxicity of h-BN-based samples is crucial. Here, we will present the synthesis and cytotoxicity study on exfoliated and functionalized hexagonal boron nitride called few-layered BN.

2.1 Synthesis methods of few-layered h-BN (fBN)

There are two typical approaches to obtain exfoliated hexagonal boron nitrogen nanosheets: top-down (exfoliation methods) or bottom-up (chemical vapor deposition (CVD) or other deposition techniques).

An example of top-down had been described by Liu et al. [25]. They used one-pot solvothermal synthesis involving mixing bulk h-BN, ethanol, and sodium hydroxide in Teflon autoclave. In this method they obtained boron nitride nanosheets and quantum dots at the same time. Marsh with co-workers found even a simpler method [26]. They produced boron nitride nanosheets (BNNSs) from bulk h-BN powders using a simple cosolvent approach. Authors used common organic solvents and water to create a mixture. It was more efficient than using the individual components to get h-BN exfoliated and suspended. They maintain that cosolvent system is inexpensive, safe to work with, and completely scalable. Han et al. [27] used 1,2-dichloroethane solution of poly[(m-phenylenevinylene)-co-(2,5-dioctoxy-p-phenylenevinylene)] to disperse and break up van der Waals forces between h-BN layers, while Zhi et al. [28] reported the large-scale fabrication of 2D h-BN nanosheets by vigorous sonication of h-BN in dimethylformamide (DMF). The choice of solvent should be optimized to overcome van der Waals forces.

The optimization to use two-step exfoliation technique combining chemical and mechanical exfoliation was also reported [29]. Chemical exfoliation of h-BN was carried out by a modified Hummer's method. h-BN was additionally delaminated mechanically. Mechanical exfoliation was performed using a tip sonicator. Chemically exfoliated h-BN was added into 1-methyl-2-pyrrolidinone (NMP) in a volume ratio of 0.5%. After the sonication, the mixture was left to evaporate the solvent. This method is simple and fast.

The most important representative of bottom-up method is chemical vapor deposition. In general, it can be divided into two types: one that requires a substrate and another which does not need it. A lot of optional substrates have been used in the process. CVD can be carried out on metals (Cu [30], Ni [31], Co [32], etc.) as well as on metal oxides (Al_2O_3) [33] or graphite [34]. The precursors can also be in different forms. Most popular are borazine [35], ammonia borane [36], and diborane [37].

Each method has its advantages and disadvantages. Exfoliation techniques ensure higher crystallinity of the material, but high-scale synthesis is very difficult. In contrast, the materials obtained from CVD give the possibility to control over the thickness or size of the sheets, but their crystallinity is lower. Therefore, the technique of material synthesis should be adapted to the requirements of a specific application.

2.2 Characterization of few-layered h-BN (fBN)

Depending on the synthesis method, a material with different properties can be expected. CVD is more suitable for large-scale synthesis in industry, but exfoliation methods have been also used for various applications, especially on a laboratory scale. Therefore, these materials cannot be clearly compared. **Table 2** presents a summary of properties of fBN such as flake size and material thickness in relation to the method of synthesis.

Following data from state of the art, it can be concluded that chemical vapor deposition provides thinner and larger layers of h-BN than in the case of exfoliation. It should be noted that in the case of exfoliation, the starting bulk material is used, while in the case of CVD, a completely new material is obtained from various molecular precursors. Mostly, the number of the obtained h-BN layers is strongly related with the used substrates. It can be also concluded that the combination of

Method	Substrates	Thickness [nm]	Flake size [μm]	Ref.
Exfoliation	Potassium permanganate Sulfuric acid 1-Methyl-2-pyrrolidinone	5	0.3–0.6	This work
Exfoliation	Ethanol Sodium hydroxide	~1	~1.2	[25]
Exfoliation	Methanol ethanol 1-Propanol 2-Propanol acetone Tert-butanol (cosolvents)	6–10	—	[26]
Exfoliation	1,2-Dichloroethane poly[(m-phenylenevinylene)-co-(2,5-dictoxy-p-phenylenevinylene)]	~1.2	Several	[27]
Exfoliation	Dimethylformamide	3–7	Smaller than pristine material	[28]
Exfoliation	Octadecylamine	1–2	0.3–0.5	[38]
Exfoliation	Zinc chloride Potassium chloride	2–6 1–3	0.5 0.2	[39]
CVD (LPCVD)	Cu foil Borazane	0.42	0.05–0.1	[30]
CVD (LPCVD)	Co film Ammonia borane	~1	> 5	[32]
CVD (LPCVD)	Al_2O_3 substrate Borazane	Temperature depending 40–228	—	[33]
CVD	Fe foil Borazine	5–15	10 × 10	[35]
CVD (AP-CVD)	Ag foil Borazine	0.7–1.3	0.1	[27]
CVD (AP-CVD)	Pt foil Borazane	0.32–0.809	1–2	[40]

Table 2.
Properties of fBN (flake size, material thickness) in relation to the synthesis method.

chemical and mechanical exfoliation is a very effective and repeatable method. **Figure 2A** presents the bulk hexagonal boron nitride. The multilayered material is clearly visible. Many flakes are aggregated and connected to each other. After the exfoliation process, even individual flakes of the material are detected (**Figure 2B**).

The exfoliation efficiency was also confirmed by atomic force microscopy (AFM). The thickness of bulk nanomaterial was estimated to be ~40 nm (**Figure 3A**). After chemical and mechanical exfoliation, the number of layers had been greatly reduced. The obtained thickness was ~5 nm, which corresponded to several layers of h-BN (**Figure 3B**).

Scanning electron microscope (SEM) was also used to analyze the flake size of fBN in greater details (**Figure 4**). The observation revealed that most of the flakes were in a size range of 0.3–1.2 μm.

Concluding this observation, using various methods the materials with similar parameters can be obtained. The issue of choosing the method of preparation should be adapted to the properties that the material should exhibit to perform the best in required applications.

2.3 Functionalization of few-layered h-BN (fBN)

Functionalization process is undertaken to provide additional/new properties. In the case of hexagonal boron nitride, the biggest challenge is to raise the materials' water solubility/dispersibility. This can be achieved by introducing the functional groups on fBN surface. One of the simplest routes is functionalization with hydroxyl groups. At the same time, as it was proved, the presence of -OH groups determines the stability of dispersion in water-based solution [41].

The procedure was easy and repeatable. Chemically and mechanically exfoliated hexagonal boron nitrides were refluxed in hydrogen peroxide for a longer time. To confirm the functionalization, FT-IR spectra were analyzed (**Figure 5**). Except for the peaks characteristic for hexagonal boron nitride (810 and 1370 cm^{-1}), clearly visible new bonds corresponding to hydroxyl groups at 2525 and 3400 cm^{-1} are detected [42].

Pristine BN nanomaterials exhibit notable hydrophobicity when interacting with water or aqueous solutions. Therefore, this functionalization allows stable dispersion in phosphate buffer solution, which is crucial for biological application [41].

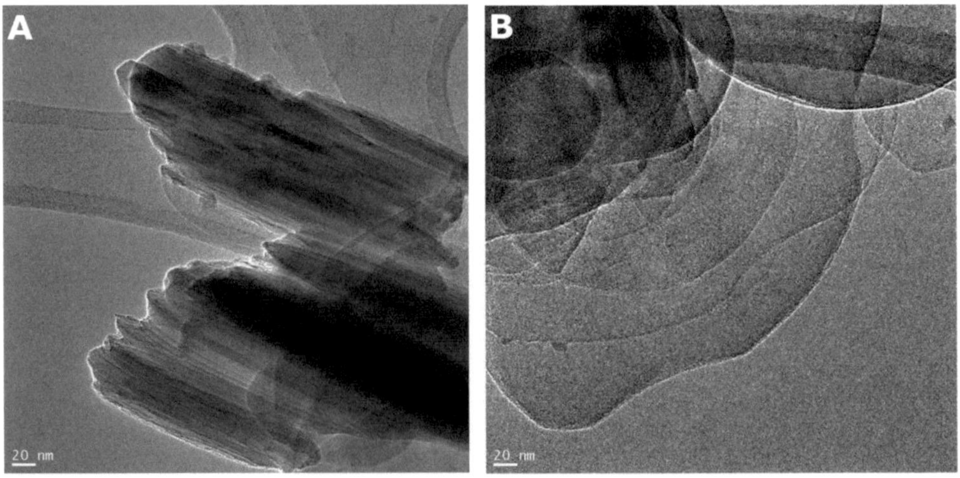

Figure 2.
Transmission electron microscope (TEM) images of bulk h-BN (A) and exfoliated fBN (B).

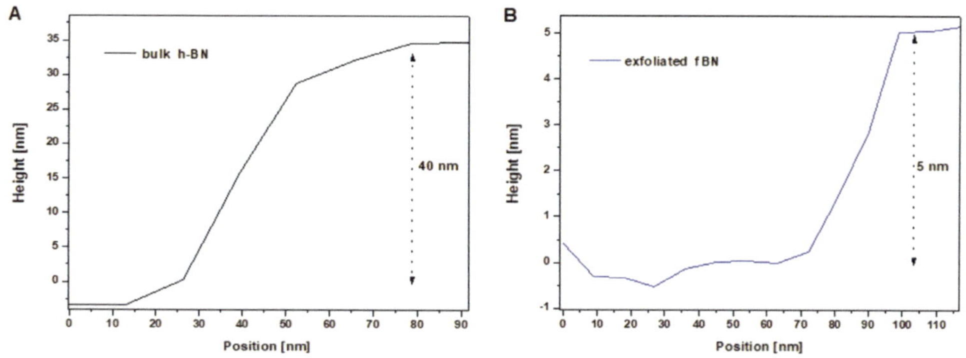

Figure 3.
Height profile of bulk h-BN (A) and exfoliated fBN (B).

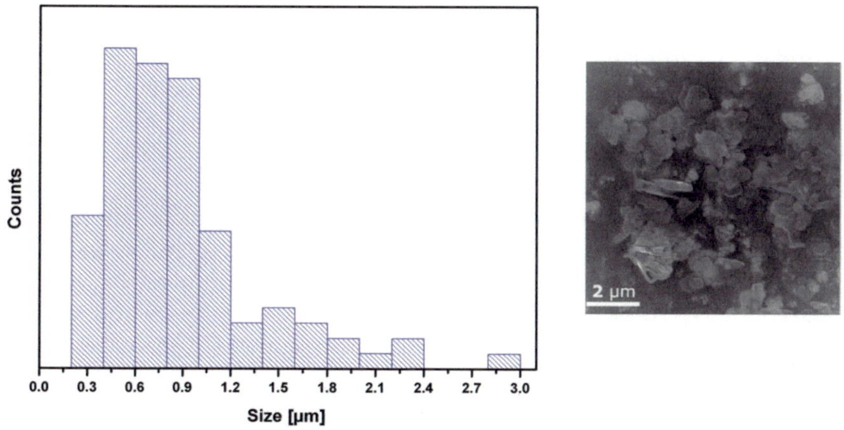

Figure 4.
Flake size distribution and SEM image of exfoliated fBN.

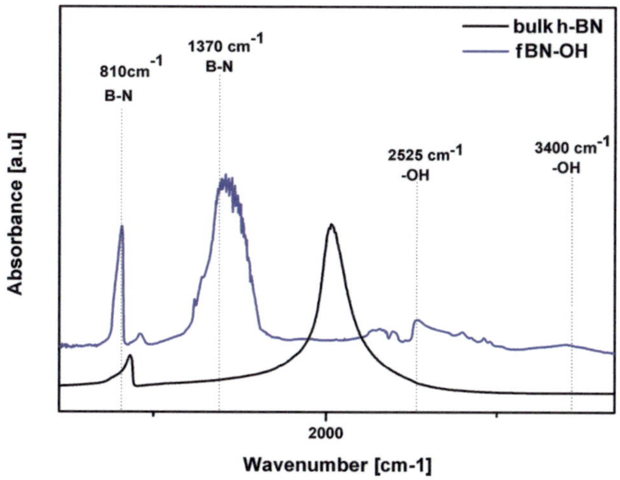

Figure 5.
FT-IR spectra of pristine and hydroxylated fBN.

Other methods for obtaining hydroxylated hexagonal boron nitride are also known. Sainsbury et al. [43] used boron nitride nanosheets with tert-butoxy groups on the surface. To induce hydroxyl groups, they mixed and sonicated piranha solution

(H_2SO_4:H_2O_2, 3:1) [43]. Moreover, the authors carried out further functionalization. They used hydroxylated material to obtain isocyanate-functionalized BNNSs. A completely different approach to obtain hydroxylated BN has been shown by Pakdel et al. [44]. Boron nitride nanostructure films were subjected to direct ion/electron bombardment in a plasma generator device. In this way they aimed to control the wetting properties of nanomaterial.

It turned out that hydroxylated h-BN can also be obtained by ball milling. Lee with co-workers [45] presented a simple ball milling of BN powders in the presence of sodium hydroxide. They connected the synergetic effect of chemical peeling and mechanical shear forces. There are many other functionalities that allow h-BN to be used in even more applications. For example, it is possible to decorate hexagonal boron nitride with metal nanoparticles. There are reports, for example, of platinum, silver, and gold decoration. Anna Harley-Trochimczyk et al. [46] described crystalline boron nitride aerogel loaded with crystalline platinum nanoparticles. They found out that this material can be used in catalytic gas sensing. Dai et al. [47] produced Ag nanoparticle coverage on porous BN microfibers and examined it for a novel pollutant-capturing surface-enhanced Raman scattering (SERS) substrate. There are already several reports on BN materials functionalized with gold; however, such a composite had not been previously tested for biological response as described below. Until now, such nanocomposite has found application in electrocatalysis [48] or hydrogen peroxide detection [49].

In research [29] simple and repeatable Au-fBN nanocomposite synthesis method was demonstrated. Briefly, exfoliated h-BN was sonicated in distilled water. The mixture was heated with gold(III) chloride trihydrate under the reflux. After a few minutes, trisodium citrate was added to the boiling mixture. The whole system was heated. **Figure 6** shows transmission electron microscope (TEM) images of the obtained nanocomposite (Au-fBN).

Based on TEM micrographs, the size of gold nanoparticles was determined (**Figure 7**). The nanoparticle size distribution was in the range from 6 to 25 nm with a majority of ~16 nm.

The presence of gold nanoparticles was confirmed by Raman spectroscopy (**Figure 8**). The peak at 1366 cm^{-1} is the most characteristic for hexagonal boron nitride. It is resulting from the E2g phonon mode and is an analogue of the G peak in graphene [50]. It is very clearly visible in the spectrum of pure material and much

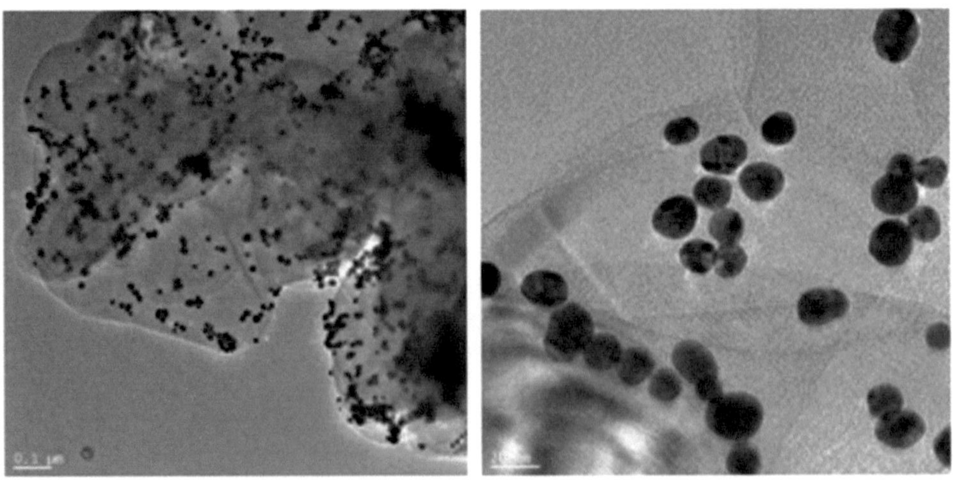

Figure 6.
TEM images of Au-fBN nanocomposite.

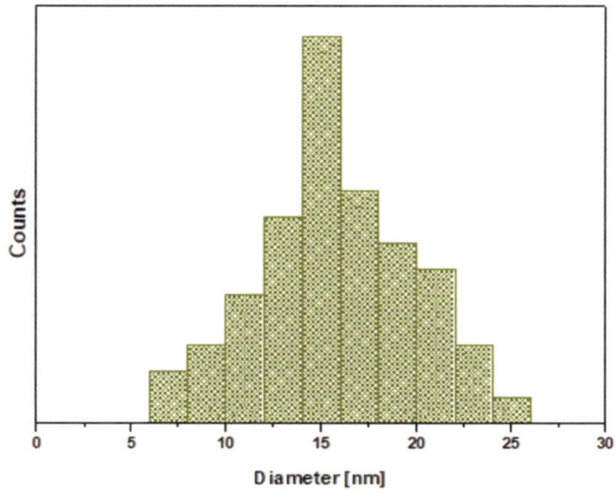

Figure 7.
Gold nanoparticle size distribution.

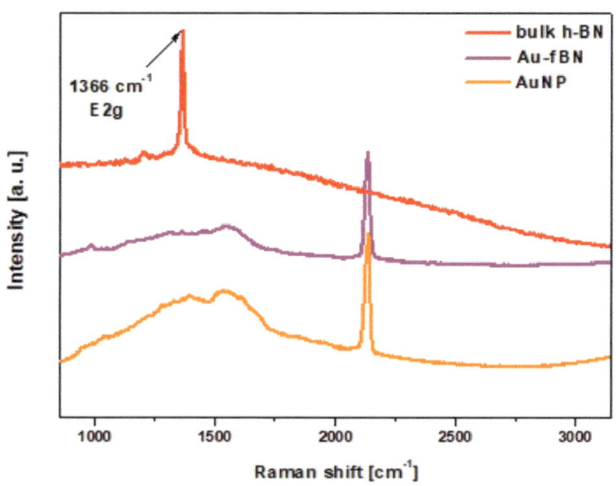

Figure 8.
Raman spectra of h-BN bulk, nanocomposite (Au-fBN), and gold nanoparticles (Au NP).

less intense in the nanocomposite. This is due to the presence of gold nanoparticles with characteristic peaks in the region from 1300 to 1600 cm^{-1} [51]. There is another intense peak in the spectrum of gold nanoparticles. It occurs at 2130 cm^{-1}, and it can also be clearly seen in the nanocomposite spectrum, which additionally ensures efficient functionalization.

Nanomaterials prepared in the method described above (fBN-OH and Au-fBN) have been subjected to biological tests, which will be discussed in further parts of the chapter.

3. The effect of few-layered BN-OH (fBN-OH) and Au-fBN nanocomposites on cellular viability

The biocompatibility of h-BN-based nanocomposites synthesized in studies [29, 41] was determined in three main steps.

The first step of the *in vitro* study was based on morphological cell analysis. This step often is omitted by the researchers, although the morphology observation is the simplest and direct method that gives possibility to identify the changes of cellular shape and adhesion ability. Both of them may be changed upon specific environmental stress [52]. **Figure 9** presents the cellular morphology and distribution of L929 and MCF-7 cells after 48-hour incubation with fBN-OH and Au-fBN nanocomposites (analysis was conducted using phase contrast microscopy, ×100, Nikon TS-100 microscope). Both cell lines grown in monolayers display typical morphology—the cells did not change shape. The cells did not show a tendency to form clusters, and the adhesion process was not impaired after 48 hours.

Moreover, in the second step, the cellular uptake and distribution of fBN-OH and Au-fBN nanocomposites were analyzed using confocal microscopy (**Figure 10**). The nanomaterials were labeled with FITC, and the presence of nanocomposites in cells was confirmed by green fluorescent signal. The internalized h-BN-based nanocomposites were accumulated in the peripheral cytoplasm and the perinuclear region, but the presence of fBN-OH and Au-fBN was not confirmed in the nucleus. The labeled nanocomposites formed small intercellular aggregates. The uptake

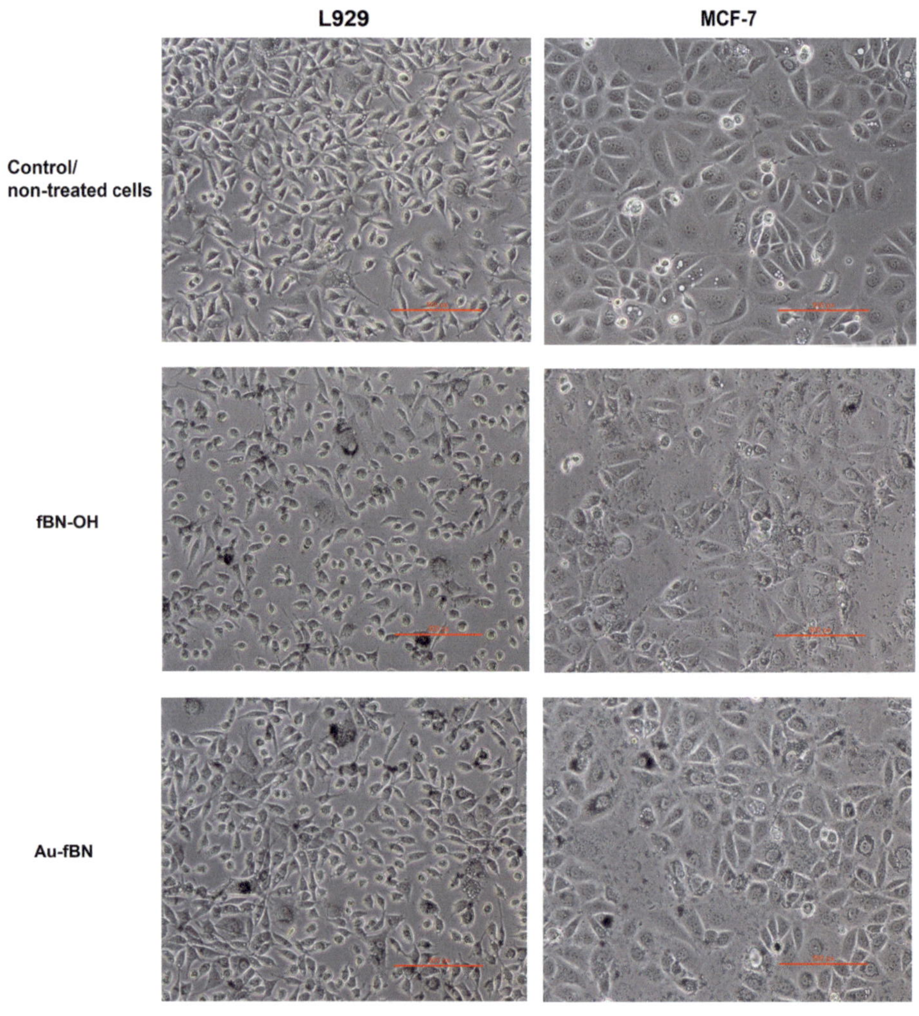

Figure 9.
Cellular morphology of cultures incubated with fBN-OH and Au-fBN nanoplates for 48 hours. Magnification ×100.

efficiency process of hexagonal boron nitride nanocomposites by normal and cancer cells was established at a similar level.

In the third step of the study, a comparison of biocompatibility results of the fBN-OH and Au-fBN nanocomposites at 3.125, 6.25, 10.0, 12.5, 25.0, 50.0, 100.0, and 200.0 μg mL^{-1} concentrations was determined using Cell Counting Kit-8 (CCK-8), neutral red uptake (NRU), and lactate dehydrogenase leaking (LDH) assays (**Figure 10**) [29]. The highest reduction of the cell viability was recorded at the concentrations of 100.0–200.0 μg mL^{-1} for fBN-OH and 200.0 μg mL^{-1} for Au-fBN in L929 cell cultures incubated for 48 hours (**Figure 10**). The MCF-7 cell cultures exhibited higher reduction of cell viability for fBN-OH at the concentration range between 12.5 and 200.0 μg mL^{-1} (**Figure 10**). The cell viability of MCF-7 cells incubated with nanocomposites loaded with gold NPs was reduced at the concentration of 10.0 and 200.0 μg mL^{-1}, in *comparison to free-grown MCF-7 control culture* (**Figure 10**).

In contrast to CCK-8 assay results, NRU assay showed higher reduction of the viability of both cell lines (**Figure 10**). Both cell lines showed higher sensitivity of

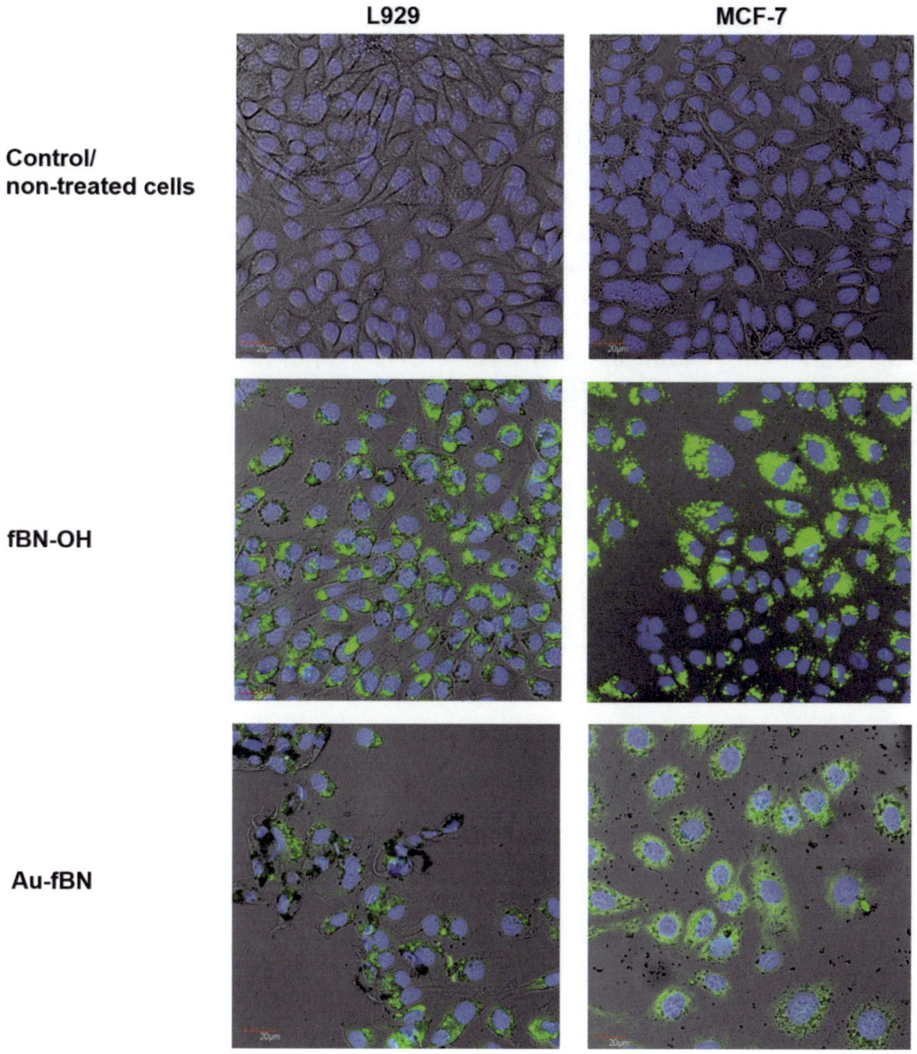

Figure 10.
Uptake of tested nanomaterials after 48-hour incubation.

neutral red dye uptake based on functional lysosomes in the presence of few-layered h-BN-based nanocomposites (**Figure 10**). In the case of fBN-OH, the L929 and MCF-7 responded to the presence of NPs in a dose-dependent manner, but MCF-7 seems to be more sensitive than L929 cell cultures. The presence of Au-fBN affected the cell viability less than the fBN-OH.

The integrity of cellular plasma membranes (analyzed via LDH leakage assay) was impaired less than the other cell's features. L929 cells as well as MCF-7 showed minimal changes in lactate dehydrogenase leakage even at the highest concentrations of fBN-OH and Au-fBN (**Figure 10**). The reduction of cell membrane integrity was the highest (to 80% vs. control cultures) for L929 and MCF-7 at concentrations of 200.0 μg mL^{-1} fBN-OH (**Figure 11**).

Pristine bulk h-BN is known to be poorly soluble in water-based solutions. Thus, the h-BN preparation (e.g., exfoliation, functionalization) should be optimized to obtain a nanomaterial that exhibits suitable properties in required applications (e.g., higher hydrophobicity that allows stable dispersion in aqueous solutions) [41]. The functionalization of the h-BN by hydroxyl groups improve h-BN hydrophobicity and allows to obtain stable dispersion in phosphate buffer solution [41] or in phosphate buffer solution supplemented with dispersant Pluronic F-127 [29]. This is crucial for cytotoxicity experimentations and biological/medical applications.

Another crucial factor in biocompatibility analysis is experiment in short- and long-term studies. In studies it was demonstrated that the effect of the fBN-OH on cells may vary depending on the species, type of cells tested, their function, and time of exposure of cells to these nanoparticles. The short-term in vitro study on L929 cell cultures and human erythrocytes as well as in vivo study on insect (*T. molitor*) hemocytes demonstrated a low cytotoxicity of this fBN-OH (dispersed in PBS), whereas a long-term study in *T. molitor* has shown a significant effect of fBN-OH on the behavior of immunocompetent cells and their function during the immune response [41].

In the preliminary study based on hexagonal boron nitride (exfoliated and functionalized with Au nanoparticles), it was found that Au-fBN nanoflakes

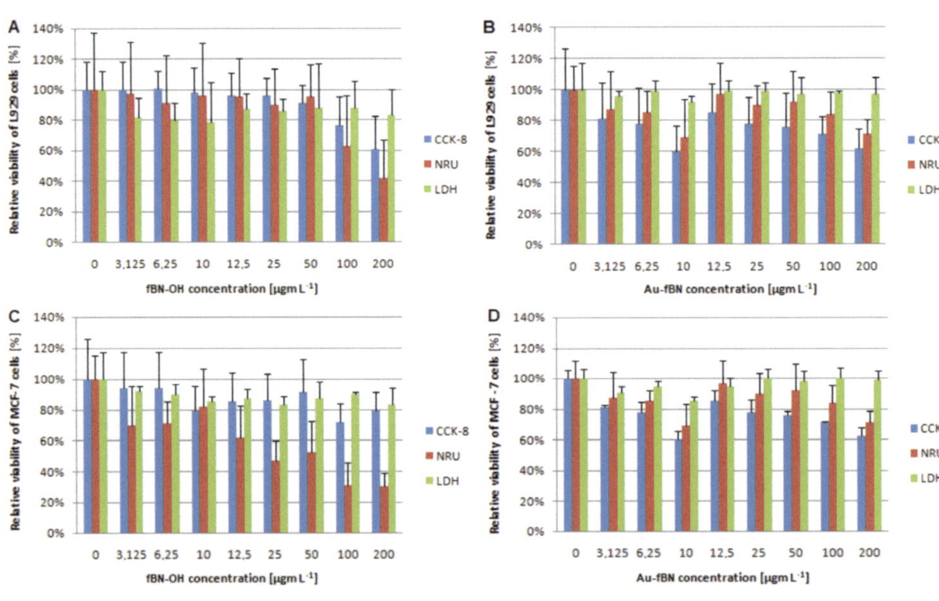

Figure 11.
Biocompatibility of fBN-OH and Au-fBN nanoplates incubated for 48 hours—L929 cell cultures (A, B) and MCF-7 cell cultures (C, D). Bars represent standard deviation.

did not affect the cellular metabolism (CCK-8) and membrane integrity (LDH assays). However, the function of lysosomes in both normal and cancer cell lines during 24-hour exposition was modified. Longer incubation, for 48 and 72 hours, affected the cell relative viability and proliferation activity of the MCF-7 cancer cell line in comparison to normal L929 cell line after 72-hour incubation period [29]. Additionally, fBN-based nanocomposites have been tested as a platform for drug delivery. Both the hexagonal boron nitride nanocomposites (fBN-OH and Au-fBN) were loaded chemically with an anticancer drug—10-hydroxycamptothecin (HCPT)—and were tested against human breast adenocarcinoma cells [53]. It was found that both nanocomposites conjugated with HCPT were effectively internalized and cumulated inside the cell cytoplasm, but not in the nuclear region of cells. Both the tested boron nitride nanocomposites loaded with 10-hydroxycomptothecin significantly reduced relative cell viability of MCF-7 cells. The slightly higher reduction was observed for Au-fBN-HCPT against human breast adenocarcinoma cells [53].

4. Conclusions

The hexagonal boron nitride (h-BN) is an attractive layered material that can be used in different industry sectors (due to its interesting physical and chemical properties). Its exfoliated form is considered as a graphene analogue. The pristine bulk h-BN is poorly soluble and exhibits a hydrophobic character in water/aqueous solutions. That is why the h-BN preparation (e.g., exfoliation, functionalization) is crucial to obtain a nanomaterial that exhibits the best properties that are required especially in in vitro and/or in vivo applications. The effect of the presented few-layered h-BN-based nanocomposites on biological environment may vary depending on the type of cells tested, their function, and time of exposure of cells to these nanoparticles. Boron nitride seems to be suitable for biomedical applications; therefore, the cytotoxicity in vitro and in vivo observations of novel few-layered h-BN-based nanocomposites are needed. The short-time studies confirmed their low cytotoxicity and suggest that h-BN can be used as a novel drug delivery system. However, medical applications need additional verification in long-term studies.

Acknowledgements

The authors are grateful for the financial support of National Science Centre within MINIATURA 2 program (no. 2018/02/X/NZ3/00161) and PRELUDIUM 11 program (no. 2016/21/N/ST8/02397).

Conflict of interest

The authors declare no conflict of interest.

Author details

Magdalena Jedrzejczak-Silicka[1*], Martyna Trukawka[2], Katarzyna Piotrowska[3*] and Ewa Mijowska[2]

1 Laboratory of Cytogenetics, West Pomeranian University of Technology, Szczecin, Poland

2 Department of Physicochemistry of Nanomaterials, West Pomeranian University of Technology, Szczecin, Poland

3 Department of Physiology, Pomeranian Medical University, Szczecin, Poland

*Address all correspondence to: mjedrzejczak@zut.edu.pl
and piot.kata@gmail.com

References

[1] Salata OV. Applications of nanoparticles in biology and medicine. Journal of Nanobiotechnology. 2004;**2**:3. DOI: 10.1186/1477-3155-2-3

[2] Fiume MM, Bergfeld WF, Belsito DV, Hill RA, Klaassen CD, Liebler DC, et al. Safety assessment of boron nitride as used in cosmetics. International Journal of Toxicology. 2015;**34**:53S-60S. DOI: 10.1177/1091581815617793

[3] Ansaloni LMS, Barros de Sousa EM. Boron nitride nanostructured: Synthesis, characterization and potential use in cosmetics. Materials Sciences and Applications. 2013;**4**:22-28. DOI: 10.4236/msa.2013.41004

[4] Su CY, Wang JC, Chen CY, Chu K, Lin CK. Spherical composite powder by coupling polymethyl methacrylate and boron nitride via spray drying for cosmetic application. Materials. 2019;**12**:706. DOI: 10.3390/ma12050706

[5] Zhu Y, Murali S, Cai W, Li X, Suk JW, Potts JR, et al. Graphene and graphene oxide: Synthesis, properties, and applications. Advances in Materials. 2010;**22**:3906-3924. DOI: 10.1002/adma.201001068

[6] Wang Y, Li Z, Wang J, Li J, Lin Y. Graphene and graphene oxide: Biofunctionalization and applications in biotechnology. Trends in Biotechnology. 2011;**29**:205-212. DOI: 10.1016/j.tibtech.2011.01.008

[7] Wu SY, An SSA, Hulme J. Current applications of graphene oxide in nanomedicine. International Journal of Nanomedicine. 2015;**10**:9-24. DOI: 10.2147/IJN.S88285

[8] Bhimanapati GR, Glavin NR, Robinson JA. 2D boron nitride: Synthesis and applications. Semiconductors and Semimetals. 2016;**95**:101-147. DOI: 10.1016/bs.semsem.2016.04.004

[9] Rathinasabapathy S, Santhosh MS, Asokan M. Significance of boron nitride in composites and its applications. In: Recent Advances in Boron Containing Materials. IntechOpen; 2019. pp. 1-11. DOI: 10.5772/intechopen.81557

[10] Ribeiro H, Luciano MA, Randow P, Vilela DN, Andrade LM. Functionalized boron nitride applications in biotechnology. In: Recent Advances in Boron Containing Materials. IntechOpen; 2019. pp. 1-15. DOI: 10.5772/intechopen.80849

[11] Kim JH, Pham TV, Hwang JH, Kim CS, Kim MJ. Boron nitride nanotubes: Synthesis and applications. Nano Convergence. 2018;**5**:17. DOI: 10.1186/s40580-018-0149-y

[12] Weng Q, Wang X, Wang X, Bando Y, Golberg D. Functionalized hexagonal boron nitride nanomaterials: Emerging properties and applications. Chemical Society Reviews. 2016;**45**:3989-4012. DOI: 10.1039/C5CS00869G

[13] Safety assessment of boron nitride as used in cosmetics. Scientific literature review for public comment. Cosmetics ingredient review. Washington, DC, USA [Internet]. 2012. Available from: https://www.cir-safety.org/sites/default/files/Boron%20Nitride_faa-final.pdf [Accessed: 25 March 2019]

[14] Haynes WM, editor. CRC Handbook of Chemistry and Physics. 92nd ed. Boca Raton, FL: CRC Press; 2011. p. 5.6

[15] Paine RT, Narula CK. Synthetic routes to boron nitride. Chemical Reviews. 1990;**90**:73-91. DOI: 10.1021/cr00099a004

[16] Golberg D, Bando Y, Huang Y, Terano T, Mitome M, Tang C, et al. Boron nitride nanotubes and nanosheets. ACS Nano. 2010;**4**:2979. DOI: 10.1021/nn1006495

[17] Wood GL, Paine RT. Aerosol synthesis of hollow spherical morphology boron nitride particles. Chemistry of Materials. 2006;**18**:4716. DOI: 10.1021/cm0602601

[18] Degrazia FW, Branco Leitune VC, Visioli F, Werner SM, Collares FM. Long-term stability of dental adhesive incorporated by boron nitride nanotubes. Dental Materials. 2018;**34**:427-433. DOI: 10.1016/j.dental.2017.11.024

[19] Bohns FR, Degrazia FW, Souza Balbinot G, Branco Leitune VC, Werner Samuel SM, García-Esparza MA, et al. Boron nitride nanotubes as filler for resin-based dental sealants. Scientific Reports. 2019;**9**:7710. DOI: 10.1038/s41598-019-44246-8

[20] Xiong SW, Pan Z, Xia Y, Fu P, Gai JG. Antimicrobial hexagonal boron nitride nanoplatelet composites for the thermal management of medical electronic devices. Materials Chemistry Frontiers. 2019;**3**:2455-2462. DOI: 10.1039/C9QM00411D

[21] Gottschalck TE, Breslawec H. International Cosmetic Ingredient Dictionary and Handbook. Washington, DC, USA: Personal Care Products Council [Internet]. 2016. Available from: http://webdictionary.personalcarecouncil.org/ctfa-static/online/FrontMatter_Vol1%20Edited%20for%20Websites.pdf [Accessed: 25 March 2019]

[22] Rasel AI, Li T, Nguyen TD, Singh S, Zhou Y, Xiao Y, et al. Biophysical response of living cells to boron nitride nanoparticles: Uptake mechanism and bio-mechanical characterization. Journal of Nanoparticle Research. 2015;**17**:441. DOI: 10.1007/s11051-015-3248-2

[23] Chen X, Wu P, Rousseas M, Okawa D, Gartner Z, Zettl A, et al. Boron nitride nanotubes are noncytotoxic and can be functionalized for interaction with proteins and cells. Journal of the American Chemical Society. 2009;**131**:890. DOI: 10.1021/ja807334b

[24] Horváth L, Magrez A, Golberg D, Zhi C, Bando Y, Smajda R, et al. In vitro investigation of the cellular toxicity of boron nitride nanotubes. ACS Nano. 2011;**5**:3800-3810. DOI: 10.1021/nn200139h

[25] Liu Q, Hu C, Wang X. One-pot solvothermal synthesis of water-soluble boron nitride nanosheets and fluorescent boron nitride quantum dots. Materials Letters. 2019;**234**:306-310. DOI: 10.1016/j.matlet.2018.09.031

[26] Marsh KL, Souliman M, Kaner RB. Co-solvent exfoliation and suspension of hexagonal boron nitride. Chemical Communications. 2015;**51**:187-190. DOI: 10.1039/C4CC07324J

[27] Han WQ, Wu L, Zhu Y, Watanabe K, Taniguchi T. Structure of chemically derived mono- and few-atomic-layer boron nitride sheets. Applied Physics Letters. 2008;**93**:223103. DOI: 10.1063/1.3041639

[28] Zhi C, Bando Y, Tang C, Kuwahara H, Golberg D. Large-scale fabrication of boron nitride nanosheets and their utilization in polymeric composites with improved thermal and mechanical properties. Advanced Materials. 2009;**21**:2889-2893. DOI: 10.1002/adma.200900323

[29] Jedrzejczak-Silicka M, Trukawka M, Dudziak M, Piotrowska K, Mijowska E. Hexagonal boron nitride functionalized with au nanoparticles—Properties and potential biological applications. Nanomaterials. 2018;**8**:605. DOI: 10.3390/nano8080605

[30] Kim KK, Hsu A, Jia X, Kim SM, Shi Y, Hofmann M, et al. Synthesis of monolayer hexagonal boron nitride on

Cu foil using chemical vapor deposition. Nano Letters. 2012;**12**:161-166. DOI: 10.1021/nl203249a

[31] Auwärter W, Kreutz TJ, Greber T, Osterwalder J. XPD and STM investigation of hexagonal boron nitride on Ni (111). Surface Science. 1999;**429**:229-236. DOI: 10.1016/S0039-6028(99)00381-7

[32] Orofeo CM, Suzuki S, Kageshima H, Hibino H. Growth and low-energy electron microscopy characterization of monolayer hexagonal boron nitride on epitaxial cobalt. Nano Research. 2013;**6**:335-347. DOI: 10.1007/s12274-013-0310-1

[33] Chen Y, Liang H, Xia X, Zhang H, Shi J, Abbas Q, et al. Growth temperature impact on film quality of h-BN grown on Al_2O_3 using non-catalyzed borazane CVD. Journal of Materials Science: Materials in Electronics. 2017;**28**:14341. DOI: 0.1007/s10854-017-7294-7

[34] Matsuda T, Uno N, Nakae H, Hirai T. Synthesis and structure of chemically vapour-deposited boron nitride. Journal of Materials Science. 1986;**21**:649-658. DOI: 10.1007/BF01145537

[35] Kim SM, Hsu A, Park MH, Chae SH, Yun SJ, Lee JS, et al. Synthesis of large-area multilayer hexagonal boron nitride for high material performance. Nature Communications. 2015;**6**:8662. DOI: 10.1038/ncomms9662

[36] Han R, Khan MH, Angeloski A, Casillas G, Yoon CW, Sun X, et al. Hexagonal boron nitride nanosheets grown via chemical vapor deposition for silver protection. ACS Applied Nano Materials. 2019;**2**:2830-2835. DOI: 10.1021/acsanm.9b00298

[37] Auwärter W. Hexagonal boron nitride monolayers on metal supports: Versatile templates for atoms, molecules and nanostructures. Surface Science Reports. 2019;**74**:1-95. DOI: 10.1016/j.surfrep.2018.10.001

[38] Lin Y, Williams TV, Xu TB, Cao W, Elsayed-Ali HE, Connell JW. Aqueous dispersions of few-layered and monolayered hexagonal boron nitride nanosheets from sonication-assisted hydrolysis: Critical role of water. Journal of Physical Chemistry C. 2011;**115**:2679-2685. DOI: 10.1021/jp110985w

[39] Gonzalez Ortiz D, Pochat-Bohatier C, Cambedouzo J, Bechelany M, Miele P. Exfoliation of hexagonal boron nitride (h-BN) in liquide phase by ion intercalation. Nanomaterials. 2018;**8**:716. DOI: 10.3390/nano8090716

[40] Gao T, Song X, Du H, Nie Y, Chen Y, Ji Q, et al. Temperature-triggered chemical switching growth of in-plane and vertically stacked graphene-boron nitride heterostructures. Nature Communications. 2015;**6**:6835. DOI: 10.1038/ncomms7835

[41] Czarniewska E, Mrówczyńska L, Jędrzejczak-Silicka M, Nowicki P, Trukawka M, Mijowska E. Non-cytotoxic hydroxyl-functionalized exfoliated boron nitride nanoflakes impair the immunological function of insect haemocytes in vivo. Scientific Reports. 2019;**9**:14027. DOI: 10.1038/s41598-019-50097-0

[42] Sudeep PM, Vinod S, Ozden S, Sruthi R, Kukovecz A, Kónya Z, et al. Functionalized boron nitride porous solids. RSC Advances. 2015;**5**:93964-93968. DOI: 10.1039/C5RA19091F

[43] Sainsbury T, Satti A, May P, Wang Z, McGovern I, Gun'ko YK, et al. Oxygen radical functionalization of boron nitride nanosheets. Journal of the American Chemical Society. 2012;**134**:18758-18771. DOI: 10.1021/ja3080665

[44] Pakdel A, Bando Y, Golberg D. Plasma-assisted interface engineering of boron nitride nanostructure films. ACS Nano. 2014;**8**:10631-10639. DOI: 10.1021/nn5041729

[45] Lee D, Lee B, Park HK, Ryu HJ, Jeon S, Hong SH. Scalable exfoliation process for highly soluble boron nitride nanoplatelets by hydroxide-assisted ball milling. Nano Letters. 2015;**15**:1238-1244. DOI: 10.1021/nl504397h

[46] Harley-Trochimczyk A, Pham T, Chang J, Chen E, Worsley MA, Zettl A, et al. Platinum nanoparticle loading of boron nitride aerogel and its use as a novel material for low-power catalytic gas sensing. Advanced Functional Materials. 2016;**26**:433-439. DOI: 10.1002/adfm.201503605

[47] Dai PC, Xue YM, Wang XB, Weng QH, Zhang C, Jiang XF, et al. Pollutant capturing SERS substrate: Porous boron nitride microfibers with uniform silver nanoparticle decoration. Nanoscale. 2014;**118**:21110-21118. DOI: 10.1039/C5NR05625J

[48] Elumalai G, Noguchi H, Lyalin A, Taketsugu T, Uosaki K. Gold nanoparticle decoration of insulating boron nitride nanosheet on inert gold electrode toward an efficient electrocatalyst for the reduction of oxygen to water. Electrochemistry Communications. 2016;**66**:53-57. DOI: 10.1016/j.elecom.2016.02.021

[49] Yang GH, Abulizi A, Zhu JJ. Sonochemical fabrication of gold nanoparticles-boron nitride sheets nanocomposites for enzymeless hydrogen peroxide detection. Ultrasonics Sonochemistry. 2014;**21**:1958-1963. DOI: 10.1016/j.elecom.2016.02.021

[50] Griffin A, Harvey A, Cunningham B, Scullion D, Tian T, Shih CJ, et al. Spectroscopic size and thickness metrics for liquid-exfoliated h-BN. Chemistry of Materials. 2018;**30**:1998-2005. DOI: 10.1021/acs.chemmater.7b05188

[51] Draz MS, Lu X. Development of a loop mediated isothermal amplification (LAMP)—Surface Enhanced Raman spectroscopy (SERS) assay for the detection of *Salmonella enterica* serotype enteritidis. Theranostics. 2016;**6**:522-532. DOI: 10.7150/thno.14391

[52] Chen S, Zhao M, Wu G, Yao C, Zhang J. Recent advances in morphological cell image analysis. Computational and Mathematical Methods in Medicine. 2012;**2012**:101536. DOI: 10.1155/2012/101536

[53] Trukawka M, Piotrowska K, Jedrzejczak-Silicka M, Mijowska E. A preliminary in vitro study of boron nitride nanocomposites loaded with 10-hydroxycamptothecin on mammalian cells. In: 5th Polish Conference Graphene and 2D Materials; 19-21 September 2019; Szczecin. Szczecin: ZUT; 2019. pp. 49-50

Section 5

Environmental Management and Risk Assessment

Chapter 10

Nanosafety

Muthuraman Yuvaraj, Venkatesan Yuvaraj,
Venugopal Arunkumar, Muthaiyan Pandiyan
and Kizhaeral Sevathapandian Subramanian

Abstract

The nanomaterials resembling nanotubes, nanospheres, nanofertilizer, nanoherbicide, nanoinsecticide, and nanosheets have the physical, chemical, biological, mechanical, electrical and thermal properties. Still, the nanoparticles have very minute dimensions, enormous area and high reactivity they need the potential ability to penetrate in living cells quite rapidly. The petite size nanoparticles contain lofty surface area may cause higher reactivity with nearby particles. It is broadly predictable that there is a critical need for more information and facts about the implications of manufactured nanomaterials on personal fitness and surroundings. Concerns about potential risks to health that may arise during the making, management, use, and discarding of these nanomaterials have been spoken over the past few years. Consequently, strong research action is being undertaken in various institutions, and industries across the world to appraise their toxicity and spread of nanoparticle.

Keywords: nanoparticle, issues of nanoparticles size, hazardous nanoparticles, guidelines, environment safety

1. Introduction

The possible risks to health from nanomaterials can be cheap by safe management and organization of the disclosure. Even as no sole part of direction can offer an ultimate, step-by-step advance to safe usage of all nanomaterials in all situations, there are some universal and exact best carry out guides that can be used in nearly all applications [1]. Nanotechnologies have speedy promoted the occasion a substitute making of smart innovative goods and processes have created an unbelievable increase latent for a huge number of industry sectors. The current dispute on the risks of nanotechnologies tends to specialize in the potential dangers of nanoparticles. A growing interest in the production and application of nanoparticles has been generated the need for appropriate safety measures [2, 3].

The protection issues with nanoparticles are not incredibly fine identified but they are possible for threat is obvious owing to the high exterior area-to-volume ratio, which can create the particles especially hasty or catalytic movement. The understanding of in what way nanomaterials relate to the alive system is imperfect [4, 5]. A toxicological study has been generated a great contract in order on the affiliation among the physical and chemical properties of nanoparticles and their difficult effect on our fitness. These artificial nanoparticles comprise nanotubes, fullerenes, nanowires, quantum dots and diverse nanoparticles used for drug release and analysis. Due to their odd shapes and high reactivity, their effect on the metabolism cannot simply be predicted [6].

IntechOpen

The inhaled nanoparticle can be deposited all through the human respiratory tract and lungs. Nanoparticles can be transferred in the lungs to added organs such as the brain, liver and maybe the fetus in pregnant women [7, 8]. Nanoparticles can get into the body during the surface of the skin, lungs, and gastrointestinal system. This force helps make free radicals, which may cause a cell to injure and break to deoxyribonucleic acid. Besides, these can pass through cell membranes in organisms and may interact with biological systems [9, 10].

2. Nano hazard identification

The detection of nano hazards is that the starts to decide risk and contact. This step involves typical nanomaterials and their connected processes that source destructive. When assessing the risks coupled with nanomaterials, particular care must be taken to spot the specific achievement of surface chemistry, shape, size and morphology on toxicity caused to diverse organs. The successive key hazard categories could also be measured when assessing risk linked to nanomaterials [11, 12] (**Figure 1**).

2.1 Surface charge

The leading exciting chemistry characteristic of nanoparticle about toxicity is that the surface charge, with toxicity rising contained by the subsequent way: neutral < anionic < cationic.

2.2 Surface chemistry

The surface chemistry of nanoparticles may require a duty inside the age group of free radicals, which influences the broad surface reactivity and toxicity of ingested particles [13].

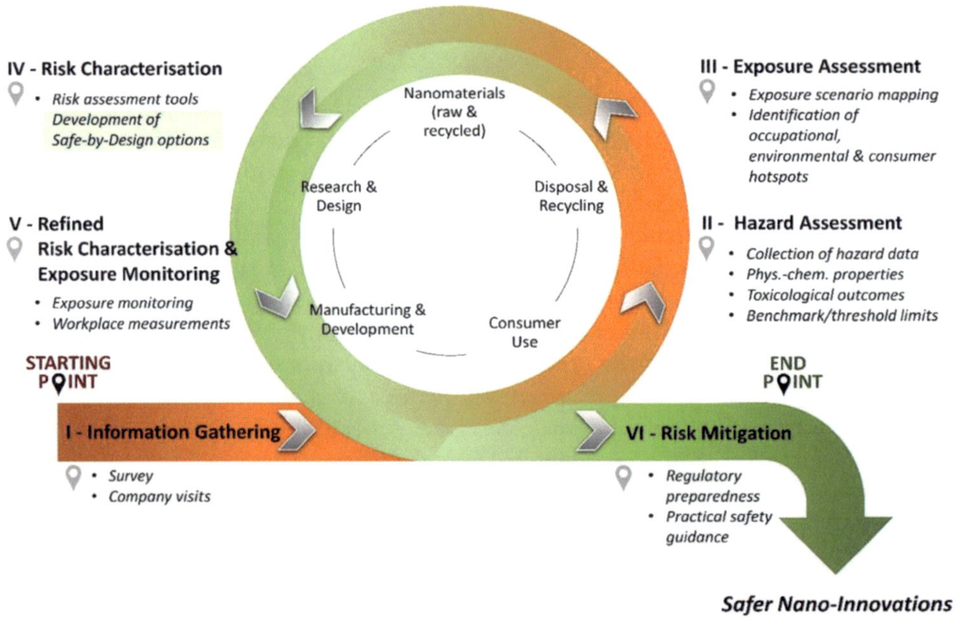

Figure 1.
Diagram of the projected safety plan.

2.3 Particle shape

Studies have recognized that contact with leathery particles like amphibole will boost the carcinogenic effect. Correspondingly the tubular formation of carbon nanotubes is supposed to cause inflammation and lesions in the lungs [14].

2.4 Particle size

Nanoparticles will go through the membrane barriers ensuing in critical compensation for occurrence particularly silver nanoparticles with size <9 nm can enter the nuclear membrane of certain human cells nucleus and cause major deoxyribonucleic acid mutation [15, 16]. Weakly soluble inhaled nanoparticles will basis aerobic stress, leading to inflammation, fibrosis, and cancer. Several research reported that considerably higher toxicity of nano metals as compared to nanoceramics that have been recognized to higher suspension rate in water [17, 18].

3. Finest practice to be pursued while using nanoparticles

3.1 Hygiene

Do not eat or store food and beverages in a nanotechnology laboratory. Do not use mouth suction for pipetting or siphoning. Wash hands regularly to reduce nanoparticle exposure during intake and dermal contact. Remove gloves when exiting the laboratory, so as not to infect doorknobs, or when handling common use objects such as phones, multiuser computers, etc.

3.2 Labeling and signage

Store in a well-sealed container, preferably one that can be opened with minimal agitation of the contents. Label all chemical containers with the identity of the contents. Hazard warning and chemical concentration information should also be included if known. Apply cautious decision when leaving operations unattended: (i) Post signs to communicate appropriate warnings and precautions, (ii) anticipate potential equipment and facility failures, and (iii) provide appropriate suppression for chance release of hazardous chemicals [19].

3.3 Clean-up measures and spills

Specifically, watch out for exposure during cleaning operations. Wear gloves and work in a fume hood while handling nanoparticle and clean the fume hood afterward. If needed, monitor the lab air nanomaterial concentrations during clean-up. Wear respiration protection when working outside a fume hood or in an open fume hood and consider overall protection [20, 21]. Materials and surfaces can be cleaned by following techniques like wiped with a wet cloth where possible, rinsing off the cloth with water or disposing of it. The vacuum cleaner is equipped with a high-efficiency particulate air filter. Monitor the exhaust of the vacuum cleaner during operation. A malfunctioning filter can increase the exposure by dispersing the nanomaterial in the air. High-efficiency particulate air filtered vacuum cleaners with a combination of wet wiping is more suitable for most nanomaterial clean-up [22, 23]. Energetic cleaning methods such as dry cleaning or the use of compressed air should be prohibited [24]. Collect spill cleanup materials in a tightly closed container. The nanoparticle spill kit containing the following items Barricade tape, Latex or nitrile gloves, Adsorbent material, Wipes, Sealable plastic bags, Walk-off mat [25].

4. Strategy for functioning with nanomaterials

Use sensible general laboratory safety practices as found in your chemical hygiene set up. Do not handle nanoparticles with your bare skin. If it is necessary to handle nanoparticle powders outside of a high-efficiency particulate air filtered to maintain exhaust streamline flow hood. Lab equipment and exhaust systems should also be evaluated before removal, remodeling, or repair [26, 27]. Given the differing artificial ways and experimental goals, no blanket recommendation will be created concerning aerosol emissions controls. Consideration should tend to the high reactivity of some nanopowder materials about potential fire and explosion hazards [28].

5. Constant monitoring of lab air

The nanoparticle detector should be installed in every lab, in which gas-phase work on nanoparticles is passed out and where the capacity of nanoparticulate material exceeds a certain limit. We advocate a limit of 1 μg/h. An instrument of this kind is commercially available as a Joint Length Monitor. This unit contains a size parting mechanism so particles <0, 1 μm area unit mostly detected [29].

6. Discarding of nanoparticles

The quantities of nanoparticles like powders, colloids exceeding the milligram range should be treated as chemical if the particle solubility in water is very small (inorganics like gold, titanium oxide). If the solubility is higher, the principles consistent with the toxicity class of the macroscopic material apply. Nanoparticle residues in water from cleaning can be poured down the drain [30] (**Table 1**).

7. Transport of nanoparticle

- Safe handling of nanomaterials and normal operation procedures
- To check the hazards and toxicity of nanoparticle
- Personal protective equipment to be kept
- Engineering controls and equipment maintenance
- Description of nanoparticles should be known
- Environmental release, shipping, customer protection
- Exposure monitoring
- Applicable regulation
- Labeling and handling of nanomaterials waste

Waste nanomaterial	Pre-treatment	Containment	Level of engineering controls	Disposal method
Dust nanoparticles	Moisten	Double	Inside a local exhausted aeration enclosure or glove box	Burning
Infected solids	Moisten if necessary	Double bag plastic, sealable	Inside a local exhausted aeration enclosure or glove box	Burning
Fluid solutions	Process solvent-soluble with the solvent waste stream. Aggregate nanoparticle will get dissolved and form ions	Drip tray or funnel vial or container or drip tray	Inside a local exhausted aeration enclosure	Burning mix with solid waste. Burn either mix with other soluble waste or dilute to drain if appropriate
Nanomaterial bound in resin or polymer	As for liquid solutions or packages a nanomaterial in a solid matrix not friable	Single containment or double containment if liquid.	General aeration	Burning or licensed landfill
Nanomaterial in a solid matrix but friable	Moisten	Double containment	Inside a local exhausted aeration enclosure	Burning or licensed landfill
Nanomaterial in a solid matrix not friable	None	Single containment	General aeration	Burning or licensed landfill

Table 1.
Handling and Disposal of Waste Nanomaterial.

8. Working place with nanoparticle

When handle nanomaterials in solutions or close substrates to reduce airborne release. While working with nanomaterials in liquids it must avoid dispersal of the liquid by operating through a spill instrumentality. Wear gloves that are suited for the liquid being handled. Avoid the dispersion of liquid droplets within the work-place air and directly close up spills, before evaporation or further spreading occurs. While working with nanomaterials in gas phase reactors add a closed reaction vessel, preferably around atmospheric or lower than atmospheric pressure [31, 32]. Make aware leak checks among runs once operating with systems under positive pressure adjust the quality safety rules for controlled vessels and place the vessel into an interior safety vessel. Clean all parts that are in touch with nanoparticles and spills after using suitable safety [33, 34].

9. Development and usage of nanomaterials

Nanomaterials must be stored and transported in sealed shatter-resistant containers. The containers must be labeled with nanomaterial or composition and near particle size, along with any known hazard warnings. Weighing and measuring of dry powders where aerosolization and discharge of nanomaterials are possible should be conducted in clear and closed areas [25]. Different processing steps such as dispersing, mixing, spraying, machining, gas-phase processing have the potential to make nanoparticles with a high concentration. Employing a closed facility to process nanomaterials will considerably reduce occupational exposure during the assembly and processing stages. Particular care to be taken to avoid disturbance of the closed liquid medium to avoid dust scattering and thus disclosure through inhalation [35, 36]. Removal of waste and by-products generated at the assembly facility should be administered with minimum exposure to humans and therefore the environment.

10. The behavior of nanopowders in the food industry

Nanotechnologies propose a diversity of possible for relevance in different areas of food technology that comprise packaging, processing, quality and shelf life, ingredients and additives. The complexity in characterizing assorted nanomaterials used the food industry and biological systems incomplete information on toxicology and lack optimal test methods the risk appraisal and supervision of nanotechnologies harder [37, 38]. A preventive advance with detailed life cycle estimation and strongly required procedures to stakeholders connecting for diverse activities as formulating best practices that will support the growth of nanotechnology in the food sector for regulating the potential risk to humans and the environment. Humans are exposed to nanomaterials using oral way during the residues present in cultivated crops, meat, and milk produced for consumption further oral contact is most significant in food processing technology and functional foods. Nanomaterial exposure from food packaging is mostly dermal, arising from the usage of such materials [39, 40].

11. Conclusions

The nanotechnology is an enables gifted technology its vast marvelous future applications. Conversely, there are a few drawbacks for example toxicity of the soil, ecological harm and human organ damage caused by nanoparticles. The vital significance provides to contain nanosafety into the occasion of novel nanotechnologies and find products of nanosafety before making a design. It has been at present identified that some engineered nanomaterials will present new and abnormal risks, but there is very little information on how these risks can be recognized, assessed and proscribed. In distinction, good working hygiene practices and existing knowledge on operational with dangerous substances provide a useful source for working safely with nanomaterials. Further, investigate to be conducted for nanosafety and discarding of the nanoparticle. Finally, in the future, many types of nanoparticles may turn out to be of less toxicity but preventative measures should be used while handling particle.

DOI: http://dx.doi.org/10.5772/intechopen.92290

Author details

Muthuraman Yuvaraj[1*], Venkatesan Yuvaraj[2], Venugopal Arunkumar[1], Muthaiyan Pandiyan[1] and Kizhaeral Sevathapandian Subramanian[3]

1 Agricultural College and Research Institute, Vazhavachanur, Tamil Nadu, India

2 Department of Physics, Arignar Anna Government Arts College, Cheyyar, Tamil Nadu, India

3 Tamil Nadu Agricultural University, Coimbatore, India

*Address all correspondence to: yuvasoil@gmail.com

References

[1] Lin S, Yu T, Yu Z, Hu X, Yin D. Nanomaterials safer-by-design: An environmental safety perspective. Advanced Materials. 2018;**17**:56-91

[2] Vithanage M, Seneviratne M, Ahmad M, Sarkar B. Contrasting effects of engineered carbon nanotubes on plants: A review. Environmental Geochemistry and Health. 2017;**39**:21-39

[3] Hol PJ, Gjerdet NR. Novel nanoparticulate and ionic titanium antigens for hypersensitivity testing. International Journal of Molecular Sciences. 2018;**19**:11-21

[4] Vietti G, Lison D, van den Brul S. Mechanisms of lung fibrosis induced by carbon nanotubes: Towards an Adverse Outcome Pathway (AOP). Particle and Fibre Toxicology. 2016;**13**:1-11

[5] Naatz S, Lin R, Li W, Jiang Z, Ji CH, Chang J, et al. Safe-by-design of CuO nanoparticles via Fe-doping, Cu-O bond lengths variation and biological assessment in cells and zebra fish embryos. ACS Nano. 2017;**11**:501-510

[6] Thomm E, Bromme R. How source information shapes lay interpretations of science conflicts: Interplay between sourcing, conflict explanation, source evaluation, and claim evaluation. Reading and Writing. 2016;**29**:1629-1652

[7] Boukhvalov DW, Yoon TH. Development of theoretical descriptors for cytotoxicity evaluation of metallic nanoparticles. Chemical Research in Toxicology. 2017;**30**:1549-1555

[8] Wang W, Sedykh A, Sun H, Zhao L, Russo DP, Zhou H, et al. Predicting nano–bio interactions by integrating nanoparticle libraries and quantitative nanostructure activity relationship modeling. ACS Nano. 2017;**11**:12641-12649

[9] Liu Z, Jiang W, Nam J, Moon J, Kim B. Immuno modulating nanomedicine for cancer therapy. Nano Letters. 2018;**18**:6655-6659

[10] Kraegeloh A, Suarez-Merino B, Sluijters T, Micheletti C. Implementation of safe-by-design for nanomaterial development and safe innovation: Why we need a comprehensive approach. Nanomaterials. 2018;**14**:4-8

[11] Pavan C, Fubini B. Unveiling the variability of quartz hazard in light of recent toxicological findings. Chemical Research in Toxicology. 2016;**30**:469-485

[12] Jeon Y-R, Yu J, Choi S-J. Fate determination of ZnO in commercial foods and human intestinal cells. International Journal of Molecular Sciences. 2020;**21**:433-439

[13] Hjorth R, van Hove L, Wickson F. What can nanosafety learn from drug development. The feasibility of "safety by design". Nanotoxicology. 2017;**113**:305-312

[14] Holman C, Piper SK, Grittner U, Diamantaras AA, Kimmelman J. Where have all the rodents gone? The effects of attrition in experimental research on cancer and stroke. PLoS Biology. 2016;**14**:25-31

[15] Lewandowsky S, Bishop D. Research integrity: Don't let transparency damage science. Nature. 2016;**529**:459-461

[16] Trinh TX, Cho J-S, Jeon H, Byun H-G, Yoon T-H, Kim J. Quasi-SMILES-based nano-quantitative structure–Activity relationship model to predict the cytotoxicity of multiwalled carbon nanotubes to human lung cells. Chemical Research in Toxicology. 2018;**31**:183-190

[17] Mulhopt S, Dilger M, Diabate S, Schlager C, Krebs T, Zimmermann R, et al. Toxicity testing of combustion aerosols at the air-liquid interface with a self-contained and easy-to-use exposure system. Journal of Aerosol Science. 2016;**96**:38-55

[18] Wang P, Voronkova M, Luanpitpong S, He X, Riedel H, Dinu C, et al. Induction of slug by chronic exposure to single-walled carbon nanotubes promotes tumor formation and metastasis. Chemical Research in Toxicology. 2017;**30**:1396-1405

[19] Prasad R, Bhattacharyya A, Nguyen QD. Nanotechnology in sustainable agriculture: Recent developments, challenges, and perspectives. Frontiers in Microbiology. 2017;**8**:1014-1019

[20] Wong JKL, Mohseni R, Hamidieh AA, MacLaren RE, Habib N, Seifalian AM. Will nanotechnology bring new hope for gene delivery. Trends in Biotechnology. 2017;**35**:434-451

[21] Malik S, Krasheninnikov AV, Marchesan S. Advances in nanocarbon composite materials. Beilstein Journal of Nanotechnology. 2018;**9**:2-10

[22] Thiruvengadam M, Rajakumar G, Chung IM. Nanotechnology: Current uses and future applications in the food industry. Biotech. 2018;**8**:74

[23] Kim DY, Kadam A, Shinde S, Saratale RG, Patra J, Ghodake G. Recent developments in nanotechnology transforming the agricultural sector: A transition replete with opportunities. Journal of the Science of Food and Agriculture. 2018;**98**:849-864

[24] Jahan S, Yusoff IB, Alias YB, Bakar AFBA. Reviews of the toxicity behavior of five potential engineered nanomaterials (ENMs) into the aquatic ecosystem. Toxicology Reports. 2017;**4**:211-220

[25] Wright MV, Matson CW, Baker LS, Castellon BT, Watkins PS, King RS. Titanium dioxide nanoparticle exposure reduces algal biomass and alters algal assemblage composition in wastewater effluent-dominated stream mesocosms. Science of the Total Environment. 2018;**626**:336-356

[26] Saint-Cricq M, Carrete J, Gaboriaud C, Gravel E, Doris E, Thielens N, et al. Human immune protein C1q selectively disaggregates carbon nanotubes. Nano Letters. 2017;**17**:3409-3415

[27] Naatz H, Lin S, Li R, Jiang W, Ji Z, Chang CH, et al. Safe-by-design CuO nanoparticles via Fe-doping, Cu-O bond length variation, and biological assessment in cells and zebrafish embryos. ACS Nano. 2017;**11**:501-515

[28] Iqbal SA, Wallach JD, Khoury MJ, Schully SD, Ioannidis JP. Reproducible research practices and transparency across the biomedical literature. PLoS Biology. 2016;**14**:12-19

[29] Truffier Boutry D, Fiorentino B, Bartolomei V, Soulas R, Sicardy O, Benayad A, et al. Characterization of photocatalytic paints: A relationship between the photocatalytic properties release of nanoparticles and volatile organic compounds. Environmental Science. Nano. 2017;**4**:1998-2009

[30] Jain N, Bhargava A, Pareek V, Akhtar MS, Panwar J. Does seed size and surface anatomy play role in combating phytotoxicity of nanoparticles. Ecotoxicology. 2017;(26):238-249

[31] Mantecca P, Kasemets K, Deokar A, Perelshtein I, Gedanken A, Bahk YK, et al. Airborne nanoparticle release and toxicological risk from metal-oxide-coated textiles: Toward a multiscale safe-by-design approach.

Environmental Science & Technology. 2017;**51**:9305-9317

[32] Starost K, Frijns E, Van Laer J, Faisal N, Egizabal A, Elizetxea C, et al. The effect of nanosilica (SiO_2) and nanoalumina (Al_2O_3) reinforced polyester nanocomposites on aerosol nanoparticle emissions into the environment during automated drilling. Aerosol Science and Technology. 2017;**51**:1035-1046

[33] Vlasova II, Kapralov AA, Michael ZP, Burkert SC, Shurin MR, Star A, et al. Enzymatic oxidative biodegradation of nanoparticles: Mechanisms, significance and applications. Toxicology and Applied Pharmacology. 2016;**299**:58-69

[34] Cobaleda-Siles M, Guillamon AP, Delpivo C, Vazquez-Campos S, Puntes VF. Safer by design strategies. Journal of Physics Conference Series. 2017;**838**:12-16

[35] Singh D, Sotiriou GA, Zhang F, Mead J, Bello D, Wohlleben W, et al. End-of-life thermal decomposition of nano-enabled polymers: Effect of nanofiller loading and polymer matrix on by-products. Environmental Science. Nano. 2016;**3**:1293-1305

[36] Lopez De Ipina JM, Hernan A, Cenigaonaindia X, Insunza M, Florez S, Seddon R, et al. Implementation of a safe-by design approach in the development of new open pilot lines for the manufacture of carbon nanotube-based nano-enabled products. Journal of Physics Conference Series. 2017;**838**:12-18

[37] Fageria L, Pareek V, Dilip V, Bhargava A, Pasha SS, Laskar IR, et al. Biosynthesized protein-capped silver nanoparticles induce ros-dependent proapoptotic signals and prosurvival autophagy in cancer cells. ACS Omega. 2017;**2**:1489-1504

[38] Bruno D, Mattos B, Tardy L, Washington LE, Magalhaes Orlando J, Rojas E. Controlled release for crop and wood protection: Recent progress toward sustainable and safe nanostructured biocidal systems. Journal of Controlled Release. 2017;**262**:139-150

[39] Reinosa JJ, Docio CMA, Ramirez VZ, Lozano JFF. Hierarchical nano ZnO-micro TiO_2 composites: High UV protection yield lowering photodegradation in sunscreens. Ceramics International. 2018;**44**:2827-2834

[40] Feliu N, Pelaz B, Zhang Q, del Pino P, Nystrom A, Parak W. Nanoparticle dosage-a nontrivial task of utmost importance for quantitative nanosafety research. Wiley Interdisciplinary Reviews: Nanomedicine and Nanobiotechnology. 2016;**8**:479-492

Chapter 11

Biological Role of *Withania somnifera* against Promiscuity of Zinc Oxide Nano Particles and Its Interaction with Macrophages

Jitendra Kumar, Chander Datt, Surya Kant Verma and Kavita Rani

Abstract

In agriculture and food industry, nanotechnology can be utilized to improve crop yield, food quality, shelf life, safety, cost and nutritional benefits. Zinc is a trace element and its deficiency causes health problems in human beings and animals. The use of zinc oxide nanoparticles (ZnO NPs) is growing exponentially in food industry, biomedicine and nanofertilizer segment. A remarkable presence of nanomaterials in ecosystem and consumer products can cause adverse effects. Hence, it is an important challenge for the use of nanoparticles in agriculture as fertilizer to enhance plant yield on one hand and their interaction with the cells of the innate immune system in animals on the other hand. So, public concern about their potential toxicity is increasing. ZnO NPs interact with cells and produce harmful effects in a dose dependent manner. The reactive oxygen species generation might be a reason for the toxicity of ZnO NPs. The toxicity is caused due to dissolved Zn^{++} ions by absorption which causes adverse effect on phagocytosis and oxidative stress by free radical while *Withania somnifera* induced the phagocytosis activity by antioxidant mechanism thus having protective effects. It is emphasized that further research is needed on the use of nanoparticles in agriculture, animal husbandry, and human health sector so that their safer levels for use could be ascertained.

Keywords: agriculture, immunotoxicity, macrophages, nanofertilizer, nanoparticles, *Withania somnifera*, zinc oxide

1. Introduction

Nanotechnology is an emerging technology which can lead to a new revolution in many fields of science [1]. Nanoparticles (NPs) are gaining importance recently due to their exciting applications in different fields like biomedical, pharmaceutical, agriculture, etc. The properties of the materials change as their size approaches the nanoscale, and nanoparticles have a very high surface area to volume ratio and high energy. Application of nanoparticle in the agriculture and food sectors is relatively new as compared to their use in health sector.

IntechOpen

In India, more than 60% of the population survive on agriculture, but unfortunately this sector is facing various global challenges. Therefore, nanotechnology has a dominant position in transforming agriculture and food industry. Nanotechnology has a great ability to transform conventional agricultural practices and boost yield and growth of corps. Zinc oxide NPs (ZnO NPs) are used as fertilizer which support their growth and improves production [2].

Zinc oxide NPs may be used as a source of Zn in supplements and functional foods [3]. ZnO NPs also act as antimicrobial agents against harmful bacteria. The antimicrobial activity of ZnO NPs has been partly attributed to their ability to penetrate into microbial cells and animal cells and generate reactive oxygen species (ROS) that damage cellular components thereby leading to cytotoxicity [4]. A single oral dose of ZnO NPs caused hepatic cell injury, kidney toxicity, and lung damage [5]. The studies in frogs showed that ZnO NPs exhibited more toxicity than a dissolved form of Zn which was attributed to their greater ability to induce oxidative damage in cells [6]. The administration of ZnO NPs increased all liver enzymes [7]. In this chapter, we attempted to explore the potential use of nanoparticles in agriculture, biological, and pharmacological significance of *Withania somnifera* against the promiscuity of zinc oxide ZnO NPs and their interaction with macrophages.

2. Use of zinc oxide nanoparticles in agriculture and animal husbandry

2.1 ZnO NPs and their potential use in agriculture

Once nanomaterials (NMs) are released to the environment, they accumulate in ecosystems and pose threats to living organisms; therefore, it is important to understand the behavior of NMs in soil and to assess the risks for arable soil ecosystems [8]. About 260,000–309,000 metric tons (MT) of NMs were produced globally in 2010 [9], and worldwide consumption of NMs is likely to grow from 225,060 to 585,000 MT during 2014–2019 [10]. The third most commonly used metal-containing NMs are ZnO NPs with an estimated global annual production between 550 and 33,400 tons [11]. The concentration of ZnO NPs in the environment was found to be 3.1–31 μg kg^{-1} and 76–760 μg L^{-1} in soil and water, respectively [12]. ZnO NPs can strongly attach to soil particles. They exhibit low mobility at various ionic strengths [13] and show higher sorption compared to ionic zinc, and possible uptake mechanism has been illustrated in **Figure 1.**

2.2 Effects of ZnO nanoparticles on animal health

Unplanned use of ZnO NPs as nanofertilizer in agriculture leads to their entry in the food chain, and ultimately nanofertilizers enter in the body directly or indirectly, and their interaction with immune cells may have deleterious effects. The effects of ZnO NPs on the immune system are not completely understood. Some researchers postulated that increased cytosolic Zn^{2+} and the generation of ROS play important roles [16]. In innate immune, cells recognize ZnO NPs via toll-like receptors (TLR) which bind to corresponding antigens ZnO NPs and activate signal transduction pathway and inflammatory response. The ZnO NPs induce apoptosis and necrosis in macrophages in relation to their important role in the clearance of entered particulates and the regulation of immune responses during inflammation.

Withania somnifera (L.) Dual (Solanaceae) Indian ginseng or Indian winter cherry is a medicinal plant. Different parts of the plant have been used in Ayurvedic medicine formulations. Withaferin A is a steroidal lactone found in the leaves and

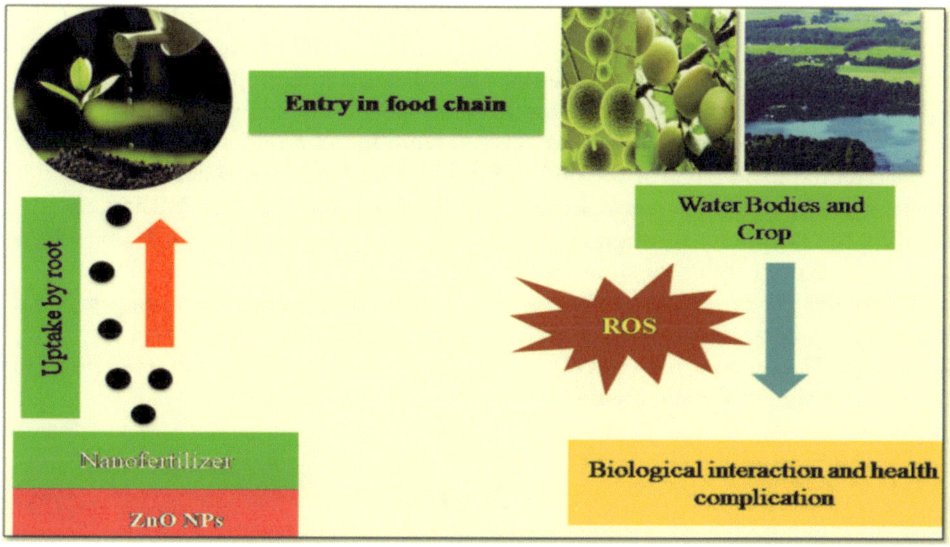

Figure 1.
Plant uptake, transport and environmental transformation mechanism of nanofertilizer (ZnO NPs) into ecosystem and entry in food chain [14, 15]. Designed by first author using Google as tool.

roots *of W. somnifera.* The biological properties of crude root extracts have been largely reported and only a few are related to the pure compound (withaferin A) as immunomodulatory function.

3. Immunological health importance of zinc as microelement

Zinc is crucial for normal development and function of cells mediating innate immunity, neutrophils, and natural killer cells (NKs). Phagocytosis, intracellular killing, and cytokine production are affected by Zn deficiency. Zinc is a micronutrient required by organisms and plays a vital role in maintaining immune and macrophage function. There is a progressive decline in immune response with the advance in aging due to the deficiency of Zn [17]. There is impairment of monocytes, reduced cytotoxicity in NK cells, and reduced phagocytosis in neutrophils [18]. Zinc is also a major intracellular regulator of lymphocyte apoptosis [19]. Impaired immune function in elderly subjects due to Zn deficiency has been shown to be reversed by an adequate Zn supplementation [18]. The beneficial effects of lower doses of Zn ($\leq$ 50 mg/d) on immune function have been reported while very high doses of Zn ($\geq$ 150 mg/d) may impair cellular immunity [20].

4. Mechanism of innate immunity in animals

The defense system is the bedrock of living systems and innate immunity is an integral part of health. It is the first line of the defense mechanism of the body from lower organism to mammals. Any alteration in innate immunity leads to disease conditions; however, adaptive immunity plays a great role in defense mechanism. Innate immunity has two arms, i.e., the afferent and efferent. The afferent arm is lipopolysaccharide (LPS) or endotoxin [21]. As to the effector arm of innate immunity, Hunter (1774) first recognized leukocytes at the site of inflammation. The cellular theory of immunity was given by Metchnikoff, 1884 [22] and must be recognized in the functional analysis of innate immune cells. Massart and Bordet had showed that injured cells secrete chemicals that attract phagocytes in 1917. The myeloid cells in invertebrates' are precursors of the innate immunity. Macrophages are professional immune cells that engulf and destroy foreign particles. Myeloid cells include mononuclear phagocytes and polymorph nuclear phagocytes. Macrophages are mononuclear phagocytes derived from blood monocytes. Macrophages are distributed in all parts of the body of the host and also present within the parenchyma of the heart, lungs, liver, brain, and peritoneal cavity. Pathogens invading the host body through any route are killed by macrophages. Macrophages have the potential ability of supervisory of innate immunity. Reactive oxygen intermediates are produced in phagosomes of neutrophils and macrophages. Superoxide radicals (O_2^-) are generated by the p91 subunit of cytochrome form (O_2) [23]. Superoxide (H2O2) is produced from O_2^- anions where superoxide dismutase is the catalytic enzyme.

$$2O_2 + \text{NADPH (oxidase)} \rightarrow 2O_2\bullet^- + \text{NADP} + H^+ \quad (1)$$

$$2H^+ + 2O_2\bullet^- = H_2O_2 + O_2 \quad (2)$$

Hypochlorous acid (HO Cl), a reactive halide, is produced from H_2O_2 by the action of myeloperoxidase. These radicals not only kill microbes directly but also generate other metabolites for this purpose, and singlet oxygen can be generated by O Cl^-, the former being strangely reactive with C: C double bands. Hydroxyl radicals can be produced where HO Cl react with superoxide.

$$Cl^- + H_2O_2 + H^+ = \text{HO Cl} + H_2O \quad (3)$$

$$O_2\bullet^- + \text{HO Cl} = O_2\bullet^- + OH\bullet + Cl^- \quad (4)$$

Therefore, hydroxyl radical (OH•) could be produced were agent using upper oxide as substrate, reactive nitrogen species (NO•) can be produced.

$$O_2\bullet^- + H_2O_2 = OH^\bullet + OH + O_2 \quad (5)$$

$$O_2\bullet^- + NO\bullet = ONOO \quad (6)$$

Complement, lactoferrin, lysozyme, and antimicrobial peptides are the humoral component of innate immunity. Lysozyme present in the saliva and tear inhibits the cell wall synthesis in bacteria. Complement is an enzymatic proton which plays an important role in innate immunity. Antimicrobial peptides and C-reactive proteins (CRP) are also having defense ability by disrupting plasma membrane.

5. Macrophages and their roles in animal health

The macrophages are mononuclear phagocytes and are committed progenitor cells in the bone marrow [24]. There are mainly two types of phagocytic cells, namely, macrophages and dendritic cells (DCs), which have similar cell surface receptors but different functional activities which are short-lived, and their life span depends on the nature of immune response [25]. All types of macrophages are differentiated from circulating monocyte and DCs by their expression of Fc, F4/80, and CD11b receptors. Macrophages are the main inducers of the adaptive T cell responses. Macrophages are skilled in scavenging dead cells, cellular debris, phagocytosis, and remodeling after tissue injury [26]. Their names and phenotypes vary based on their anatomical location. Physiological characters and significant roles of macrophages are listed in **Table 1** [27].

Sr.No.	Characteristic	Macrophages
1.	Precursor cells and origin of macrophages	Progenitor myeloid cell of bone marrow
2.	Maturation Site of macrophages	All tissues of body
3.	Phenotypic difference	CD68+,F4/80+ (mouse) or EMR1+ (human), CD107b+,(Mac-3+)
4.	Mature macrophages cells in circulation	No (or very less)
5.	Mature cells recruited into tissues from circulation	No
6.	Proliferative ability of mature cells	May vary by subpopulation (M_2 macrophages can proliferate)
7.	Mature cells normally present	Connective tissues
8.	Life span	7 to 30 days
9.	Detection of pathogens and initiation of inflammation	Have ability
10.	Inflammation	Increase
11.	Antigen presentation	Main cell for this work
12.	Detoxification of animal venom	Have ability

Table 1.
Physiological characters and significant roles of animal macrophages.

There are three main subtypes of macrophages: one is classically activated M_1 macrophages which play an important role in host defense and antitumor immunity, while another one is M_2 macrophages, the suppressor and regulator of wound healing. Third type is M_3 which are phagocytic cells that continuously express different types of receptors that facilitate removal of necrotic tissue, aged red blood cells, and toxin molecules from the circulation. Macrophages maintain tissue homeostasis, while macrophages and DCs act as sentinel cells for the immune response [26]. Neutrophils are recruited and inflammation is promoted by mediators as indicated by macrophages [28]. Last main classes of macrophages are known as regulatory macrophages and are similar to suppressive M_2 macrophages [29]. Regulatory macrophages are induced by toll-like receptor (TLR) agonist in the presence of prostaglandin, apoptotic cells, and immunoglobulin G (IgG) immune complexes and defined the release of the immunosuppressive cytokines IL-10 and TGF-1 [29]. Regulatory macrophages are poor antigen-presenting cells (APCs) and have the inclination to induce T_{H2} and regulatory T cell responses that can further suppress antitumor and chronic inflammatory responses.

5.1 Significance of macrophages in innate immunity

The macrophages are important cells of immune system that function in innate and adaptive immunity and can play major role in the protective and pathogenic activity. Different types of pattern recognition receptors including biosensor like C-type lectin receptors, helicase RIG like receptors, NOD-like receptors and TLRs are expressed in macrophages.

The invading pathogens, foreign substances (ZNFs, silica, and stone dust particle), microbes and dead and dying cells are recognized by these receptors as a danger signal [30]. Adaptors induced signaling causes myeloid differentiation and regulation of inflammatory vesicle formation activity. This cascade further triggers antimicrobial activity of M_1 macrophages by stimulating the production of cytokines TNF and IL-1 [31]. Apart from innate immunity, macrophages also play an important role in wound healing [32].

5.2 Promiscuity and interaction of zinc oxide nanoparticles with macrophages

The ZnO NPs have been engineered, synthesized, and commonly used in products including sunscreens, cosmetic products, food and medical materials. These play a significant role in the biomedical area for disease diagnosis and therapy [33].

ZnO NPs are also widely used in the food industry and as nanofertilizer in agriculture. The wide application of ZnO NPs increased the chance of human and animal's exposure [34]. They can be absorbed into the body and redistributed into various organs after environmental exposure [34]. Hence, the safety assessment of nanoparticle is mandatory. The ZnO NPs can influence the immune system and affect the process of diseases and the emergency responses of immunity governed by macrophages [35]. ZnO NPs are foreign particles, and the macrophages play an important role in the recognition, processing, and removal of ZnO NPs [36]. The ZnO NPs interact with soluble proteins to form a halo corona that affects NP activity. The composition of protein coronas varies according to the size of NPs [37]. Protein coronas of NP surface have two layers including hard corona nearer to the NP surface and soft corona composed of reversibly adsorbed materials and large-size NPs phagocytized by macrophages through nanoparticle protein complexes corona. ZnO NPs deflate phagocytosis of macrophages and show cytotoxic and bactericidal activities by enhancing oxidative stress which may disrupt bacterial outer cell membrane and causes cell apoptosis. The ZnO NPs also inhibit nitric oxide (NO) production through the NF-Kβ signaling. NO reduces ZnONPs toxicity in rice seedlings by regulating oxidative damage and antioxidant defense systems [38].

5.3 Mechanism of ZnO NPs induced toxic effects on cells of immune system

The effects of ZnO NPs on the immune system depend on their physicochemical properties [39]. A nanotoxicological effect of NPs depends on the size, size distribution, surface area, electrostatic charge, and solubility [40]. The ZnO NPs are more water-soluble which result in more dissolution of toxic ions and ROS production [41]. ZnO NPs undergo endocytosis into the macrophages cells, dissolve into bioavailable zinc ion, and increase oxidative stress through ROS which cause immunotoxicity. The important factor for the immunotoxicity of ZnO NPs is ROS. Intracellular ROS production has at least some contribution in cell death induced by ZnO NPs [42, 43].

6. Effect on epithelial barriers of innate immunity

The important components of the innate immune system are epithelial barriers, phagocytic cells (dendritic cells, polymorphonuclear leukocytes, monocytes/macrophages), phagocytic leukocytes, basophils, mast cells, eosinophils, natural killer cells, circulating plasma proteins. TLR is the main signaling in the innate immunity which induce expression of inflammatory gene. Metal oxide nanoparticles trigger the TLR signaling pathway.

7. The innate immune system and role of TLRS signaling pathway

The innate immune system relies on the recognition of pathogen-associated microbial particles (PAMPs) through a limited number of germ line-encoded pattern recognition receptors belonging to the family of TLRs [44]. The activation of TLR signaling induces cytokines production and phagocytosis of macrophages along with catalytic activity of NK cells. More importantly, TLR signaling activation can also enhance antigen presentation via upregulating the expression of major histocompatibility complex (MHC) and co-stimulatory molecules (CD80 and CD86) on dendritic cells leading to adaptive immunity activations. Nanoparticles enhanced TLR signaling pathways which act as adjuvants [45]. The TLR antagonists or inhibitors that reduced the inflammatory response would have beneficial therapeutic effects in autoimmune diseases and sepsis [46].

7.1 Effect of NPs on TLR signaling of innate immunity health

The TLR is a type I transmembrane receptors which contain an N-terminal domain (leucine-rich repeat) and a C-terminal toward cytoplasm. When macrophage receptors recognized PAMP, TLRs recruit a TIR domain such as MyD88 and TRIF and initiate signaling events called downstream signaling by the secretion of different inflammatory molecules (chemokines, inflammatory cytokines, and IFNs I) [47]. The TLR signaling is responsible for the transcription of inflammatory and immune responses genes [48]. ZnO nanoparticles induced MyD88-dependent proinflammatory cytokines via a TLR signal pathway [49]. The TLRs may have important roles in NP uptake and for their cellular response which is directly proportional to the size of NPs.

7.2 Effects of NPs on phagocytic cells

Macrophages and dendritic cells have phagocytic activity; hence they readily uptake nanoparticles. Therefore, magnetic nanoparticles and nanoparticles-based PET agents were usually used for the visualization of macrophages in human diseases (cancer, atherosclerosis, myocardial infarction, aortic aneurysm, and diabetes).

8. Indian ayurvedic medicinal plant: *Withania somnifera*

Withania somnifera (Ashwagandha), an Indian Ayurvedic medicinal plant, is a green shrub and belongs to the Solanaceae family. For over 3000 years, Indians cultivated and applied its whole plant extract or separate constituents in Ayurvedic and indigenous medicine [50]. It was shown to have anti-inflammatory, antitumor, anti-stress, antioxidant, immuno-modulatory, hematopoietic, and rejuvenating properties thus benefiting the endocrine, cardiopulmonary, and central nervous systems [51]. It inhibits immunologically induced inflammation and a variety of pharmacological effects in *Babl/c mice* [52]. Various mechanisms have been proposed to explain the antitumor activity of Ashwagandha including potent anti-inflammatory, anti-angiogenic, anti-metastatic, pro-apoptotic, and radio-sensitizing properties [53]. An extract of *W. somnifera* showed immunological activity in *Balb/c mice*. Treatment with different doses of *W. somnifera* root extract (20 mg/dose/animal; i.p.) enhanced the total WBC counts. *W. somnifera* extract along with sheep red blood cell antigen (SRBC) increased antibody titer in circulation and plaque-forming cell numbers (PFC) in the spleen and reduced the delayed-type hypersensitivity reaction in mice model. Withania extract improved in phagocytic activity of macrophages when compared to untreated mice. The immunomodulatory effects of *W. somnifera* against ZnO NP-mediated toxicity in *Balb/c* mice study showed a dose-dependent reduction in phagocytosis, an increase in the levels of NO production along with upregulation of *TLR6, and arginase* gene. However, the adverse effect of ZnO NP on macrophages was reduced by *W. somnifera* extract and withaferin A with decreased *TLR6* overexpression and improved phagocytic activities [14].

8.1 Pharmacological and medicinal activities of withaferin a

Withaferin A is the key withanolide prototype which has been shown to have anti-inflammatory [54], antitumor [55], anti-angiogenesis [56], radio-sensitizing activity, and chemopreventive [57] and immunosuppressive [58] properties. Withaferin A is highly reactive because of the ketone containing unsaturated

A ring, the epoxide in B ring, and unsaturated lactone ring. In another study, withaferin A inhibited NF-κB at a very low concentration by targeting the ubiquitin-mediated proteasome pathway in endothelial cells. In vitro experiments demonstrated that withaferin A interfered with TNF-induced NF-κB activation at the level or upstream of IKKβ [57]. Withaferin A inhibited the expression of iNOS in the lipopolysaccharide (LPS)-stimulated murine macrophage cell line [59]. Withaferin-A inhibited, LPS-induced COX-2 expression and PGE2 production in BV_2 murine microglial cells [60]. Both pre and post-treatment of astrocytes with Withaferin-A attenuated LPS-induced production of tumor necrosis factor-α and the expression of COX-2 with expression of induced nitric oxide synthase by blocking the NF-κB activity [61]. Treatment with withaferin A increased SOD, catalase, and glutathione peroxidase activity in rat brain frontal cortex and striatal concentrations [62].

9. Conclusions

Nanoparticles are gaining importance recently due to their exciting applications in different fields like agriculture, human health, and livestock sector. Increased application of ZnO NPs is clearly indicating the adverse effect on immunity. It is, therefore, necessary to explore safety level of ZnO NPs and their role in humans and animals. The future work must be placed in the context of current risk assessments which must be associated with ZnO NPs toxicity and safety level and their uses. Further research work is emphasized for elucidating the nature of ZnO nanoparticles and their fate in living and non living matrices which can serve as to safeguard the ecosystem functioning. The ecosystem strengthening should be in term of agriculture and livestock particularly concerns production, food resource, immune and health status of animals. The role of *W. somnifera* as an antidote to immune complication induced by ZnO NPs exposure needs further research.

Conflict of interest

The authors declare no competing interest.

Notes/thanks/other declarations

We would like to acknowledge the support from the Director, ICAR-National Dairy Research Institute, Karnal-132,001, Haryana, India.

Author contributions

The authors' responsibilities were as follows: Dr. Jitendra Kumar, Dr. Chander Datt, Suryakant Verma and Kavita Rani conceived and designed the chapter.

Author details

Jitendra Kumar[1]*, Chander Datt[2], Surya Kant Verma[1] and Kavita Rani[1]

1 Division of Animal Biochemistry, ICAR-National Dairy Research Institute, Karnal, Haryana, India

2 Division of Animal Nutrition, ICAR-National Dairy Research Institute, Karnal, Haryana, India

*Address all correspondence to: jitoperon@gmail.com

References

[1] Rico CM, Majumdar S, Duarte-Gardea M, Peralta-Videa JR, Gardea-Torresdey JL. Interaction of nanoparticles with edible plants and their possible implications in the food chain. Journal of Agricultural and Food Chemistry. 2011;**59**(8):3485-3498

[2] Liu R, Lal R. Potentials of engineered nanoparticles as fertilizers for increasing agronomic productions. Science of the Total Environment. 2015;**514**:131-139

[3] Wang Y, Yuan L, Yao C, Ding L, Li C, Fang J, et al. A combined toxicity study of zinc oxide nanoparticles and vitamin C in food additives. Nanoscale. 2014;**6**(24):15333-15342

[4] Sirelkhatim A, Mahmud S, Seeni A, Kaus NHM, Ann LC, Bakhori SKM, et al. Review on zinc oxide nanoparticles: Antibacterial activity and toxicity mechanism. Nano-Micro Letters. 2015; **7**(3):219-242

[5] Li CH, Shen CC, Cheng YW, Huang SH, Wu CC, Kao CC, et al. Organ biodistribution, clearance, and genotoxicity of orally administered zinc oxide nanoparticles in mice. Nanotoxicology. 2012;**6**(7):746-756

[6] Bacchetta R, Moschini E, Santo N, Fascio U, Del Giacco L, Freddi S, et al. Evidence and uptake routes for zinc oxide nanoparticles through the gastrointestinal barrier in Xenopus laevis. Nanotoxicology. 2014;**8**(7): 728-744

[7] Saman S, Moradhaseli S, Shokouhian A, Ghorbani M. Histopathological effects of ZnO nanoparticles on liver and heart tissues in wistar rats. Advances in Bioresearch. 2013;**4**(2):83-88

[8] Shrestha B, Acosta-Martinez V, Cox SB, Green MJ, Li S, Cañas-Carrell JE. An evaluation of the impact of multi-walled carbon nanotubes on soil microbial community structure and functioning. Journal of Hazardous Materials. 2013;**261**:188-197

[9] Yadav T, Mungray AA, Mungray AK. Fabricated nanoparticles. Reviews of Environmental Contamination and Toxicology. 2014;**230**:83-110

[10] BCC Research. Global Markets for Nanocomposites, Nanoparticles, Nanoclays, and Nanotubes; 2014. Available form: https://www.bccresearch.com/market-research/nanotechnology/nanocompositesmarketnan021f.html?vsmaid=203/. [Accessed: 19 October 2017]

[11] Peng YH, Tsai YC, Hsiung CE, Lin YH, Shih Y. Influence of water chemistry on the environmental behaviors of commercial ZnO nanoparticles in various water and wastewater samples. Journal of Hazardous Materials. 2017;**322**:348-356

[12] Boxall ABA, Chaudhry Q, Sinclair C, Jones A, Aitken R, Jefferson B. et al. Current and future predicted environmental exposure to engineered nanoparticles. Report by the Central Science Laboratory (CSL) York for the Department of the Environment and Rural Affairs (DEFRA), UK; 2007. Available from: wwTv.de-fra.gov.uk/science/Project_Data/Document Library/CB01098/CB01098_627()_FRP.pdf

[13] Zhao L, Peralta-Videa JR, Ren M, Varela-Ramirez A, Li C, Hernandez-Viezcas JA, et al. Transport of Zn in a sandy loam soil treated with ZnO NPs and uptake by corn plants: Electron microprobe and confocal microscopy studies. Chemical Engineering Journal. 2012;**184**:1-8

[14] Kumar J, Mitra MD, Hussain A, Kaul G. Exploration of

immunomodulatory and protective effect of Withania somnifera on trace metal oxide (zinc oxide nanoparticles) induced toxicity in Balb/c mice. Molecular Biology Reports. 2019;**46**: 2447-2459

[15] Adams LK, Lyon DY, Alvarez PJ. Comparative eco-toxicity of nanoscale TiO2, SiO2, and ZnO water suspensions. Water Research. 2006;**40**(19):3527-3532

[16] Sahu D, Kannan GM, Vijayaraghavan R, Anand T, Khanum F. Nanosized zinc oxide induces toxicity in human lung cells. International Scholarly Research Notices: Toxicology. 2013;**2013**:316075

[17] Dardenne M. Zinc and immune function. European Journal of Clinical Nutrition. 2002;**56**(S3):S20

[18] Shankar AH, Prasad AS. Zinc and immune function: The biological basis of altered resistance to infection. The American Journal of Clinical Nutrition. 1998;**68**(2):447S-463S

[19] Ibs KH, Lothar R. Zinc-altered immune function. The Journal of Nutrition. 2003;**133**(5):1452S-1456S

[20] Chandra RK. Excessive intake of zinc impairs immune responses. JAMA. 1984;**252**(11):1443-1446

[21] Pfeiffer R. Untersuchungen uber das Choleragift. Medical Microbiology and Immunology. 1892;**11**(1):393-412

[22] Metchnikoff E. Ueber eine sprosspilzkrankheit der daphnien. Beitrag Zur Lehre Über Den Kampf Der Phagozyten Gegen Krankheitserreger. Archiv für pathologische Anatomie und Physiologie und für. 1884;**96**(2): 177-195

[23] Wentworth P, Wentworth AD, Zhu X, Wilson IA, Janda KD, Eschenmoser A, et al. Evidence for the production of trioxygen species during antibody-catalyzed chemical modification of antigens. Proceedings of the National Academy of Sciences. 2003;**100**(4):1490-1493

[24] Doulatov S, Notta F, Eppert K, Nguyen LT, Ohashi PS, Dick JE. Revised map of the human progenitor hierarchy shows the origin of macrophages and dendritic cells in early lymphoid development. Nature Immunology. 2010;**11**(7):585-593

[25] Geissmann F, Manz MG, Jung S, Sieweke MH, Merad M, Ley K. Development of monocytes, macrophages, and dendritic cells. Science. 2010b;**327**(5966):656-661

[26] Gordon S, Taylor PR. Monocyte and macrophage heterogeneity. Nature Reviews Immunology. 2005;**5**(12): 953-964

[27] Galli SJ, Borregaard N, Wynn TA. Phenotypic and functional plasticity of cells of innate immunity: Macrophages, mast cells and neutrophils. Nature Immunology. 2011;**12**(11):1035

[28] Cros J, Cagnard N, Woollard K, Patey N, Zhang SY, Senechal B, et al. Human CD14 dim monocytes patrol and sense nucleic acids and viruses via TLR7 and TLR8 receptors. Immunity. 2010; **33**(3):375-386

[29] Mosser DM, Edwards JP. Exploring the full spectrum of macrophage activation. Nature Reviews Immunology. 2008;**8**(12):958-969

[30] Geissmann F, Gordon S, Hume DA, Mowat AM, Randolph GJ. Unravelling mononuclear phagocyte heterogeneity. Nature Reviews Immunology. 2010a;**10** (6):453-460

[31] Martinon F, Burns K, Tschopp J. The inflammasome: A molecular platform triggering activation of inflammatory caspases and processing of proIL-β. Molecular Cell. 2002;**10**(2):417-426

[32] Wynn TA, Barron L. Macrophages: Master regulators of inflammation and fibrosis. Seminars in Liver Disease. 2010;**30**(03):245-257

[33] Mahapatro A, Singh DK. Biodegradable nanoparticles are excellent vehicle for site directed in-vivo delivery of drugs and vaccines. Journal of Nanobiotechnology. 2011; **9**(1):55

[34] Newman MD, Stotland M, Ellis JI. The safety of nanosized particles in titanium dioxide and zinc oxide-based sunscreens. Journal of the American Academy of Dermatology. 2009;**61**(4): 685-692

[35] Laskin DL, Sunil VR, Gardner CR, Laskin JD. Macrophages and tissue injury: Agents of defense or destruction? Annual Review of Pharmacology and Toxicology. 2011;**51**: 267-288

[36] Dobrovolskaia MA, McNeil SE. Immunological properties of engineered nanomaterials. Nature Nanotechnology. 2007;**2**(8):469-478

[37] Lundqvist M, Stigler J, Elia G, Lynch I, Cedervall T, Dawson KA. Nanoparticle size and surface properties determine the protein corona with possible implications for biological impacts. Proceedings of the National Academy of Sciences. 2008;**105**(38): 14265-14270

[38] Chen J, Liu X, Wang C, Yin SS, Li XL, Hu WJ, et al. Nitric oxide ameliorates zinc oxide nanoparticles-induced phytotoxicity in rice seedlings. Journal of Hazardous Materials. 2015; **297**:173-182

[39] Zolnik BS, Gonzalez-Fernandez A, Sadrieh N, Dobrovolskaia MA. Minireview: Nanoparticles and the immune system. Endocrinology. 2010; **151**(2):458-465

[40] Brun NR, Lenz M, Wehrli B, Fent K. Comparative effects of zinc oxide nanoparticles and dissolved zinc on zebrafish embryos and eleuthero-embryos: Importance of zinc ions. Science of the Total Environment. 2014; **476**:657-666

[41] Magdolenova Z, Collins A, Kumar A, Dhawan A, Stone V, Dusinska M. Mechanisms of genotoxicity. A review of in vitro and in vivo studies with engineered nanoparticles. Nanotoxicology. 2014; **8**(3):233-278

[42] Xia T, Kovochich M, Brant J, Hotze M, Sempf J, Oberley T, et al. Comparison of the abilities of ambient and manufactured nanoparticles to induce cellular toxicity according to an oxidative stress paradigm. Nano Letters. 2006;**6**(8):1794-1807

[43] Song W, Zhang J, Guo J, Zhang J, Ding F, Li L, et al. Role of the dissolved zinc ion and reactive oxygen species in cytotoxicity of ZnO nanoparticles. Toxicology Letters. 2010;**199**(3): 389-397

[44] Takeda K, Akira S. TLR signaling pathways. Seminars in Immunology. 2004;**16**(1):3-9

[45] Tamayo I, Irache JM, Mansilla C, Ochoa-Repáraz J, Lasarte JJ, Gamazo C. Poly (anhydride) nanoparticles act as active Th1 adjuvants through toll-like receptor exploitation. Clinical and Vaccine Immunology. 2010;**17**(9): 1356-1362

[46] Tse K, Horner AA. Update on toll-like receptor-directed therapies for human disease. Annals of the Rheumatic Diseases. 2007;**66**(suppl 3): iii77-iii80

[47] Kawai T, Akira S. The role of pattern-recognition receptors in innate immunity: Update on toll-like receptors.

Nature Immunology. 2010;**11**(5): 373-384

[48] Lafferty EI, Qureshi ST, Schnare M. The role of toll-like receptors in acute and chronic lung inflammation. Journal of Inflammation. 2010;7(1):57

[49] Chang H, Ho CC, Yang CS, Chang WH, Tsai MH, Tsai HT, et al. Involvement of MyD88 in zinc oxide nanoparticle-induced lung inflammation. Experimental and Toxicologic Pathology. 2013;**65**(6): 887-896

[50] Mirjalili MH, Moyano E, Bonfill M, Cusido RM, Palazón J. Steroidal lactones from Withania somnifera, an ancient plant for novel medicine. Molecules. 2009;**14**(7):2373-2393

[51] Mishra L, Mishra P, Pandey A, Sangwan RS, Sangwan NS, Tuli R. Withanolides from Withania somnifera roots. Phytochemistry. 2008;**69**(4): 1000-1004

[52] Davis L, Girija K. Suppressive effect of cyclophosphamide-induced toxicity by Withania somnifera extract in mice. Journal of Ethnopharmacology. 1998; **62**(3):209-214

[53] Yu SM, Kim SJ. Production of reactive oxygen species by withaferin a causes loss of type collagen expression and COX-2 expression through the PI3K/Akt, p38, and JNK pathways in rabbit articular chondrocytes. Experimental Cell Research. 2013; **319**(18):2822-2834

[54] Sabina EP, Chandal S, Rasool MK. Inhibition of monosodium urate crystal-induced inflammation by withaferin a. Journal of Pharmacy & Pharmaceutical Sciences. 2008;**11**(4):46-55

[55] Devi PU, Sharada AC, Solomon FE. In vivo growth inhibitory and radiosensitizing effects of withaferin a on mouse Ehrlich ascites carcinoma. Cancer Letters. 1995;**95**(1–2):189-193

[56] Mohan R, Hammers H, Bargagna-Mohan P, Zhan X, Herbstritt C, Ruiz A, et al. Withaferin a is a potent inhibitor of angiogenesis. Angiogenesis. 2004; **7**(2):115-122

[57] Manoharan S, Panjamurthy K, Balakrishnan S, Vasudevan K, Vellaichamy L. Circadian time-dependent chemopreventive potential of withaferin-a in 7, 12-dimethyl-benz [a] anthracene-induced oral carcinogenesis. Pharmacological Reports. 2009b;**61**(4):719-726

[58] Shohat B, Kirson I, Lavie D. Immunosuppressive activity of two plant steroidal lactones withaferin a and withanolide E. Biomedicine. 1978;**28**(1): 18-24

[59] Oh JH, Lee TJ, Park JW, Kwon TK. Withaferin a inhibits iNOS expression and nitric oxide production by Akt inactivation and down-regulating LPS-induced activity of NF-κB in RAW 264.7 cells. European Journal of Pharmacology. 2008;**599**(1):11-17

[60] Choi MJ, Park EJ, Min KJ, Park JW, Kwon TK. Endoplasmic reticulum stress mediates withaferin A-induced apoptosis in human renal carcinoma cells. Toxicology In Vitro. 2011;**25**(3): 692-698

[61] Martorana F, Guidotti G, Brambilla L, Rossi D. Withaferin a inhibits nuclear factor-κB-dependent pro-inflammatory and stress response pathways in the astrocytes. Neural Plasticity. 2015;**38**:1964

[62] Bhattacharya SK, Satyan KS, Ghosal S. Antioxidant activity of glycowithanolides from Withania somnifera. Indian Journal of Experimental Biology. 1997;**35**:236-239

Chapter 12

Polycyclic Aromatic Hydrocarbons (PAHs) and Their Influence to Some Aquatic Species

Ayoub Baali and Ahmed Yahyaoui

Abstract

Polycyclic aromatic hydrocarbons (PAHs) are ubiquitous environmental pollutants generated primarily during the incomplete combustion of organic materials (e.g., coal, oil, petrol, and wood). Many PAHs have toxic, mutagenic, and/or carcinogenic functions. PAHs are highly lipid soluble which lead to a fast absorption by the gastrointestinal tract of marine mammals. They are immediately distributed in a vast variety of tissues with a notable tendency for localization in body fat. Metabolism of PAHs is obtained via the cytochrome P450-mediated mixed function oxidase system with oxidation or hydroxylation as the first step. PAHs are environmental contaminants that pose significant risk to health of fish. The effect of PAHs on fish is a topic of rising attention in a lot of countries. Different studies using the bile metabolites separated by high-performance liquid chromatography with fluorescence detection were presented. The aim is to compare the levels of PAH metabolites in fish from different areas and fish species. The major metabolite present in all fish was 1-hydroxypyrene. The data confirm the importance of 1-hydroxypyrene as the key PAH metabolite in fish bile and suggest that the European eel is an ideal species for monitoring PAHs.

Keywords: PAHs, organic pollutants, metabolism, fish, 1-hydroxypyrene, European eel

1. Introduction

Aquatic ecosystems are susceptible to receiving and accumulating contaminants [1]. In particular, polycyclic aromatic hydrocarbons (PAHs) have been identified as general causes of the deterioration of aquatic ecosystems in recent decades [2].

Polycyclic aromatic hydrocarbons (PAHs) are ubiquitous and persistent environmental contaminants found in sediments and associated waters of urbanized estuaries and coastal areas [3–5]. They are a class of compounds found in crude oil and are everywhere in the aquatic ecosystem [6–12]. PAHs are the most toxic pollutants of crude oil and are remembered by the United States Environmental Protection Agency (EPA) as priority toxic components because of its persistence in the environment and are toxic to fishes [13, 14]; thus, PAHs are of special interest following oil spills and in environmental control. They come from natural and anthropogenic sources. The latter can be associated to pyrolysis and incomplete combustion of organic element [15]. Wastewater, atmospheric deposition, and petroleum spillage are some of the most important PAH sources. PAHs and their intermediate degradation products have the potential to generate toxic or mutagenic effects in fish [16–18] and humans [19]. PAH metabolites in the bile fluid are generally accepted as measures for PAH exposure in fish because of the rapid metabolism of PAH in most vertebrates [3]. Therefore, PAH metabolites in fish are recommended as monitoring parameters in European seas [20, 21].

In this chapter, we briefly review the origin, toxicity, and transformation of PAHs in the aquatic environment, highlighting their efficient metabolism in fish. We also review the presence of PAHs on fish bile and the works reported on that.

2. Organic contamination by polycyclic aromatic hydrocarbons (PAH)

2.1 PAH origin

PAHs are mainly formed during the incomplete combustion of organic matter and during the slow maturation of organic matter accumulated in deep sedimentary environments. These two origins present distinct formation mechanisms that are realized with different kinetics and induce variable molecular distributions (related to stability) [22].

2.1.1 Pyrolytic origin

Pyrolytic PAHs are generated by processes of incomplete combustion of organic matter at high temperatures. The mechanisms involved in their formation involve the production of free radicals by pyrolysis at high temperature (≥500°C) of the fossil material (oils, fuel oil, organic matter, etc.) under oxygen-deficient conditions. PAHs of pyrolytic origin come from the combustion of automotive fuel, domestic combustion (coal, wood, etc.), industrial production (steelworks, aluminum smelters, etc.), and energy production (power stations operating on oil or coal) or incinerators [23].

2.1.2 Petrogenic origin

The process of diagenesis can give rise to petroleum and other fossil fuels containing the so-called petrogenic PAHs. These PAHs are formed at low temperatures (150°C) over long periods of time. They result from exposure of organic matter to adequate conditions of temperature and pressure. The proportion of PAHs in oils varies according to their origin and level of refinement. In general, petrogenic PAH mixtures are marked by a predominance of low molecular weight PAHs, three cycles or less, and substituted PAHs [22].

PAHs represent between 20 and 40% by weight of crude oils which are mainly composed of saturated hydrocarbons. However, they are less than a few percent of the composition of refined gasoline (<0.5% by mass) or kerosene [24].

2.1.3 Biological origin

PAHs can also be formed by microorganisms from biogenic precursors such as diterpenes and triterpenes, steroids, pigments, or quinones in sediments or recent soils [25, 26]; these precursors can come from terrestrial or aquatic biological tissues (plants, animals, bacteria, macro- and microalgae) [27, 28].

2.2 PAH toxicity

The toxicity of several PAHs is a phenomenon that is well-known. Research has been conducted by several environmental groups such as the US Environmental Protection Agency-Toxic Substances Control Act (US EPA-TSCA) and the International Agency for Research on Cancer (IARC). The toxicity of PAHs to aquatic species is affected by metabolism and photooxidation. They are generally harmful in the presence of ultraviolet light. PAHs have moderate to high acute toxicity to aquatic organisms and birds. Mammals can absorb PAHs by various routes, e.g., dermal contact, inhalation, and ingestion [14, 29, 30]. The concentrations of PAHs found in fish are expected to be much higher than in the environment from which they were taken because of their bioaccumulation. Withal, metabolism of PAHs is sufficient to prevent biomagnifications [31, 32].

Teleost fish have an immense capacity to metabolize PAHs because of the enzymes cytochrome P450 in their tissues that oxidatively biotransform PAHs to hydroxylated metabolites [33].

The half-life times of PAHs in various biological tissues (bivalves, crustaceans, and fish) are of the order of a few days to 10 days and are about five times higher for heavy PAHs relative to lower PAHs.

The environmental matrices are moreover complex, containing numerous endogenous or exogenous, mineral or organic molecules between which interactions can take place. Synergistic toxic effects have been observed in particular between metals and PAH quinones [34].

Indeed, the carcinogenic nature of some of these molecules alone or in mixtures is proven. Twelve of these are classified by the International Agency for Research on Cancer (IARC) as probably carcinogenic to humans [35]. After contamination by these substances, they are biotransformed in the liver into different (poly)hydroxy-PAHs.

The risks of PAHs to fish and other aquatic organisms in natural systems are highly uncertain due to the occurrence of complex, incompletely characterized mixtures of these chemicals, large spatial heterogeneity in exposure concentrations, incomplete understanding of the importance of UV-activated PAH toxicity, the biological and physical controls on fish exposure to UV light, and the bioaccumulation of PAHs. These uncertainties are especially great for early-life-stage fish, which might be particularly susceptible to UV-activated because of their small size, lack of protective pigmentation and gill coverings, and ready accumulation of PAHs.

3. Transformations of PAHs in marine ecosystem

3.1 Physical and chemical degradation

Sediments contaminated with PAHs pose a real threat to all living organisms, even those that feed on the benthic prey.

PAHs with a low molecular weight can be found in all environmental matrices, since higher molecular weight compounds are more deeply associated (physically and chemically) with sediments/soils and particles than the other abiotic sample types. PAHs in air can be modified via chemical oxidation and photochemical processes [8], whereas in sediments/soils and the uppermost portion of the water column, degradation of PAHs, particularly lower molecular weight PAHs, occurs via photooxidation [6, 36]. In addition to parent PAHs, oxygenated PAH metabolites formed during these degradation processes can persist associating with sediments up to 6 months after initial addition to the water column and thus can endure in the environment for extended periods of time [37]. In water samples and sediment, some microorganisms (e.g., fungi, bacteria) have been demonstrated to mineralize PAHs under aerobic conditions, particularly those compounds that contain two- and three-fused rings (e.g., fluorene, naphthalene), to their basic elements or to biodegrade these compounds to more polar degradation products [3, 8]. More information on PAH microbial degradation pathways and identification of degradation can be found in Cerniglia and Heitkamp [38], Juhasz and Naidu [39], and Bamforth and Singleton [40]. Part of research studies have proved that pyrene can be mineralized by certain strains of bacteria (e.g., *Mycobacterium*) under optimum growing conditions in the laboratory, but it is uncertain if this occurs in the natural environment [41, 42]. In contrast, other higher molecular weight PAHs (e.g., five- and six-ring compounds) are not readily degraded by microbes and thus are more likely to accumulate in these environmental media (particularly in fine-grained sediments with high organic carbon content) [3, 39]. Under anoxic conditions, PAHs persist in sediments, particularly in organic sediments [42].

3.2 Biotransformation in the aquatic food web

Pyrolytic PAHs are the most common in aquatic environments. After the emission of pyrolytic PAHs into the atmosphere, the molecules fall back and settle on the surface of the water or soil [23]. Under the action of soil leaching, PAHs are transported to water bodies. These hydrophobic molecules then associate with other particles of the column of water and accumulate in the sediment [23].

In aquatic organisms, exposure to PAHs can occur through dermal exposure, respiration, or consumption of contaminated prey (e.g., annelids, crustaceans) or sediment [43]. Biotransformation of PAHs in aquatic organisms occurs to varying degrees depending on a number of factors, including the rate of uptake, metabolic capability, physical condition, feeding strategy, and age [43, 44]. Invertebrates are capable of PAH uptake from their environment and have been shown to have varying levels of PAH-metabolizing capability [44]. Mollusks generally have lower PAH-metabolizing capability than certain species of polychaetes, crustaceans, and fish [3].

PAH metabolism in fish is mainly conducted by inducible enzymes of the cytochrome P450 family, in particular CYP1A. These enzymes are localized in the membranes of the smooth endoplasmic reticulum, located mainly in the liver, but are also present in other organs. They are expressed and functional from the earliest stages of fish development. These enzymes catalyze the addition of an oxygen atom to the PAH molecule through an NADPH-dependent reaction. CYP1A protein is induced during exposure of the body to PAHs. CYP1A induction is rapid, and activity levels are often increased by a factor of 100 a few hours after exposure. These highly polar conjugated metabolites are then excreted into urine or the bile for rapid rejection over the gastrointestinal tract [14, 43, 45, 46]. Concerning the result of this rapid metabolism in fish, concentrations of parent PAHs are insignificant in muscle and other tissues. Thus, to determinate a recent exposure to PAHs in teleost fish, bile and urine are used, with the preference of bile because of its easy sampling. Otherwise, differences in the metabolism of benzo[a]pyrene (BaP), including differences in the types and proportions of metabolites formed, have been shown between two fish of freshwater [47, 48]. These differences could contribute to variations in susceptibility to these carcinogenic compounds among fish species. Differences in glutathione-S-transferases may also help explain differential susceptibility to chemically induced carcinogenesis among fish species [46]. A number of analytical methods have been developed to measure PAH metabolites in fish bile and are reviewed in [14]. Oil spills, including the Deepwater Horizon (DWH) spill in the Gulf of Mexico in 2010, show the necessity of the need for additional methods to determine PAH exposure in seafood or protected species (e.g., marine mammals) where species cannot be lethally collected. For example, a rapid, sensitive HPLC-fluorescence method was developed by the US Food and Drug Administration [49] during the DWH spill and was used by federal and Gulf state analytical laboratories as part of the seafood safety response [50]. The development of new analytical methods like those can provide important information on PAH exposure in aquatic organisms.

4. Effects of PAHs on aquatic species

PAHs are an important factor of contamination in the environment but also a risk to human health. In fact, the dangers related to PAHs vary according to their toxicity on the one hand and the many sources of exposure on the other. It has also been proven that carcinogenic and mutagenic effects related to a single compound of PAHs were found. A large number of effects have been identified [51]. In fact, genotoxicity and tumorigenesis observed in fish are linked to the presence of metabolites. Beyond genotoxicity, there are many other effects observed, for example, in behavior, reproduction, and growth.

Benzo[a]pyrene, for example, which is highly studied, leads to a decrease in weight [52] and growth [53], an increase in the gonado-somatic index (GSI) in Japanese medaka (*Oryzias latipes*) [52], DNA breaks in oysters (*Crassostrea gigas*) [54], and DNA adducts in zebrafish and on human liver cells (HepG2) [55]. Teratogenic effects in particular on the heart of sardine (*Clupea pallasii*) [56] and zebrafish [57, 58] have been observed as well as anemia in scorpion fish (*Sebastes schlegelii*) [59]. Benzo[a]pyrene affects the reproduction of isopods (*Oniscus asellus* and *Asellus porcellio scaber*) [53] and accumulates in oocytes in catfish (*Ictalurus punctatus*) [60]; it disrupts the expression of the aromatase (enzyme necessary for the conversion of androgen such as estrogen isosterone) in female mummichog (*Fundulus heteroclitus*) [61] and inhibits the synthesis of testosterone and estradiol in flounder (*Platichthys flesus* L.) [62].

The toxicity of a compound can be enhanced or reduced by endogenous and exogenous factors. For example, in fish, hypoxia [63], geographical origin and fish life history [64], and/or the various PAH compounds [65] can cause variations. The penetration time in the fish embryo and the depuration time can vary considerably. In addition, the effects produced by these molecules, tested individually, do not necessarily follow a dose-effect relationship [52].

4.1 Effects of PAHs on the survival

Survival is a commonly used variable. This variable has made it possible to develop standardized tests in toxicology such as LD50 (lethal dose) or LC50 (lethal concentration) calculations. Although protected in their chorions, fish eggs and then larvae are particularly exposed because, in most cases, they are unable to flee contaminated areas during their early-life stages [66]. It is during development, during the establishment of all organs and systems, that contaminants can pass this barrier. They can affect the development and have long-term consequences. Exposure to PAHs can lead to decreased survival in aquatic organisms during acute exposures. For example, there has been a decrease in survival after early exposure of salmon (*Oncorhynchus gorbuscha*) to dissolve PAHs [67].

In the case of chronic exposure in the early stages, similar effects can be observed. Impairment in survival has been observed in salmon (*Oncorhynchus gorbuscha*) exposed to crude oil [68], in minnow (*Pimephales promelas*) exposed to contaminated sediment [69], in *Chanos chanos* and capelin (*Mallotus villosus*) exposed to dissolved PAHs (anthracene, B[a]P, pyrene and heavy fuel oil) [66, 70], and in shrimp (*Palaemonetes pugio*) exposed to the pyrene feed which also shows reduced survival [71]. In other studies, survival is not affected by PAHs. This is the case, for example, in terrestrial isopods, where oral administration does not have significant effects on survival [53]. It is also not affected after exposure to BaP in mummichog (*Fundulus heteroclitus*) [72]. PAHs can affect survival in some cases and not in others. This extreme variable may not be the most sensitive for all species or all types of exposure.

4.2 Malformations and growth

PAHs induce malformations during development. They lead to a decrease in skeletal mineralization in bass (*Dicentrarchus labrax*) [73] and craniofacial deformities in scorpion fish (*Sebastiscus marmoratus*) [74]. Jaw malformations [75] in this same fish as well as in zebrafish [58] were also observed. The number of edemas is also increased in scorpion fish (*Sebastes schlegelii*), salmon (*Oncorhynchus gorbuscha*) [67, 76], and medaka (*Oryzias latipes*) [77], as well as the occurrence of hemorrhages in trout (*Oncorhynchus mykiss*) [78]. The impact of PAHs on growth is frequently reflected in a reduction in size and/or weight [67, 79, 80]. This reduction in growth is observed regardless of the mode of administration of PAHs, the concentrations used, and the duration of exposure [59, 70, 81]. Weight reduction is often proportional to contamination [81]. Unfortunately, these are not the only visible damage. A decrease in lipid reserves may be observed and result in a decrease in energy reserves [10, 79].

4.3 Metabolism and osmoregulation

In a PAH study, fish were exposed to the soluble fraction of a crude oil mixture. Structural lesions and morphological differences are noted on the gill [82]. These differences would be related to a metabolism aimed at reducing contact with the pollutant, which would reduce the gill surface and oxygen supply. A reduction in oxygen uptake could compromise the fish metabolism [82].

Osmoregulation problems following exposure of *Sebastiscus marmoratus* to dissolve PAHs have been observed [75]. PAHs would inhibit Na^+/K^+ activity in a dose-dependent manner and play a role in osmoregulation.

4.4 Effect on behavior

The behavioral response of an animal following exposure to stress and/or contaminant (s) is increasingly studied [83–87].

The behavior makes it possible to discriminate a large number of integrating variables from the changes induced by PAHs. Swimming activity can be assessed as well as other aspects such as lethargy, anxiety, social communication, eating behavior, flight response, learning, or reproductive behavior.

A reduced swimming activity in seabream (*Sparus aurata*) was observed following a 4 days of exposure to dissolved PAHs [88, 89]: phenanthrene, fluorine, and pyrene [89]. An increase in lethargy and a reduction in the number of surface surges have also been observed following exposure to dissolved PAHs in this species [88, 89].

These variables can also be used to evaluate the neurotoxic effects of a contaminant. The reduction of social interactions following exposure to phenanthrene [89] is proven.

The escape response, in the presence of fluoranthene, has been demonstrated in control fish [90]. The fish are placed in a double flow aquarium. A flow of control water and a flow of water containing fluoranthene are present. Fish that have never been exposed are fleeing fluoranthene. On the other hand, fish that have been previously exposed to a high dose of fluoranthene no longer leak the molecule [90].

Learning and exploration abilities are diminished after exposure to PAHs. For example, discrimination of a familiar object is altered in mice exposed to BaP. In the same vein, dietary exposure of the mother to a mixture containing the 16 priority PAHs of the USEPA leads to behavioral alteration in the next generation, especially in a new environment. The reproductive behavior can also be disturbed. The ability of a male to find a female can be altered, as is the case in amphipods, for example [91].

4.5 Effect on reproduction

PAHs are lipophilic molecules that are transported and found in the ovaries via vitellogenin and/or lipovitellin [60]. They can also result in inhibition of vitellogenin synthesis, as has already been shown in trout after exposure to β-naphthoflavone [92]. This exposure compromises the maturation of the ovaries and causes an increase in apoptosis in gonadal cells [91]. These pollutants lead, for example, to reproductive inhibition in shrimp exposed to pyrene [71]. A decrease in fecundity, number of breeding cycles, and larval survival is observed in different fish species. In mussels, gametes are deformed and are present in small numbers [91].

Females are not the only ones to be affected. Male sperm quality can also be altered after exposure to benzo[b]fluoranthene, as is the case in mice exposed via breast milk [59]. Sperm quality is reduced, and there is also an increase in testicular apoptosis.

5. PAHs in eels

High-performance liquid chromatography (HPLC) is generally used for the determination of PAH metabolites in considerable fish species [93–98] and has been covered by an intercalibration exercise [22].

Although bile metabolites have been measured in many species of fish [13], those selected for biomonitoring programs tend to be common, long-lived species at the top of the food chain, with relatively sedentary life styles and benthic habits [99]. Consequently, the common eel (*Anguilla anguilla*) has been used in studies of PAH contamination [100, 101]. Pleuronectid flatfish are also well-suited to biomonitoring, and the European flounder (*Pleuronectes flesus*), an abundant flatfish in most European estuaries, has been frequently chosen to assess PAH contamination [102, 103].

The study conducted by Ruddock et al. [104] in the Severn Estuary showed that from the six metabolites of polycyclic aromatic hydrocarbons (PAHs) identified and quantified from the bile of *Anguilla anguilla*, *Pleuronectes flesus*, and *Conger conger* collected during 1997, the main metabolite present in all fish was 1-hydroxypyrene with lower proportions of 1-hydroxychrysene and 1-hydroxyphenanthrene and small concentration of three benzo[a]pyrene derivatives. The results approve the importance of 1-hydroxypyrene as the important PAH metabolite in fish bile and suggest that the *A. anguilla* is an excellent species for monitoring PAHs in estuarine ecosystems. 1-Hydroxypyrene is invariably the major metabolite present in the bile of fish exposed to PAH-contaminated sediments [105], and this was confirmed by the results of this work for fish in the Severn Estuary. Pyrene is produced by many petrogenic and pyrolytic processes [43] and has been detected in significant number in sewage outfalls [106]. It is regarded the best general indicator of PAH exposure in fish [100, 107]. The contribution of 1-OH-Phen to the total metabolites detected ranged from approximately 2% in flounders and conger eels to 8% in common eels.

Phenanthrenes are released to the atmosphere during the combustion of fossil fuels, particularly coal, oil, and its refined products [43]. Like all PAHs with two to four benzene rings, phenanthrenes can remain suspended in airborne particles for long periods [108]. Compared to the other PAHs detected, BaP has a very low solubility in water and low bioavailability, but metabolites of BaP are especially important because of their potent mutagenic and carcinogenic properties [109–111].

A recent study conducted by Baali et al. [2] on bile metabolites of PAHs in 18 European eels (*Anguilla anguilla*), 7 moray (Muraenidae), and 28 conger eels (*Conger conger*) from Moroccan waters (Moulay Bousselham lagoon and Boujdour) shows the presence of two polycyclic aromatic hydrocarbon (PAH) metabolites, 1-hydroxypyrene (1-OH-Pyr) and 1-hydroxyphenanthrene (1-OH-Phen). The high-performance liquid chromatography with fluorescence detection method was used to separate the bile metabolites.

The goals of the present study were to compare the levels of PAH metabolites in eels from the lagoon and sea and also to compare levels of PAH metabolites between the different eels.

In this study the PAH metabolites (1-OH-Pyr and 1-OH-Phen) were detected in all species. The results of this investigation show that the concentration of 1-OH-Pyr was high for *Anguilla anguilla* than the other species (**Figure 1**). The conger eels represent the species with the lower concentration of 1-OH-Pyr. This result reflects the low degree of contamination in Boujdour coast (**Figure 1**). Thus, the presence of high concentration of 1-OH-Pyr and 1-OH-Phen in the bile of the European eels and morays reflects the high degree of contamination in the lagoon which is due to the anthropogenic activity in Moulay Bousselham lagoon. From the comparison between the contamination of the European eels and morays belonging to Moulay Bousselham lagoon, the results show that the first species present a higher concentration of PAH metabolites than the second one (**Figure 1**). This conclusion confirms that the *Anguilla anguilla* is more suitable species for monitoring PAH contamination. The European eels spend most of their life in muddy sediment which usually present a high PAH concentration levels. The pollutants in sediment are easily accumulated [112–114]. Accordingly, it is recognized that sediment contamination has a particular interest with regard to aquatic ecosystem quality. Sediment is an important source of pollutants and the factor with the high impact on the deterioration of the water quality. Although the feeding habit of the European eels may result in higher exposure to PAHs whence the high concentration of 1-OH-Pyr and 1-OH-Phen in the bile of this species [115], the accumulation of PAHs from the surrounding water is considered more efficient than impacted food [116]. The level of PAH metabolites in fish bile varies according to the area. The results show that Boujdour Sea is not a polluted site [117]. Moulay Bousselham lagoon is a semi-closed area; the concentration of pollutants in this site is higher than Boujdour Sea because of its lower water circulation. In the lagoon PAHs are easily accumulated than that in the sea [112]. Our results confirm that 1-OH-Pyr is the major metabolite present in fish bile [104, 105] and the best indicator of PAH exposure in fish [100, 107]. It was found that 1-OH-Pyr is the dominant compound in eel bile [118–120]. The results show that the levels of PAHs in Morocco are lower than those obtained in the other regions. As a conclusion of this study, the possible health risk of PAH contamination in Boujdour coast and Moulay Bousselham lagoon might be low compared to the other European sites.

The concentration of 1-OH-Pyr varies significantly with length ($p < 0.05$) for each species. The results obtained in this study [2] show that the concentration of PAH metabolites does not always increase with the size; there are obviously factors which can affect the exposure of this pollutant such as species differences, age, sex, maturity, and diet.

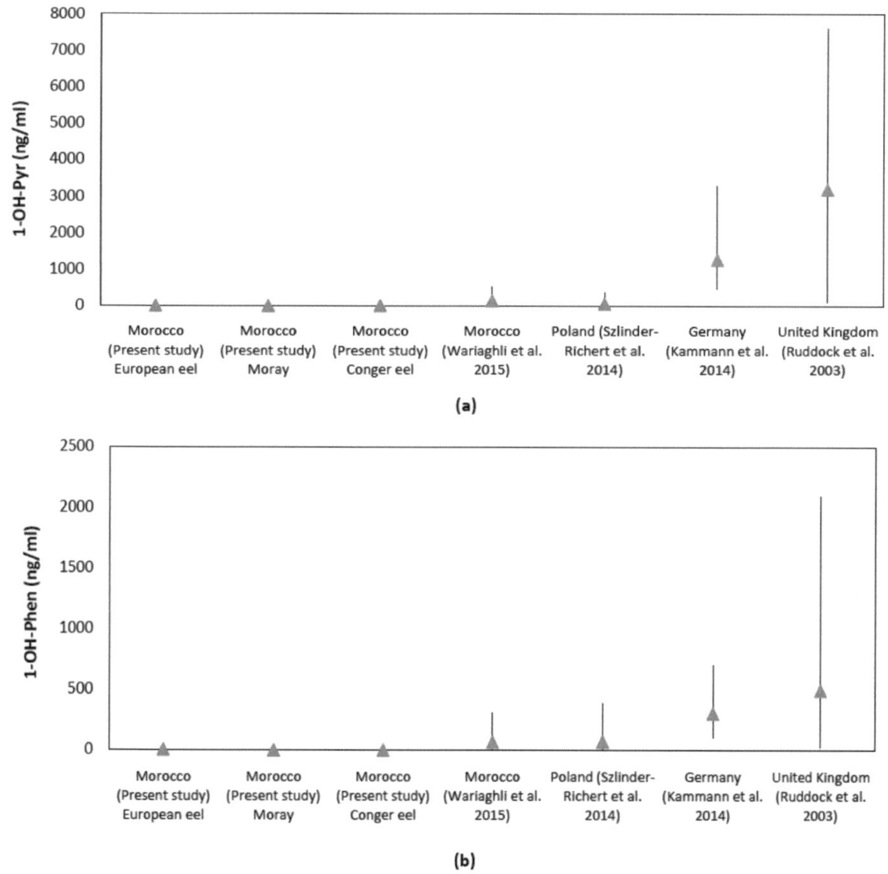

Figure 1.
Bile metabolite 1-hydroxypyrene (a) and 1-hydroxyphenanthrene (b) concentrations detected in European eels (Anguilla anguilla) collected from different areas and eels from Morocco (conger, moray, and European eel) as mean (triangles) and range (panels).

6. Conclusion

PAHs are originally organic compounds that are created from the partial combustion of organic elements or pyrolysis of organic material. These compounds are associated to the treatment of wood, oil, coal, and gas in order to produce the energy.

PAHs are transferred in the air in gas or particle aspect, and they are accumulated by wet and dry deposition. The transported elements play important role in the chemistry of the atmosphere. These particles also have significant impact in human health, because many PAHs are classified as probable human carcinogens.

The other faculty of PAHs is the capacity of degrading microorganism such as bacteria, fungi, and algae. It concerns the failure of organic compounds through biotransformation into less complex metabolites and through mineralization into inorganic minerals.

In this chapter, many effects on the biology of species following exposure to PAHs have been demonstrated. At the end of these organic studies on fish, it has been shown that the PAH biliary metabolites studied have the potential to describe the state of exposure of fish to organic pollutants (PAHs).

The study of a possible contamination of eels from different countries shows that 1-hydroxypyrene (1-OH-Pyr) is the dominant pollutant present in fish bile and is the best general indicator of PAH contamination.

Of the different eels investigated, European eels (*Anguilla anguilla*) contained the highest metabolite concentrations. This species looks like the most suitable for monitoring PAH contamination in the environment.

Using the studies conducted by several authors, we found that the rivers and lagoon contain PAH concentrations much higher than the coastal waters. These results appear normal in view that there is low water exchange in the rivers and lagoon ecosystems.

Finally we conclude that the quantification and identification of the metabolites in fish bile can give a rapid indication on the level of PAH contamination.

Conflict of interest

The authors declare that they have no competing interests.

Author details

Ayoub Baali* and Ahmed Yahyaoui
Laboratory of Biodiversity, Ecology and Genome, Faculty of Science, Mohammed V University in Rabat, Rabat, Morocco

*Address all correspondence to: ayoubbaali22@gmail.com

References

[1] Ahmad I, Pacheco M, Santos A. *Anguilla anguilla* L. oxidative stress biomarkers: An in situ study of freshwater wetland ecosystem (Pateira de Fermentelos, Portugal). Chemosphere. 2006;**65**:952-962

[2] Baali A, Kammann U, Hanel R, El Qoraychy I, Yahyaoui A. Bile metabolites of polycyclic aromatic hydrocarbons (PAHs) in three species of fish from Morocco. Environmental Sciences Europe. 2016;**28**:25. DOI: 10.1186/s12302-016-0093-6

[3] Meador J, Stein J, Reichert W, Varanasi U. Bioaccumulation of polycyclic aromatic hydrocarbons by marine organisms. Reviews of Environmental Contamination and Toxicology. 1995;**143**:79-165

[4] Woodhead RJ, Law RJ, Matthiessen P. Polycyclic aromatic hydrocarbons in surface sediments around England and Wales, and their possible biological significance. Marine Pollution Bulletin. 1999;**38**:773-790

[5] Blahová J, Havelková M, Kružíková K, Hilscherová K, Halouzka R. Assessment of contamination of the Svitava and Svratka rivers in the Czech Republic using selected biochemical markers. Environmental Toxicology and Chemistry. 2010;**29**(3):541-549

[6] McElroy AE, Farrington JW, Teal JM. Bioavailability of PAH in the aquatic environment. In: Varanasi U, editor. Metabolism of Polycyclic Aromatic Hydrocarbons in the Aquatic Environment. Boca Raton, FL: CRC Press; 1989. pp. 1-40

[7] Ramesh A, Walker SA, Hood DB, Guillén MD, Schneider K, Weyand EH. Bioavailability and risk assessment of orally ingested polycyclic aromatic hydrocarbons. International Journal of Toxicology. 2004;**23**(5):301-333

[8] Lima ALC, Farrington JW, Reddy CM. Combustion-derived polycyclic aromatic hydrocarbons in the environment—A review. Environmental Forensics. 2005;**6**:109-131

[9] Hylland K. Polycyclic aromatic hydrocarbon (PAH) ecotoxicology in marine ecosystems. Journal of Toxicology and Environmental Health, Part A. 2006;**69**:109-123

[10] Meador JP, Sommers FC, Ylitalo GM, Sloan CA. Altered growth and related physiological responses in juvenile Chinook salmon (*Oncorhynchus tshawytscha*) from dietary exposure to polycyclic aromatic hydrocarbons (PAHs). Canadian Journal of Fisheries and Aquatic Sciences. 2006;**63**:2364-2376

[11] Meador JP, Buzitis J, Bravo CF. Using fluorescent aromatic compounds in bile from juvenile salmonids to predict exposure to polycyclic aromatic hydrocarbons. Environmental Toxicology and Chemistry. 2008;**27**(4):845-853

[12] Yanagida GK, Anulacion BF, Bolton JL, Boyd D, Lomax DP, Olson OP, et al. Polycyclic aromatic hydrocarbons and risk to threatened and endangered Chinook salmon in the lower Columbia River estuary. Archives of Environmental Contamination and Toxicology. 2012;**62**(2):282-295

[13] Tuvikene A. Responses of fish to aromatic hydrocarbons. Annales Zoologici Fennici. 1995;**32**:295-309

[14] Beyer J, Jonsson G, Porte C, Krahn MM, Ariese F. Analytical methods for determining metabolites of polycyclic aromatic hydrocarbon (PAH) pollutants in fish bile: A review. Environmental Toxicology and Pharmacology. 2010;**30**:224-244

[15] Eisler R. Eisler's Encyclopedia of Environmentally Hazardous Priority Chemicals. 1st ed. Amsterdam: Elsevier; 2007. 986 p

[16] Brinkmann M, Hudjetz S, Cofalla C, Roger S, Kammann U, Zhang X, et al. A combined hydraulic and toxicological approach to assess re-suspended sediments during simulated flood events. Part I-multiple biomarkers in rainbow trout. Journal of Soils and Sediments. 2010;**10**:1347-1361

[17] Brinkmann M, Eichbaum K, Kammann U, Hudjetz S, Cofalla C, Buchinger S, et al. Physiologically-based toxicokinetic models help identifying the key factors affecting contaminant uptake during flood events. Aquatic Toxicology. 2014;**152**:38-42

[18] Monteiro PRR, Reis-Henriques MA, Coimbra J. Plasma steroid levels in female flounder (*Platichthys flesus*) after chronic dietary exposure to single polycyclic aromatic hydrocarbons. Marine Environmental Research. 2000a;**49**:453-467

[19] Chen SC, Liao CM. Health risk assessment on human exposed to environmental polycyclic aromatic hydrocarbons pollution sources. Science of the Total Environment. 2006;**366**:112-123

[20] OSPAR Commission. Co-ordinated environmental monitoring programme (CEMP). 2008. Available from: http://www.ospar.org/content/content.asp?menu=00900301400000 [Accessed: 27 December 2015]

[21] HELCOM. Core indicators final report of the HELCOM CORESET project. Baltic Sea Environment Proceedings No. 136. 2013. 71 p. http://www.helcom.fi/Lists/Publications/BSEP136.pdf#search=core%20set [Accessed: 26 December 2015]

[22] Wariaghly F. Etude écotoxicologique et parasitologique chez l'Anguille (*Anguilla anguilla* L.) dans les estuaires marocains : Sebou et Loukkos (Atlantique) [thesis]. Rabat: Université Mohammed V-Agdal, Faculté des Sciences; 2013

[23] Abdel-shafy HI, Mansour MSM. A review on polycyclic aromatic hydrocarbons: Source, environmental impact, effect on human health and remediation. Egyptian Journal of Petroleum. 2016;**25**:107-123

[24] Cole GM. Assessment and Remediation of Petroleum Contaminated Sites. 1st ed. Lewis Publishers; 1994. 384 p

[25] Laflamme RE, Hites RA. The global distribution of polycyclic aromatic hydrocarbons in recent sediments. Geochimica et Cosmochimica Acta. 1978;**42**(3):289-303

[26] Wakeham SG, Schaffner C, Giger W. Polycyclic aromatic hydrocarbons in recent lake sediments-I. Compounds having anthropogenic origins. Geochimica et Cosmochimica Acta. 1980;**44**:403-413

[27] Ventakesan MI. Occurrence and possible sources of perylene in marine sediments—A review. Marine Chemistry. 1988;**25**(1):1-27

[28] Wang X, Hong HS, Mu JL, Lin JQ, Wang SH. Polycyclic aromatic hydrocarbon (PAH) metabolites in marine fishes as a specific biomarker to indicate PAH pollution in the marine coastal environment. Journal of Environmental Science and Health, Part A. Toxic/Hazardous Substances and Environmental Engineering. 2008;**43**:219-226

[29] Dong C, Chen C, Chen C. Determination of polycyclic aromatic hydrocarbons in industrial harbor

sediments by GC-MS. International Journal of Environmental Research and Public Health. 2012;**9**:2175-2188

[30] Veltman K, Huijbregts MAJ, Rye H, Hertwich EG. Including impacts of particulate emissions on marine ecosystems in life cycle assessment: The case of offshore oil and gas production. Integrated Environmental Assessment and Management. 2011;**7**:678-686

[31] Inomata Y, Kajino M, Sato K, Ohara T, Kurokawa J, Ueda H, et al. Emission and atmospheric transport of particulate PAHs in Northeast Asia. Environmental Science & Technology. 2012;**46**(9):4941-4949. DOI: 10.1021/es300391w

[32] Tudoran MA, Putz MV. Polycyclic aromatic hydrocarbons: From in cerebro to in silico eco-toxicity fate. Chemical Bulletin of Politehnica University of Timisoara. 2012;**57**(71):50-53

[33] Choi MS. Effects of tributyltin (TBT) on the expression of cytochrome P4501A, aryl hydrocarbon receptor and vitellogenin genes[Master's thesis]. Sunmoon University; 2012

[34] El Morhit M, Fekhaoui M, Elie P, Girard P, Yahyaoui A, El Abidi A, et al. Heavy metals in sediment, water and the European glass eel *Anguilla anguilla* (Osteichthyes: Anguillidae), from Loukkos River estuary (Morocco, eastern Atlantic). Cybium. 2009;**33**:219-228

[35] AESN (Agence de l'Eau Seine Normandie). Guide des profils de vulnérabilité des eaux de baignade. 2009. p. 84

[36] McElroy AE, Farrington JW, Teal JM. Bioavailability of polycyclic aromatic hydrocarbons in the aquatic environment. In: Varanasi U, editor. Metabolism of Polycyclic Aromatic Hydrocarbons in the Aquatic Environment. Boca Raton, Florida: CRC Press, Inc.; 1989. pp. 2-33

[37] Hinga KR, Pilson MEQ. Persistence of benz[a]anthracene degradation products in an enclosed marine ecosystem. Environmental Science & Technology. 1987;**21**:648-653

[38] Cerniglia CE, Heitkamp MA. Microbial degradation of polycyclic aromatic hydrocarbons (PAH) in the aquatic environment. In: Varanasi U, editor. Metabolism of Polycyclic Aromatic Hydrocarbons in the Aquatic Environment. Boca Raton, FL: CRC Press; 1989. pp. 41-68

[39] Juhasz AL, Naidu R. Extraction and recovery of organochlorine pesticides from fungal mycelia. Journal of Microbiological Methods. 2000;**39**:149-158

[40] Bamforth SM, Singleton I. Bioremediation of polycyclic aromatic hydrocarbons: Current knowledge and future directions. Journal of Chemical Technology and Biotechnology. 2005;**80**(7):723-736

[41] Heitkamp MA, Franklin W, Cerniglia CE. Microbial metabolism of polycyclic aromatic hydrocarbons: Isolation and characterization of a pyrene-degrading bacterium. Applied and Environmental Microbiology. 1988;**54**:2549-2555

[42] Heitkamp MA, Cerniglia CE. Polycyclic aromatic hydrocarbon degradation by a *Mycobacterium* sp. in microcosms containing sediment and water from a pristine ecosystem. Applied and Environmental Microbiology. 1989;**55**:1968-1973

[43] Varanasi U, Stein JE, Nishimoto M. Biotransformation and disposition of polycyclic aromatic hydrocarbons in fish. In: Varanasi U, editor. Metabolism of Polycyclic Aromatic Hydrocarbons in the Aquatic Environment. Boca Raton, FL: CRC Press; 1989. pp. 93-149

[44] James MO. Biotransformation and disposition of PAH in aquatic invertebrates. In: Varanasi U, editor. Metabolism of Polycyclic Aromatic Hydrocarbons in the Aquatic Environment. Boca Raton, FL: CRC Press; 1989. pp. 70-88

[45] Roubal WT, Collier TK, Malins DC. Accumulation and metabolism of carbon-14 labeled benzene, naphthalene, and anthracene by young coho salmon (*Oncorhynchus kisutch*). Archives of Environmental Contamination and Toxicology. 1977;**5**:513-529

[46] Carls MG, Holland L, Larsen M, Collier TK, Scholz NL, Incardona JP. Fish embryos are damaged by dissolved PAHs, not oil particles. Aquatic Toxicology. 2008;**88**:121-127

[47] Pangrekar J, Kandaswami C, Kole P, Kumar S, Sikka HC. Comparative metabolism of benzo(a)pyrene, chrysene and phenanthrene by brown bullhead liver microsomes. Marine Environmental Research. 1995;**39**:51-55

[48] Sikka HC, Steward AR, Kandaswami C, Rutkowski JP, Zaleski J, Kumar S, et al. Metabolism of benzo(a) pyrene and persistence of DNA adducts in the brown bullhead (*Ictalurus nebulosus*). Comparative Biochemistry & Physiology. 1991;**100C**(1-2):25-28

[49] Gratz S, Mohrhaus A, Gamble B, Gracie J, Jackson D, Roetting J, et al. Screen for the presence of polycyclic aromatic hydrocarbons in select seafoods using LC-fluorescence. Laboratory Information Bulletin. 2010;**4475**:1-39

[50] Ylitalo GM, Krahn MM, Dickhoff WW, Stein JE, Walker CC, Lassitter CL, et al. Federal seafood safety response to the Deepwater Horizon oil spill. Proceedings of the National Academy of Sciences of the United States of America. 2012;**109**(50):20274-20279

[51] Hansen D, Di Toro D, McGrath J, Swartz R, Mount D, Burgess R, editors. Procedures for the Derivation of Equilibrium Partitioning Sediment Benchmarks (ESBs) for the Protection of Benthic Organisms: PAH Mixtures. Narragansett, RI: Duluth, MN: Newport, Or: USEPA; 2003. p. 175

[52] Chikae M, Hatano Y, Ikeda R, Morita Y, Hasan Q, Tamiya E. Effects of bis(2-ethylhexyl) phthalate and benzo[a]pyrene on the embryos of Japanese medaka (*Oryzias latipes*). Environmental Toxicology and Pharmacology. 2004;**16**:141-145

[53] Van Brummelen TC, Van Gestel CAM, Verweij RA. Long-term toxicity of five polycyclic aromatic hydrocarbons for the terrestrial isopods *Oniscus Asellus* and *Porcellio Scaber*. Environmental Toxicology and Chemistry. 1996;**15**:1199-1210

[54] Wessel N, Rousseau S, Caisey X, Quiniou F, Akcha F. Investigating the relationship between embryotoxic and genotoxic effects of benzo[a] pyrene, 17[alpha]-ethinylestradiol and endosulfan on *Crassostrea gigas* embryos. Aquatic Toxicology. 2007;**85**:133-142

[55] Miranda CL, Chung WG, Wang-Buhler JL, Musafia-Jeknic T, Baird WM, Buhler DR. Comparative in vitro metabolism of benzo[a]pyrene by recombinant zebrafish CYP1A and liver microsomes from [beta]-naphthoflavone-treated rainbow trout. Aquatic Toxicology. 2006;**80**:101-108

[56] Incardona JP, Carls MG, Day HL, Sloan CA, Bolton JL, Collier TK, et al. Cardiac arrhythmia is the primary response of embryonic Pacific herring (*Clupea pallasi*) exposed to crude oil during weathering. Environmental Science & Technology. 2009;**43**:201-207

[57] Hicken CE, Linbo TL, Baldwin DH, Willis ML, Myers MS, Holland L, et al. Sublethal exposure to crude oil

during embryonic development alters cardiac morphology and reduces aerobic capacity in adult fish. Proceedings of the National Academy of Sciences of the United States of America. 2011;**108**:7086-7090

[58] Incardona JP, Collier TK, Scholz NL. Defects in cardiac function precede morphological abnormalities in fish embryos exposed to polycyclic aromatic hydrocarbons. Toxicology and Applied Pharmacology. 2004;**196**:191-205

[59] Kim SG, Park DK, Jang SW, Lee JS, Kim SS, Chung MH. Effects of dietary benzo[a]pyrene on growth and hematological parameters in juvenile rockfish, Sebastes schlegeli (Hilgendorf). Bulletin of Environmental Contamination and Toxicology. 2008;**81**:470-474

[60] Montverdi GH, Di Giulio RT. In vitro and in vivo association of 2,3,7,8-tetrachlorodibenzo-p-dioxin and benzo[a]pyrene with the yolk-precursor protein vitellogenin. Environmental Toxicology. 2000;**19**(10):2502-2511. DOI: 10.1002/etc.5620191016

[61] Patel MR, Scheffler BE, Wang L, Willett KL. Effects of benzo(a) pyrene exposure on killifish (*Fundulus heteroclitus*) aromatase activities and mRNA. Aquatic Toxicology. 2006;**77**(3):267-278

[62] Rocha Monteiro PR, Reis-Henriques MA, Coimbra J. Polycyclic aromatic hydrocarbons inhibit in vitro ovarian steroidogenesis in the flounder (*Platichthys flesus* L.). Aquat. Toxicology. 2000;**48**:549-559

[63] Matson CW, Timme-Laragy AR, Di Giulio RT. Fluoranthene, but not benzo[a]pyrene, interacts with hypoxia resulting in pericardial effusion and lordosis in developing zebrafish. Chemosphere. 2008;**74**:149-154

[64] Diekmann M, Nagel R. Different survival rates in zebrafish (*Danio rerio*) from different origins. Journal of Applied Ichthyology. 2005;**21**:451-454

[65] Djomo JE, Garrigues P, Narbonn JF. Uptake and depuration of polycyclic aromatic hydrocarbons from sediment by the zebrafish (*Brachydanio rerio*). Environmental Toxicology and Chemistry. 1996;**15**:1177-1181

[66] Frantzen M, Falk-Petersen IB, Nahrgang J, Smith TJ, Olsen GH, Hangstad TA, et al. Toxicity of crude oil and pyrene to the embryos of beach spawning capelin (*Mallotus villosus*). Aquatic Toxicology. 2012;**108**:42-52

[67] Carls MG, Rice SD, Hose JE. Sensitivity of fish embryos to weathered crude oil: Part I. Low-level exposure during incubation causes malformations, genetic damage, and mortality in larval pacific herring (*Clupea pallasi*). Environmental Toxicology and Chemistry. 1999;**18**:481-493

[68] Heintz RA, Short JW, Rice SD. Sensitivity of fish embryos to weathered crude oil: Part II. Increased mortality of pink salmon (*Oncorhynchus gorbuscha*) embryos incubating downstream from weathered Exxon valdez crude oil. Environmental Toxicology and Chemistry. 1999;**18**:494-503

[69] Colavecchia MV, Backus SM, Hodson PV, Parrott JL. Toxicity of oil sands to early life stages of fathead minnows (*Pimephales promelas*). Environmental Toxicology and Chemistry. 2004;**23**:1709-1718

[70] Palanikumar L, Kumaraguru AK, Ramakritinan CM, Anand M. Toxicity, feeding rate and growth rate response to sub-lethal concentrations of anthracene and benzo[a]pyrene in milkfish *Chanos chanos* (Forskkal). Bulletin of

Environmental Contamination and Toxicology. 2013;**90**:60-68

[71] Oberdörster E, Brouwer M, Hoexum-Brouwer T, Manning S, McLachlan JA. Long-term pyrene exposure of grass shrimp, *Palaemonetes pugio*, affects molting and reproduction of exposed males and offspring of exposed females. Environmental Health Perspectives. 2000;**108**(7):641-646

[72] Dong W, Wang L, Thornton C, Scheffler BE, Willett KL. Benzo(a) pyrene decreases brain and ovarian aromatase mRNA expression in *Fundulus heteroclitus*. Aquatic Toxicology. 2008;**88**:289-300

[73] Danion M, Deschamps MH, Thomas-Guyon H, Bado-Nilles A, Le Floch S, Quentel C, et al. Effect of an experimental oil spill on vertebral bone tissue quality in European sea bass (*Dicentrarchus labrax* L.). Ecotoxicology and Environmental Safety. 2011;**74**:1888-1895

[74] Shi X, He C, Zuo Z, Li R, Chen D, Chen R, et al. Pyrene exposure influences the craniofacial cartilage development of *Sebastiscus marmoratus* embryos. Marine Environmental Research. 2012;**77**:30-34

[75] Li R, Zuo Z, Chen D, He C, Chen R, Chen Y, et al. Inhibition by polycyclic aromatic hydrocarbons of ATPase activities in *Sebastiscus marmoratus* larvae: Relationship with the development of early life stages. Marine Environmental Research. 2011;**71**:86-90

[76] Jee JH, Park KH, Keum YH, Kang JC. Effects of 7,12 dimethylbenz(a) anthracene on growth and haematological parameters in Korean rockfish, *Sebastes schlegeli* (Hilgendorf). Aquaculture Research. 2006;**37**:431-442

[77] Le Bihanic F, Clérandeau C, Morin B, Cousin X, Cachot J. Developmental toxicity of PAH mixtures in fish early life stages. Part I: Adverse effects in rainbow trout. Environmental Science and Pollution Research. 2014;**21**:13720-13731. DOI: 10.1007/s11356-014-2804-0

[78] Sundberg H, Ishaq R, Åkerman G, Tjärnlund U, Zebühr Y, Linderoth M, et al. A bio-effect directed fractionation study for toxicological and chemical characterization of organic compounds in bottom sediment. Toxicological Sciences. 2005;**84**:63-72

[79] Gilliers C, Claireaux G, Galois R, Loizeau V, Le Pape O. Influence of hydrocarbons exposure on survival, growth and condition of juvenile flatfish: A mesocosm experiment. Journal of Life Sciences. 2012;**4**:113-122

[80] Gundersen DT, Kristanto SW, Curtis LR, Al-Yakoob SN, Metwally MM, Al-Ajmi D. Subacute toxicity of the water-soluble fractions of Kuwait crude oil and partially combusted crude oil on *Menidia beryllina* and *Palaemonetes pugio*. Archives of Environmental Contamination and Toxicology. 1996;**31**:1-8

[81] Moles A, Rice SD. Effects of crude oil and naphthalene on growth, caloric content, and fat content of pink salmon juveniles in seawater. Transactions of the American Fisheries Society. 1983;**112**:205-211

[82] Agamy E. Impact of laboratory exposure to light Arabian crude oil, dispersed oil and dispersant on the gills of the juvenile brown spotted grouper (*Epinephelus chlorostigma*): A histopathological study. Marine Environmental Research. 2013;**86**:46-55

[83] Ali S, Champagne DL, Richardson MK. Behavioral profiling of zebrafish embryos exposed to a panel of 60 water-soluble compounds. Behavioural Brain Research. 2012;**228**(2):272-283. DOI: 10.1016/j.bbr.2011.11.020

[84] Chen TH, Wang YH, Wu YH. Developmental exposures to ethanol or dimethylsulfoxide at low concentrations alter locomotor activity in larval zebrafish: Implications for behavioral toxicity bioassays. Aquatic Toxicology. 2011;**102**:162-166

[85] Egan RJ, Bergner CL, Hart PC, Cachat JM, Canavello PR, Elegante MF, et al. Understanding behavioral and physiological phenotypes of stress and anxiety in zebrafish. Behavioural Brain Research. 2009;**205**:38-44

[86] López-Patiño MA, Yu L, Cabral H, Zhdanova IV. Anxiogenic effects of cocaine withdrawal in zebrafish. Physiology & Behavior. 2008;**93**:160-171

[87] Sackerman J, Donegan J, Cunningham C, Nguyen N, Lawless K, Long A, et al. Zebrafish behavior in novel environments: Effects of acute exposure to anxiolytic compounds and choice of *Danio rerio* line. Journal of Comparative Psychology. 2010;**23**:43-61

[88] Correia AD, Goncalves R, Scholze M, Ferreira M, Reis-Henriques MA. Biochemical and behavioral responses in gilthead seabream (*Sparus aurata*) to phenanthrene. Journal of Experimental Marine Biology and Ecology. 2007;**347**:109-122

[89] Goncalves R, Scholze M, Ferreira AM, Martins M, Correia AD. The joint effect of polycyclic aromatic hydrocarbons on fish behavior. Environmental Research. 2008;**108**:205-213

[90] Farr AJ, Chabot CC, Taylor DH. Behavioral avoidance of fluoranthene by fathead minnows (*Pimephales promelas*). Neurotoxicology and Teratology. 1995;**17**:265-271

[91] Vignet C. Altération de la physiologie des poissons exposés à des hydrocarbures aromatiques polycycliques (HAP): Comportement et reproduction [thesis]. France: Université de La Rochelle; 2014

[92] Anderson MJ, Miller MR, Hinton DE. In vitro modulation of 17-b-estradiolinduced vitellogenin synthesis: Effects of cytochrome P4501A1 inducing compounds on rainbow trout (*Oncorhynchus mykiss*) liver cells. Aquatic Toxicology. 1996;**34**:327-350

[93] Holth TF, Nourizadeh-Lillabadi R, Blaesbjerg M, Grung M, Holbech H, Petersen GI, et al. Differential gene expression and biomarkers in zebrafish (*Danio rerio*) following exposure to produced water components. Aquatic Toxicology. 2008;**90**:277-291

[94] Pikkarainen A. Ethoxyresorufin-O-deethylase (EROD) activity and bile metabolites as contamination indicators in Baltic Sea perch: Determination by HPLC. Chemosphere. 2006;**65**:1888-1897

[95] Pj V, Keinänen M, Vuontisjärvi H, Barsiene J, Broeg K, Förlin L, et al. Use of biliary PAH metabolites as a biomarker of pollution in fish from the Baltic Sea. Marine Pollution Bulletin. 2006;**53**:479-487

[96] Kammann U, Lang T, Vobach M, Wosniok W. Ethoxyresorufin-O-deethylase (EROD) activity in dab (*Limanda limanda*) as biomarker for marine monitoring. Environmental Science and Pollution Research. 2005;**12**:140-145

[97] Harman C, Thomas K, Tollefsen KE, Meier S, Bøyum O, Grung M. Monitoring the freely dissolved concentrations of polycyclic aromatic hydrocarbons (PAH) and alkylphenols (AP) around a Norwegian oil platform by holistic passive sampling. Marine Pollution Bulletin. 2009;**58**:1671-1679

[98] Zm T, Amb G, Hansen R, Andersen O. 1-Hydroxypyrene as a biomarker of PAH exposure in the marine polychaete Nereis diversicolor. Marine Environmental Research. 2009;**67**:38-46

[99] McMaster ME, Van Der Kraak GJ, Munkittrick KR. An epidemiological evaluation of the biochemical basis for steroid hormonal depressions in fish exposed to industrial wastes. Journal of Great Lakes Research. 1996;**22**:153-171

[100] Van der Oost R, Beyer J, Vermeulen NPE. Fish bioaccumulation and biomarkers in environmental risk assessment: A review. Environmental Toxicology and Pharmacology. 2003;**13**:57-149

[101] Pointet K, Milliet A. PAHs analysis of fish whole gall bladders and livers from the Natural Reserve of Camargue by GCy MS. Chemosphere. 2000;**40**:293-299

[102] Eggens ML, Opperhuizen A, Boon JP. Temporal variation of CYP1A indices, PCB and 1-OH pyrene concentration in flounder, *Platichthys flesus*, from the Dutch Wadden Sea. Chemosphere. 1996;**33**:1579-1596

[103] Hylland K, Sandvik M, Skasre JU, Beyer J, Egaas E, Goksøyr A. Biomarkers in flounder (*Platichthys flesus*): An evaluation of their use in pollution monitoring. Marine Environmental Research. 1996;**42**:223-227

[104] Ruddock PJ, Bird DJ, McCalley DV. Bile metabolites of PAHs in three species of fish from the Severn Estuary. Ecotoxicology and Environmental Safety. 2002;**51**:97-105

[105] Ariese F, Kok SJ, Verkaik M, Gooijer C, Velthorst NH, Hofstraat JW. Synchronous fluorescence spectrometry of fish bile: A rapid screening method for the biomonitoring of PAH exposure. Aquatic Toxicology. 1993;**26**:273-286

[106] Zhou JL, Fileman TW, Evans S, Donkin P, Llewellyn C, Readman JW, et al. Fluoranthene and pyrene in the suspended particulate matter and surface sediments of the Humber Estuary, UK. Marine Pollution Bulletin. 1998;**36**:587-597

[107] Lin ELC, Cormier SM, Racine RN. Synchronous fluorometric measurement of metabolites of polycyclic aromatic hydrocarbons in the bile of brown bullhead. Environmental Toxicology and Chemistry. 1994;**13**:707-715

[108] Neff JM. Sources of PAH in the aquatic environment. In: Polycyclic Aromatic Hydrocarbons in the Aquatic Environment. London: Applied Science Publishers; 1979. pp. 7-43

[109] Cavalieri E, Rogan E. Role of radical cations in aromatic hydrocarbon carcinogenesis. Environmental Health Perspectives. 1985;**64**:69-84

[110] Johnston EP, Baumann PC. Analysis of fish bile with HPLC fluorescence to determine environmental exposure to benzo(a)pyrene. Hydrobiologia. 1989;**188**(1):561-566

[111] Penning TM, Burczynski ME, Hung CF, McCoull KD, Palackal NT, Tsuruda L. Dihydrodiol dehydrogenases and polycyclic aromatic hydrocarbon activation: Generation of reactive and redox active O-quinones. Chemical Research in Toxicology. 1999;**12**:1-18

[112] Hisano T, Hayase T. Countermeasures against water pollution in enclosed coastal seas in Japan. Marine Pollution Bulletin. 1991;**23**:479-484

[113] Moriarty C. Eels: A Natural and Unnatural History. Londres: David & Charles; 1978. 192 p

[114] Van Schooten FJ, Maas LM, Moonen EJC, Kleinjans JCS, van der Oost R. DNA dosimetry in biological indicator species living on PAH-contaminated soils and sediments. Ecotoxicology and Environmental Safety. 1995;**30**(2):171-179

[115] Wheeler A. The eels. The Fishes of the British Isles and North-West Europe. London: Macmillan & Co.; 1969. pp. 223-230

[116] Sandvik M, Horsberg TE, Skaare JU, Ingebrigtsen K. Comparison of dietary and waterborne exposure to benzo[a]pyrene: Bioavailability, tissue disposition and CYP1A1 induction in rainbow trout (*Oncorhynchus mykiss*). Biomarkers. 1998;**3**:399-410

[117] Kammann U, Akcha F, Budzinski H, Burgeot T, Gubbins MJ, Lang T, et al. PAH metabolites in fish bile: From the Seine Estuary to Iceland. Marine Environmental Research. 2017;**124**:41-45. DOI: 10.1016/j.marenvres.2016.2.014

[118] Kammann U, Brinkmann M, Freese M, Pohlmann JD, Stoffels S, Hollert H, et al. PAH metabolites, GST and EROD in European eel (*Anguilla anguilla*) as possible indicators for eel habitat quality in German rivers. Environmental Science and Pollution Research. 2014;**1**:2519-2530

[119] Ruddock PJ, Bird DJ, McEvoy J, Peters LD. Bile metabolites of polycyclic aromatic hydrocarbons (PAHs) in European eels *Anguilla anguilla* from United Kingdom estuaries. Science of the Total Environment. 2003;**301**:105-117

[120] Wariaghli F, Kammann U, Hanel R, Yahyaoui A. PAH metabolites in bile of European Eel (*Anguilla anguilla*) from Morocco. Bulletin of Environmental Contamination and Toxicology. 2015;**95**(6):740-744